KT-484-217

To my daughters, Jessica and Kayla,
who distracted me from my typing and editing
on a frequent basis and allowed me to remember,
while playing with them, why I do work so hard.

Contents

Preface

Anyone who has studied strength and conditioning has come in contact with an abundance of prepackaged information in a cookbook format. This material is based on the philosophy that any athlete can fit in any program. *Athletic Body in Balance,* on the other hand, adopts the philosophy that a program should be built around the athlete.

I designed the system in this book based on my experience as an orthopedic and sports physical therapist and strength and conditioning specialist. I've had the unique opportunity to witness the human body perform through all angles of the physical spectrum. I've seen amazing feats of athletic accomplishment as well as intense struggles in recuperation and rehabilitation. This book has evolved from my experience, mistakes, and success. I am on a continual quest to develop a model to refine athletic conditioning, prevent injuries, improve performance, and simplify the assessment and problem-solving process.

Throughout my journey, two key words have emerged—*efficient* and *effective.* In my mind, these two words dance around each other in a yin-and-yang waltz. *Efficient* describes action without wasted movement or unnecessary energy expenditure. It's best described as the level at which a champion actually gets to enjoy being a champion. At the height of their careers, the great ones are relaxed and enjoy themselves in the midst of constant chaos and challenge.

Take, for example, Jack Nicklaus, Michael Jordan, Wayne Gretzky, and countless other professional and amateur athletes who played long enough to relax and enjoy competition. The word *relax* in no way implies taking competition lightly or giving less than 100 percent. It means to compete without anxiety. These elite athletes embody the confidence that can come only from training as one should train and playing as one should play. This is the result of time and self-criticism. With this competitive maturity come wisdom and perspective for oneself and the game. Perspective and experience affect preparation by reducing wasted energy in training. With continually refining training, a subtle confidence emerges and reduces the anxious feeling that preparation may not be complete. These individuals become efficient in exercise.

Efficiency removes the fluff and fanfare from exercise, disregards the gimmicks and trends, and gets to the heart of the movements that create improvement and keep everything in tune.

Effective simply means yielding results. If a workout is trimmed to save time but is not helping the athlete achieve performance goals, the workout—although efficient—is not *effective* at improving or refining performance. This book will help you create a balanced dance of efficient and effective exercise suited to your needs, breaking down the fundamental factors of consistent performance and putting them into an assessment sequence that will allow you to customize a training program. *Efficiency and effectiveness* is the underlying theme of training suggestions throughout this book.

Every great coach clings to a fundamental system. The basic principles of the system provide a way to test new techniques and exercises to make sure they fit into the system before incorporating them into the athlete's program. The system prevents the coach from incorporating trendy exercises or techniques that may be counterproductive or potentially dangerous. The principles of the system do not change even as new techniques and exercises are introduced. Systems provide structure and feedback. If new fads and exercise trends don't fit within the structure, they are not implemented. If they do not provide the necessary feedback, they cannot be effectively used.

The system in this book includes tests for each phase of conditioning. The scores on these tests will reveal strengths and weaknesses. Step by step, the athlete will work to overcome weaknesses. Many of the concepts and strategies in this book will seem familiar. Many may be alien or seem like a waste of time. However, they have been included specifically because they work and, just as important, they work in a specific sequence. Don't skip a step or work on a different aspect of conditioning. Using the chapters in this book out of sequence or outside of their intended progression will not yield efficient and effective long-term results.

Throw away any ideas about a quick fix or a fast track. Trends and fads usually are created to sell something. We want things better and faster than humanly possible, but something always suffers when we try to rush natural processes. Training and conditioning require a conscious balance of body systems. Good training is about implementing effective assessment strategies and being in touch with specific needs at every stage of physical development. Conditioning decisions should not be made on a whim. Nor should exercises be randomly deleted just because they don't result in immediately perceptible benefits. Many excellent conditioning programs have been changed or trashed right before the results would have been apparent. An efficient and effective system will provide structure and feedback even when immediate changes aren't seen or felt.

Early in the book, I use automobiles and computers as metaphors because, although few of us are experts on either, most of us depend on their technology. Even if you can't program a computer or tune an automobile, you should still be an educated consumer. To the extent that you understand the workings and systems of automobiles or computers, you can save time and be more productive (that is, be more efficient and more effective).

A basic knowledge of automobiles and computers can save time and money and keep someone from falling victim to schemes and ads that prey on ignorance. In the same way, the more educated an athlete becomes about the workings of the body, with all its limitations and potential, the less intimidated and insecure the athlete will be when making decisions about training. Many athletes waste time dabbling in different training methodologies, trying to discover their personal formulas. This book provides a glimpse into the human body and its function in a format that is not intimidating or confusing.

Injury prevention is an important theme in this book. By adopting efficient and effective training systems early, many injuries caused by an unbalanced approach and poor problem-solving techniques can be prevented. Injury prevention is not a glamorous subject, and it's a hard issue to research and prove (much harder than performance enhancement). Steps have been taken in the assessment and exercise sections of this book to focus on early indicators and warning signs of potential injuries. Not all injuries can be avoided, because sport and competition sometimes push the body beyond its limits. However, many injuries can be prevented, especially those that occur in training and conditioning. An injury can change the outcome of an athlete's career—costing an athlete a scholarship, a sign-on bonus, or even a starting position.

The goal of this program is to be as complete and holistic as possible. Many programs may provide quick results in one aspect of performance but neglect another. My hope is that you are not in a rush and will take the information in this book and slowly blend it into your current routine. I also hope that you will not overlook the secret to success—consistency and hard work. It is best if the consistency and hard work are applied in the right direction. *Athletic Body in Balance* will serve as a quiet coach. It will consistently remind you to stay focused on your goals and to be patient as you work through the system.

Welcome to the journey. I hope it's a positive one.

Acknowledgments

I am not a writer. I am an orthopedic physical therapist and a strength and conditioning specialist who enjoys all aspects of sports medicine and training. My experience and love for my work have helped me develop into a lecturer and a teacher. This book was an opportunity for me to write down what I have been talking about for a few years. For that opportunity, I would like to thank Martin Barnard from Human Kinetics for recognizing the message I was trying to convey in my lectures.

I would also like to thank Stephanie Montgomery of Reebok® University, who has given me one of the greatest opportunities of my life and allowed me to work closely with Reebok® to develop conditioning programs in both fitness and sports. I have truly enjoyed my experiences with Reebok® and all of the enthusiastic and creative people at Reebok® University who have given me support and encouragement.

I would like to thank Margaret Dykstra, whose editing skills allowed me to actually say in writing what I was thinking. I would also like to thank Nancye Payne who originally transcribed this entire text and who has since encouraged me to study punctuation and spelling in greater depth.

My thanks to Mike Voight, Paul Hughes, Pete Draovitch, Steve McGee, and Jim Meadows who have been colleagues, mentors, and friends and have each in their own way shown me how to think outside the box.

When I moved back to my hometown of Danville, Virginia, I truly felt that my career had come full circle. I feel that my best work has been done in the same place I grew up. I would like to thank Howard Dunn, Charlie Smith, and the entire staff at Rehabilitation Services of Danville, past and present, for welcoming me home to practice physical therapy and truly supporting me both as a professional and a friend. The information in this book is the result of many hours of brainstorming, working with athletes, presenting lectures and workshops, and enjoying road trips with a team of professionals whose friendship I cherish.

Keith Fields, Kyle Kiesel, Lee Burton, and Joe Van Allen gave up many weekends and weeknights to help me develop and refine this material. I would like to take this opportunity to thank them for their commitment, criticism, praise, and friendship.

I would like to thank my family, who has always been there for me in my personal and professional development.

Introduction

This is not just another training and conditioning book. What makes it unique is its focus on building a program around the athlete, rather than the other way around. The athlete is the best resource in developing a sound conditioning program. Why is that so important?

Exercise fads and trends will keep coming. Some will work; some will not. Many athletes try things because their friends, training partners, teammates, or favorite pros say that they work. They read magazine articles that recycle and repackage exercises for every ailment, problem, and body part. They buy equipment because they think that in this age of technology there may be a secret way to train better or faster. But even if an athlete does stumble onto what seems to be the right workout, how can the athlete be sure something isn't being left out? What type of assessment is used to decide what needs to be done? The claimed value of an exercise is often based on nothing more than how much a particular muscle burns when a particular movement is performed. It may seem like science, but it's not.

Many exercise and conditioning programs are a mix of fact, fiction, biased opinions, advertising, media hype, and personal anecdotes. Ultimately, athletes and trainers have to wade through all these options to decide how to spend training time. This book will provide the tools for an effective assessment and build a philosophy of balance that will act as a guide through the confusion of training and conditioning. You will learn to refine movement and explore potential. You will learn to base exercise practices on what assessments show. You will assess your movement patterns and train accordingly. Movement, not muscles, will be a constant guide throughout this book.

So, here you are at the beginning. This can be a daunting place to be. Think of it as a trip. Dr. Steven Covey, author of *The Seven Habits of Highly Effective People,* describes a trip in terms of both *efficient* and *effective* travel. You need both a clock and a compass to make sure the journey is efficient and effective. If you look at the clock but not the compass, you may make great time but arrive at the wrong place. If you look only at the compass, you may eventually arrive at the right place but it may take too long.

For your trip, first you must create a map. Second, you must correctly read and interpret the map. Finally, you must consistently execute the necessary steps in the correct sequence in order to physically travel the journey.

To create a map for personal physical conditioning, you must understand and follow some physical laws and allow for your personal limitations. The physical laws that govern the human body and the neuromuscular system dictate how the body responds to conditioning. These laws must be taken into account as you develop your map. Every athlete has physical limitations with regard to time, space, and ability. Proper assessment tools will help you understand where you are and then set objective and attainable goals. This book will help you understand the tools and techniques to be used and where they will be effective during the journey.

To read the map, you need consistent and objective feedback and should follow a specific sequential approach. This is about pacing. Strength and conditioning professionals call this *periodization:* it's a way to make sure the athlete peaks at the necessary time, usually at a point of vital competition. It's easy to make mistakes by misinterpreting the map or by rushing through one leg of the journey only to be hindered in another leg by poor planning.

The steps of your journey must be executed in the proper sequence. The journey itself is about the physical act of taking the daily steps necessary to progress forward and attain conditioning goals.

This book presents efficient and effective methods for enhancing performance by addressing the fundamentals of human conditioning. It offers assessments for key fitness parameters and introduces basic building blocks of human performance that are often overlooked. These fundamental parameters explain why some injuries linger and others quickly disappear and why some athletes get better sports performance through weight training while others simply get bigger with no change or even a decline in sports performance.

Most programs are developed without all of the necessary information, leaving more to chance than necessary. Driving without a complete map may be fun, but it is not likely to get you where you want to go. The assessments in this book will help set a baseline (the accurate information needed to draw a complete map) and help identify your strengths and weaknesses. The majority of the time will be spent on improving weaknesses. Many sports and conditioning philosophies advocate maximizing strengths, but it is better to confront weaknesses and move through problem areas.

Either nature or competition will find an overlooked weakness, so failing to address your weaknesses is simply not a good idea. This book will explain how and why a weak link can increase the potential for injury and negatively influence performance. Fix the problems when you find them, and remember that there are no shortcuts to greatness.

The stages, or levels, of conditioning provided in this book dictate where to start the program. The sequential approach will help you understand how to move through each level, maintaining gains and modifying the program to address specific needs. You get control, keep control, and, most important, understand why.

PART I

ATHLETIC MOVEMENT

1

Mind and Movement

An ancient Greek story about an Olympic hero named Milo is an apt illustration of modern principles of athletic conditioning and preparation. Unlike today's athletes, Milo did not use steel weights as resistance, nor did he use a specific exercise apparatus. Every day, Milo lifted a small calf into his arms and carried the calf a certain distance. As the calf grew into a bull, Milo continued his training. On the first day of the Olympics, Milo walked the length of the track while carrying a full-grown bull. This story contains a few lessons for us today.

First, *training should be progressive.* Milo didn't start by carrying a full-grown bull. His training intensity increased as the calf grew. I'm sure that some days he was tired or felt that he could have worked harder. Each day he completed his task, his body was introduced to greater amounts of stress. He made the necessary physical adaptation to accomplish an amazing feat by the end of his training cycle, his Olympic debut.

Second, *training must progress toward a time or event.* Milo planned his training to build to a peak for the Olympics. He also may have made the necessary arrangements to find a calf that would be fully grown at or around that date. This demonstrated foresight and goal setting. The world's best conditioning program will provide nothing in competition if peak performance is not available at the time of competition.

Periodization is commonly used by strength coaches to plan training and conditioning programs to progress to a future time or event. Training usually runs in cycles, following the season of the sport. Usually there is an offseason, preseason, and season. Through periodized training, physical conditioning and sport skills are maximized when they are needed most—in competition. Although one can maintain good conditioning throughout life, no one can physically or mentally maintain peak condition without a break. Look at training as a cycle of building, competing, and rebuilding.

Third, *good training requires vision.* Milo had vision but also was objective in his training. Milo started by lifting a calf, not a bull. It is almost inconceivable to think of lifting a bull, much less walking while carrying the bull. On the other hand, it is completely within reach to lift a small calf and walk. Milo did not have the physical or mental capacity to lift a bull on the first day of his training, but he had confidence and dedication. Each day he did not think about how heavy the bull would be or how long he would walk. He just looked at the calf, a calf that looked very much like it did the day before and much the same as it would look the next day. Milo was not intimidated by his training; therefore, he trained as just another part of his daily activities.

So there you have it. Training includes a physical load that needs to be disbursed across a period of time to allow growth, development, and conditioning to complete a task (progressive training). You've got to plan and know how and when to perform your best (periodization). Psychology is as important as physiology. How you feel about training and what you are willing to do in your program (vision) are as important as what you do in training. You have to believe in your training program. Seeing may be believing, but you cannot see the results of training until you first use preparation, time, and effort effectively. So do you have to see to believe, or do you first have to believe to see? Learn from Milo. He first believed, and then he accomplished something no one had seen before.

Know thyself.

—Inscription on the Temple of Apollo in Delphi, 6th century B.C.

The Human Body

Athletic movement is first and foremost about human movement. A general understanding of the human body and its systems is necessary to make the most of the conditioning information in the chapters that follow. Because the tests and exercises in this book are based on the way the body creates, recognizes, and refines movement, a basic understanding of the body will give each test and exercise purpose.

The most common mistake I have seen in professional and collegiate conditioning is one of emphasis. Athletes know more about their programs or conditioning routines than they do about their own bodies and the way they move. That is the medical equivalent of a patient knowing more about the medication than the disease it is supposed to cure or treat.

Many of the common assessment tools and tests used in sports do not directly affect the conditioning program. Data are used to create records for each athlete but not to modify or individualize that athlete's performance program. An athlete who is not aware of his individual test results has no way to check progress and modify the program accordingly.

The chapters that follow will explain new ways to use test information to maximize the benefits of conditioning. Test data will be grouped so that the athlete will understand what the results reveal. The chapters will present programs that address each group of tests. In other words, the cure can be found only if the disease is diagnosed.

Motor Programs

In computer terminology, there is an important distinction between hardware and software. This distinction can help demonstrate how the body creates, recognizes, and refines movement. *Hardware* refers to the components of the actual machine; *software* refers to the programs (commands or instructions) that allow the machine to fulfill the task requested of it. When we discuss the human body, including the muscles, joints, ligaments, and everything else physical, we are referring to the body's hardware. When we discuss motor programs, we are referring to the body's software.

Motor programs are simply ways that the brain stores information about movement. For example, when you ride a bicycle, swing a golf club, or shoot a free throw,

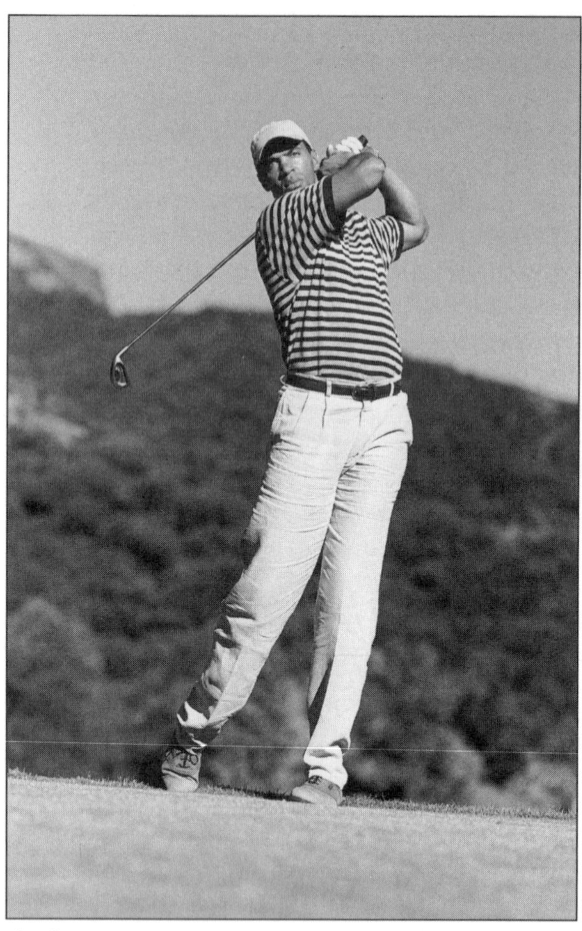

The brain creates a motor program out of a sequence of movements, such as a golf swing, so the athlete can access the movement sequence in a more efficient way.

you develop a motor program that allows you to do this activity again without having to relearn the mechanics.

The motor program is the body's way to conserve energy and storage space. The brain creates a specific programmed sequence of movements unique to the body and activity. That way, you don't have to put together all the individual parts of the movement each time you want to use that movement. For example, each time you go to the driving range, you can access the brain file on the golf swing without having to put together the individual parts of the swing. The more a motor program is used, the more efficient and refined it becomes. Professional athletes develop motor programs that are so refined they can perform effectively under varying conditions and high levels of physical and mental stress.

So all practice is good, right? Not necessarily. If an activity is practiced with poor form, the poor form will be part of the information recorded in the motor program. Practice does not make perfect; perfect practice makes perfect.

Motor programs can be general or specific. General, or basic, motor programs are almost like a common or standard operating system; specific programs relate to particular activities. Infants share common movements necessary to develop their minds and bodies. Almost all infants follow the same path or sequence to move from crawling to walking. The general motor program is common to all individuals; but specific motor programs are unique, based on age and experience. The basic motor program (general human movement) creates a platform for specific motor programs (sport-specific human movement). The general system is a frame of reference for basic movement and contains such information as

- maximum reach,
- center of gravity (center of mass),
- limits in twisting right and left,
- walking stride,
- running stride,
- how squatting feels,
- how lunging feels, and
- balance.

Motor programs are first used when an infant starts to move, whether rolling, crawling, or walking. Most children learn to walk long before they can effectively communicate with words and before they develop the observational skills to simply mimic such a complex movement. Therefore, walking is learned through *feel,* not through verbal communication or observation. It is important to understand this because as an athlete tries to learn a new movement pattern, a coach or training partner often will use words or demonstrate the movement rather than use feel. But the language of movement is written through feel. This feel is called *proprioception* or *body awareness;* it's the way the body senses both touch and movement. This is not to say that words and observations cannot refine and even help athletic movement. However, it is important whenever possible to learn movement through moving.

When there is a problem with movement, consider the hardware and software. It is common to assume that with enough practice the software or motor program can be refined and improved. This may be true if the hardware is functioning optimally. However, it is wrong to assume that an athlete is in optimal shape just because she works out and trains hard. The athlete may develop muscle and improve endurance, but what are her movement patterns like?

The way an athlete moves, not the way an athlete looks, defines the athlete. For example, modern weight-training practices often have more in common with bodybuilding than with sport performance or movement enhancement. An athlete must develop sound movement patterns long before worrying about performance enhancement. These movement patterns are not possible in the presence of poor flexibility or poor body control—that is, poor mobility and stability.

Sport-Specific Conditioning

John Wooden, the famous UCLA basketball coach, did not have a formal conditioning program. In his practices he set up many stations that trained some part of basketball skill. Each station featured short bursts of activity to force his athletes to execute proper technique while focusing on the fundamentals of the sport and consistency of performance. When the whistle blew, players sprinted to another station, arriving winded and fatigued only to have to perform a high-level skill again and again as they rotated from station to station.

John Wooden's approach is the fundamental element that has often been forgotten in sports today. We compartmentalize training: We have a weight-training session, a sprint session, a speed session. We get sports massages and think about stretching every now and then. At another time, we work on technique or simulate competitive situations. This confuses the brain. In competition, the athlete needs to have it all together and needs it now. An athlete cannot compartmentalize training and expect the brain to put it all together in competition.

John Wooden added conditioning during and between skill sessions. This is the essence of coaching—creating conditioning under the guise of skill training and using competitive situations to create greater training intensity. Wooden was extremely intuitive and efficient. He was quoted as saying, "If we meet an equally skilled team, we will always prevail because we are better conditioned." They were not better conditioned because they spent more time running wind sprints and logged more weight room hours. They were better conditioned because they ran, sprinted, and quickly moved from one skill to another and still were able to perform the skill. This erases the line between conditioning and training sport skill. It incorporates into training the many breaks that are automatically part of competition—breaks to be used to actively rest, focus, and recover. It teaches time management: Take a breath when you can; relax whenever possible. In the words of John Wooden, "Be quick but don't hurry."

Physical Systems

Although human joints move like hinges, no axis or pin holds the joint together so that it rotates around a central point. A joint has two forms of support that hold it together: the ligament and the muscles surrounding the joint. Usually there is a ligament to support the joint in each direction the joint naturally moves. The joint is completely surrounded and protected by the *joint capsule.* The *synovial fluid* within the capsule serves both to lubricate and to nourish the cartilage, the soft material on the end of each bone in the joint.

The second support structure, the complex network of muscles surrounding that joint, falls into two main categories: muscles that primarily stabilize the joint and muscles that primarily move the joint. Stabilizing muscles usually are the first layer of muscle surrounding the joint (or, anatomically speaking, the deepest layer of muscle). These muscles can be said to squeeze the joint together and give it instantaneous support when the joint is moved or loaded. They are often referred to as *postural muscles* because they maintain body posture or joint position during activity. After they perform their role, the larger muscles (or prime movers) then pull the joint in a certain direction as the muscles shorten.

An extremely complex communication system exists among the joint, ligaments, and muscles that work together to protect the joint. The ligaments are aligned in the direction of stress for two reasons. First, ligaments protect the joint by providing tensile strength to keep the joint from separating. Second, within the ligaments are small sensors that monitor the tension so that when it reaches a certain point, the muscles activate to protect the joint.

The sensors in the joint capsule and in the cartilage provide information to the brain about the feel or position of the joint as well as the speed and direction of the movement. Muscles also have sensors called *muscle spindles.* These sensors keep the muscle in a state of readiness and awareness by constantly monitoring tension so that the muscle can be relaxed (or contracted) to allow for proper movement. All this occurs automatically in the form of reflex activity, which does not require conscious thought. It is the same system that causes the knee-jerk reflex when your knee is struck with a reflex hammer. The joints and muscles function automatically to protect the body and make movement efficient. The information they provide is a critical factor in proprioception and body awareness.

Body awareness comes from the sensory system. The sensory system not only helps you feel what's going on but also allows your body to function automatically. Many of the muscles in the body react automatically. They are completely dependent on how the sensory system functions.

For a long time, the body was considered a vehicle for movement. Now we know the body is also extremely sensitive to input. It is one big sensory organism that makes fine adjustments as it receives information. When the body does not function optimally, when muscles are tight or weak, or when joints are stiff or unstable, this information gets distorted so that automatic reactions are distorted. This can hurt performance, increase fatigue, and expose the body to unnecessary stress.

The tests and exercises in this book will help you become more aware of how the body works. Eventually this will help you teach yourself how best to train your body. Know the rules, then play the game.

2

Identifying Weak Links

Overcoming adversity is a common theme in athletics. In defeat and injury, which all athletes will experience, athletes are either created or destroyed. Objectivity, reason, and action are the keys to turning defeat and injury into opportunities to discover weaknesses and learn more about yourself. Every sport has stories of young, small, or average athletes who are forced to practice with older, bigger, or better players. These athletes confront their weakness every day, which can be overwhelming. But an athlete who uses a little objectivity and reasoning in these situations can prevail.

For example, a basketball player goes against an opponent of equal size and strength but superior skills and achievements. As expected, the less-skilled player gets beat at every scrimmage. Initially he gets discouraged, but then he realizes discouragement is not productive. He gets smart and looks at the situation objectively.

His opponent has a better vertical leap, but their shuttle run stats and quickness are equal. He recognizes a 10 percent difference between them in offensive abilities and a 20 percent difference in defensive abilities during the first and second quarters, but a 40 percent difference in offensive abilities and a 50 percent difference in defensive abilities during the third and fourth quarters. So a significant problem seems to be fatigue. With this information in mind, the basketball player plans an aggressive conditioning program. First he adds interval training using a jump rope and wind sprints. He adds skill drills between sprint and jump rope routines. Not only does his endurance improve, but offensive and defensive skills also begin to improve. Eventually a well-rounded, mentally and physically strong athlete emerges. By confronting his weaknesses, the athlete was able to overcome them.

It's the way that creates the warrior.

—Dan Millman

Weak Links

Coaches and athletes probably misunderstand weak links and energy leaks more than any other topic in sports and conditioning. Everyone understands the injury that is caused when an athlete slips or when two athletes collide, but athletes and coaches are constantly perplexed when an athlete's shoulder slowly starts to hurt more and

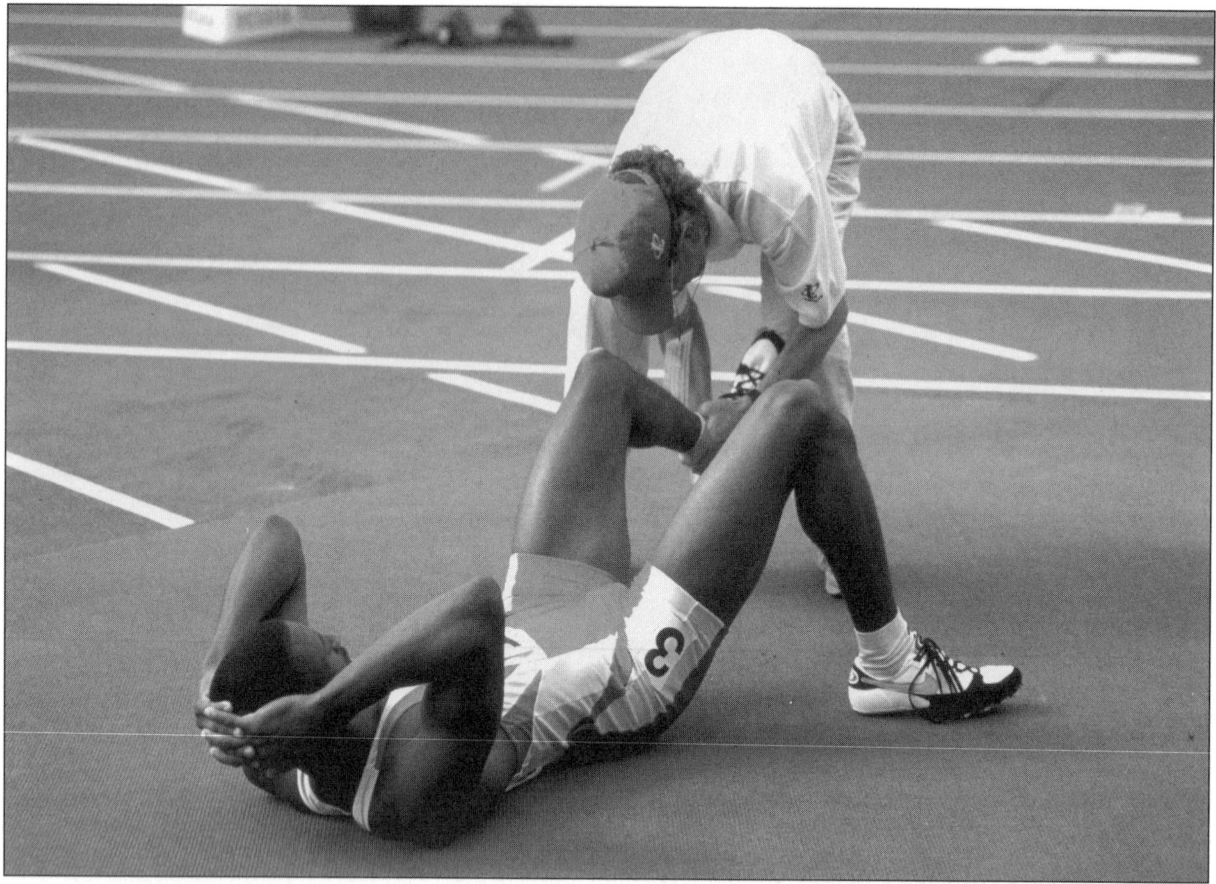

Aches and pains that have no identifiable external cause may be due to microtrauma.

more or when low back pain starts to occur daily in training. Barring any disease or deformity, such pain is usually the result of microtrauma.

Microtrauma results from small amounts of stress imposed on the body over time caused by poor biomechanics and overtraining. Both cause excessive strain on the body, but each has distinct potential as a cause of microtrauma. *Poor biomechanics* refers to movement mistakes in which the body compensates and uses suboptimal joint alignment, muscle coordination, and posture. These little mistakes often cannot be observed by the untrained eye and don't immediately hurt performance. They manifest as fatigue and appear when the fundamentals of conditioning and technique are not observed. Because these tiny errors often don't hurt performance, the athlete is usually not aware of the problem. *Overtraining* is not about movement mistakes. In fact, overtraining can result from too much of the right thing. Any type of training in excess is a loss of perspective.

To get at the heart of the problem, one must decide whether the microtrauma is a result of too much of the right thing or too much of the wrong thing. Most blame microtraumas on overtraining and not enough rest and recovery, but this often is not the case. For example, imagine an athlete who has increased her running distance, added more plyometrics to her training routine, and added speed and agility work. Suddenly, her right knee starts to hurt. Overtraining is an easy scapegoat, but the left knee did just as much work. Why doesn't it hurt, too?

The term *weak link* does not mean simply a muscle weakness; it can be used to identify any physical limitation. It also can be used to identify inadequate movement patterns, poor endurance, faulty coordination, limited sport skill, or a lack of flexibility. An athlete starting or restarting a conditioning program will have many goals and aspirations, many things he wants to change and fix or improve. It is best to focus on a single component that needs improvement.

Many athletes think they already know what their weakest links are. However, it is extremely difficult for an athlete to evaluate herself without some objective tool or standard criteria. Opinions, emotions, likes, and dislikes about training and conditioning, as well as the chosen sport or recreational activity, are all key factors.

As a rule, strength, flexibility, endurance, power, and speed programs are discussed and practiced as though the components were separate and independent. The truth is, they are interrelated. Separating them makes as much sense as individually training each finger and thumb and hoping they will work together when it's time to catch or throw a ball.

Testing for weak links is done in phases. Movement is considered the root. On top of movement is physical conditioning; on top of physical conditioning is skill. First, you test movement. Then you test physical conditioning. Finally, you appraise skill with the help of coaching, video analysis, and records of past and present performance. At this point, movement and physical conditioning should be the focus because they are the foundation of skill. It is important to strengthen, or at least balance, the foundation before reassessing skill. This may seem like common sense, but athletes at all levels fail to practice this principle.

Balance is a key factor in elite training programs. Strength, flexibility, speed, and stamina must be balanced. Without balance, efficiency is sacrificed. When efficiency is lost, so is power.

An athlete needs to be open and willing to test objectively and train accordingly, to administer the tests and do what those tests say to do. An athlete may desperately want to improve speed, but if the test reveals that speed is adequate (although in need of improvement) but flexibility is the weakest link, then he must be committed to work on flexibility first and progress to a speed workout only when speed is the weakest link. This requires discipline. If flexibility is the weakest link, then speed training could potentially cause injury or biomechanical stress over time. High-level speed training requires maximum range of motion and flawless body awareness. Both of these things are significantly limited when flexibility is limited.

Energy Leaks

Energy leaks can result from weak links. The term *energy leak* indicates poor efficiency as well as stress. An energy leak occurs when all of the energy generated to perform a certain task or movement does not go specifically into that task or movement. Science tells us the energy must go somewhere. Usually, the energy creates stress within the body. The stress can take many forms. It may cause unnecessary work or movement in another part of the body, placing greater stress on certain muscles and tendons (strains). It may create unnatural motion of the spine or limbs, placing greater stress on joints and ligaments (sprains). This movement can create stress and trauma that may go unnoticed for weeks or months. Eventually the athlete will pay the price if the stress continues. For example, consider an athlete who is generally stiff throughout the hips. Testing identifies flexibility to be the weakest link, but the athlete continues to insist that strength and endurance are what he needs to work on. His training could have many energy leaks. Let's say he chose to run hills instead of focusing on flexibility. Hill running requires the athlete to lift the knee as high as possible. Hill running promotes acceleration, leg strength, and good sprinting form, but an athlete who attempts hill running without optimal hip flexibility will use some other form of movement to help gain the stride length necessary for hill training. The brain and body will compensate for the lack of flexibility and use alternative movement patterns. This athlete is not working *through* the weak link; he is working *around* it and is creating an energy leak in doing so. Poor form almost always results in an energy leak.

It is possible for an athlete to perform well even when poor form is used, but eventually the athlete will experience breakdown, inconsistency, fatigue, soreness, and even injury. It should be the goal of the training program to create efficient movement in the activity. This will conserve energy, keep the athlete relaxed, and allow the athlete to practice more and compete with less stress.

The problem is that poor form may be easier, more familiar, and more comfortable, and it may even seem to take less energy than proper form. Proper form, however, will take far less energy in the long run. Poor form, even if it leads to some initial success, will eventually rob the athlete and cost far more time and effort than what is required to fix the weak links. Poor form can incorporate less overall muscle activity and therefore seem easier, but don't confuse this feeling with efficiency. Muscles are accustomed to generating the desired movement and maintaining optimal body position. To be efficient, the athlete must fulfill both criteria and then demonstrate the ability to reproduce the activity without a decline in quality. The athlete who understands this will be more efficient and will develop the muscles that were designed to perform the activity.

Microtrauma can be the result of overtraining, but multiple factors are associated with microtrauma—inadequate warm-up and cool-down, lack of body awareness, poor nutrition and hydration, as well as suboptimal biomechanics. Preferential training, in which the athlete practices one form of training to the point of neglecting others, can also play a role. Do what is necessary; there's no way to avoid it. If testing shows a weakness in one area, that is the area that must be trained. When testing reveals improvement in that area, another area can be addressed. But until that point, work on the weakest link.

The purpose of this program is to find the weak links. Once a weak link is identified, the program provides a systematic approach to train the weakest link and then retest the link to find improvements. Retesting should identify the next weak link, and so on. This can get tricky. Realize that completely getting rid of a weak link is not a destination—it's a journey.

Many athletes feel that coaches hold them back or redirect their attention to unnecessary fundamentals, technical basics, and activities that seem to have little or no relevance to what they want to do. This, however, is the true art of coaching. Knowing when to advance, change, and modify training should be based on many factors and not simply the athlete's desire to move ahead.

The art of coaching or self-coaching is maximizing benefits while minimizing risks. Now, more than ever before, we want to believe in the quick fix, believe that hard work, discipline, and dedication can be avoided in favor of some innovative fast track that will still lead to the winner's circle time and time again. That's simply not the case. No matter how good you are, you will always have at least one weakness that must be consistently confronted, trained, polished, and reevaluated. The true champion will spend more time working on weakness than showing off strength. You need to know more about your weakness than any opponent could ever discover or any condition or situation could ever expose. It has been said that the only person who is truly objective is the one who knows that he is not. It is so hard to be objective about oneself. This book will help identify the weakest link and train it accordingly. Objectivity is built into the system.

3

Analyzing Movement

Movement is ultimately what defines great athletes. It certainly is what defined Barry Sanders. At 5 feet 8 inches and 203 pounds, Barry had a relatively average, if not small, body for the NFL. Many wondered whether he could survive the punishment meted out in professional football. But Barry's ability to move was unique. He was compact and quick. He demonstrated a perfect balance of control and quickness. He soon quieted his critics. But his physique didn't define his career; his movement did.

To be ignorant of motion is to be ignorant of nature.

—*Aristotle*

Modern science tells us that the brain does not recognize individual muscle activity—it doesn't need to. Instead, the brain looks at movement patterns and creates coordination between all the muscles needed. This coordination is called a *motor program.*

Isolated muscle development does not play a major role in motor pattern development. Don't confuse form with function. Weight training with muscle isolation is popular in bodybuilding because bodybuilding is about form. Muscle size and symmetry are the goals. But most sports are about movement. Speed, quickness, agility, power, control, coordination, and stamina are the keys to success. The goal of training is not to change how the body looks, but to improve how the body moves. Therefore, sport training should focus on movement patterns rather than individual muscles. Muscles will develop naturally as different movement patterns are worked, so most athletes will look as if they have done some bodybuilding. But the focus is on *function;* great form is just a by-product.

Many activities in sports, recreation, and fitness have the same basic movement patterns. Throwing a baseball and serving in tennis rely on some of the same motor programs of shifting weight from one foot to another and rotating the body to develop a rotary speed in the hips and shoulders to accelerate the arm. Although golf and baseball are very different sports, swinging a baseball bat and swinging a golf club use some of the same motor programs when energy is transferred from a hip turn to a shoulder turn to an arm swing. The brain does not have to remember millions of independent activities because many of them overlap and are interrelated. This conserves memory space in the brain and allows quick access to movement information for learning and refinement.

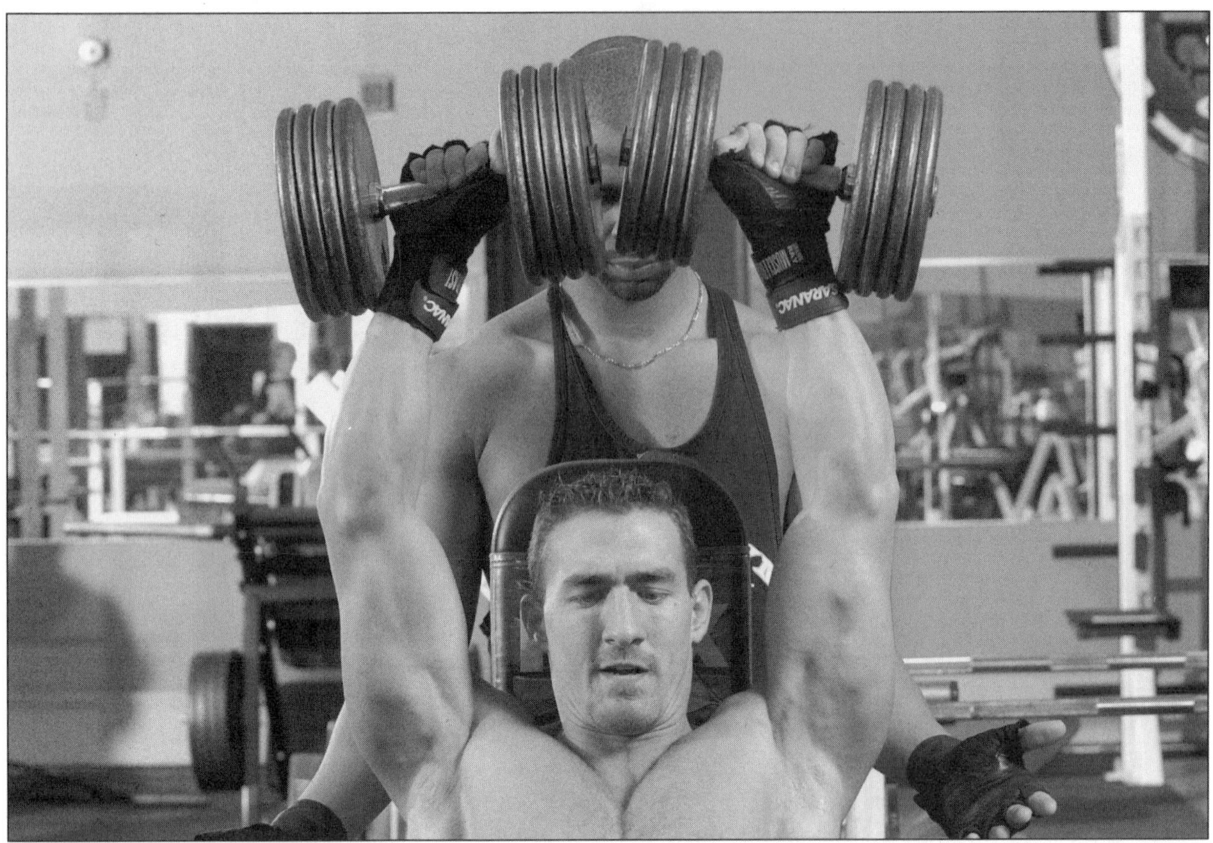

Bodybuilders focus on isolating certain muscles in order to build bulk. Athletes should focus on improving movement patterns in order to improve performance.

The *performance pyramid* is a simple diagram constructed to provide a mental image and understanding of human movement. It is made of three rectangles of diminishing size to demonstrate how one type of movement builds on another. Each rectangle represents a certain type of movement. The pyramid must always be constructed from the bottom up and must always have a tapered appearance (a broad base and a narrow top).

The first level represents the foundation: mobility and stability, or the ability to move through fundamental patterns. It is not concerned with in-depth technical analysis of every possible movement, but evaluates each movement as *optimal, passing,* or *failing.*

The second level is related to performance. Once ability to move is established, the efficiency of movements is evaluated. More specifically, power is evaluated—not specific power but general power (also called *gross athleticism*).

The vertical leap is a good example of a test of gross athleticism. First, because gravity affects all bodies equally, the vertical leap does not discriminate unfairly against body size, as other tests do. Second, even though jumping is very important in some sports (such as basketball and volleyball) and rarely considered in others (such as cycling and marathon running), it demonstrates the ability to produce or generate power.

From a training standpoint, it is very important to be able to compare individuals of different sports in a general format. The first two levels of the pyramid allow us to make this comparison so that athletes can learn from each other and from different training regimens. It is important not to get sport specific with testing at this level of the performance pyramid. That will reduce the ability to compare athletes of different sports and learn from each other. It also is important not to do too many tests at this level. The more tests performed, the more complicated it can get. A few simple movements will show how efficient an athlete is at generating power.

The last level of the pyramid is specific skill. A battery of tests assesses ability to do a given activity, participate in a specific sport, or play a specific position within that sport. This level also looks at competition statistics and any specific testing relative to one's sport.

When evaluating the pyramid, we look at its shape. The four basic profiles are the *optimum* performance pyramid, the *overpowered* performance pyramid, the *underpowered* performance pyramid, and the *underskilled* performance pyramid. Of course, these are simply generalizations to serve as examples for some of the most common problems seen in sports today.

Optimum Performance Pyramid

The optimum performance pyramid (figure 3.1) has a broad base with a slightly smaller level in the middle and an even smaller level on top. This illustrates an athlete who has appropriate or optimal functional movement. This athlete possesses the ability to explore a full range of movement, demonstrating body control and movement awareness throughout numerous positions.

The athlete also has demonstrated a requisite amount of power. Compared to average athletic performance statistics, this athlete also has demonstrated average or above-average general power production. The athlete uses well-coordinated linking movements or kinetic linking. This means that during a test such as the vertical leap, the athlete loads the body in a crouched position, throws the arms, slightly extends the trunk, and then explodes through the legs in a well-timed, well-coordinated effort so that no movement is wasted and optimal efficiency is reached. This athlete has the potential to learn other kinetic linking movements and power production movements with appropriate time, practice, and analysis.

The third level illustrates an average or optimal amount of sport-specific or activity-specific skill. Note how the broad base creates a buffer zone for the middle level and the middle level creates a buffer zone for the top pillar. This buffer zone is extremely important. The absence of a buffer zone should raise a red flag. Without the buffer zone, potential for injury exists. At the least, the absence of buffer zones compromises power and efficiency. The buffer zone is a sign that the athlete's functional movements are more than adequate to handle the amount of power he can generate. The power generated (the middle of the pyramid) can more than control the skill that the athlete possesses.

The optimum performance pyramid is the pyramid in which movement patterns, movement efficiency, and sport skill are balanced and adequate. This does not mean that they cannot be improved, but any improvement should not upset the balance and appearance of the pyramid.

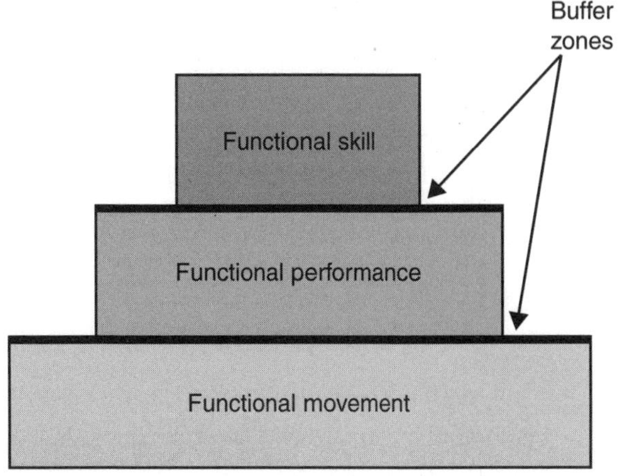

Figure 3.1 The optimum performance pyramid.

Overpowered Performance Pyramid

The overpowered performance pyramid (figure 3.2) represents the athlete who scores very poor on mobility and stability tests (the first level), very high on power production (the second level), and adequate in skill (the third level). The athlete's ability to move freely in simple and basic positions is limited by poor flexibility or poor stability in some movement patterns. This causes the athlete to have a suboptimal functional movement score, which appears as a smaller level at the base of the pyramid.

The overpowered athlete is not necessarily too strong; her ability to generate power exceeds her ability to move freely. This athlete needs to improve movement patterns while maintaining her current level of power. This athlete's diagram does not really look like a pyramid. The base (functional movement) and the top (functional performance) are nearly the same size. This athlete generates a significant amount of power but has many restrictions and limitations in functional movement. Many highly skilled and well-trained athletes appear this way. This athlete may never have experienced an injury and may be performing better than ever, but in training she should focus on functional movement patterns. Removing the limitations to functional movement will provide a broader base and create a greater buffer zone.

The athlete may not see an immediate tangible improvement in performance. In fact, sport-specific performance and power production may remain the same or even go down slightly as mobility and stability improve. However, it is unlikely that this athlete will improve in general power production or sport-specific skill to any large degree without first improving general fundamental basic movement patterns. Therefore, whether this athlete targets functional movement patterns for injury prevention or as a way to realize untapped performance, she will eventually see improvement.

To improve flexibility, the overpowered athlete should adopt a specific flexibility program based on weak links as discovered through testing. Generally yoga and Pilates are good choices, but look for small gains rather than big changes. After four weeks, retest to check for progress. The overpowered athlete needs a longer warm-up session before training and competition than other athletes. The body needs plenty of time to become loose and flexible. Massage may help improve movement patterns and flexibility.

In weight training, the overpowered athlete needs to think less about weight and more about range of motion. She should try using dumbbells instead of barbells for upper-body exercises because spiral movements have a greater range of motion. Cable columns are another excellent choice.

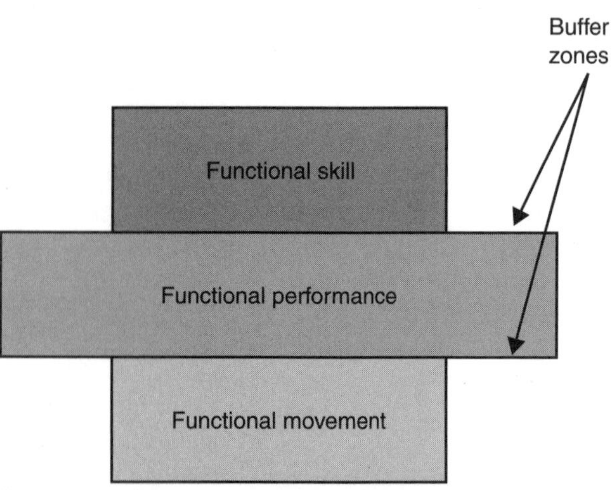

Figure 3.2 The overpowered performance pyramid.

Underpowered Performance Pyramid

The underpowered performance pyramid (figure 3.3) represents the athlete who demonstrates a broad base and optimal movement patterns with very poor power production at the middle of the pyramid and adequate skill in a specific movement. This athlete has the requisite movement patterns to perform multiple tasks, activities, and sport skills but lacks gross athleticism or the ability to produce power in simple movement patterns.

The underpowered athlete has excellent freedom of movement, but efficiency is poor and power could be improved. The training and conditioning program for this athlete should focus on efficiency and power without negatively affecting movement patterns. This athlete would benefit from power training, plyometrics training, or weight training. It is important that the athlete maintain functional movement patterns while gaining strength, power, endurance, and speed. This reserve of power will create the buffer zone for sport-specific skill. It will also improve efficiency.

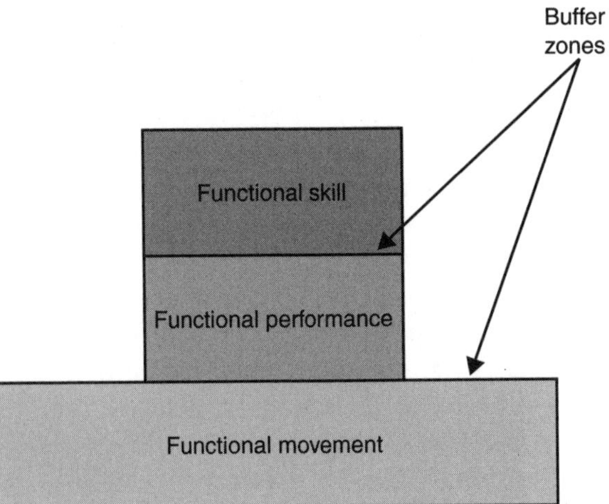

Figure 3.3 The underpowered performance pyramid.

Consider the example of a young pitcher who has extremely good mobility and stability and has honed his pitching skills through video analysis and expert instruction. In order to pitch effectively, he must use a very high level of energy expenditure for a short amount of time. He does not need to be on a mobility or stability program and probably does not need to tinker with pitching mechanics to improve his pitching. This athlete should create better strength, power, and endurance reserves within the body and therefore improve gross athleticism to create a buffer zone between the second and third levels of the pyramid. This buffer zone allows the athlete to pitch at the same level of effectiveness with a higher level of efficiency or a lower level of energy expenditure. As this athlete improves his power, his maximum pitching speed may not change at all. However, under normal circumstances he can expect improvement between pitching bouts in consistency, endurance, and recovery.

The underpowered athlete needs a workout plan that will wake up the neurological system and get it ready to react and control the great movement patterns he is capable of. User-friendly exercises such as wind sprints, jogging, rope jumping, pushups, and even martial arts can be used to improve the ability to direct and control power. Progress should be slow but consistent.

In the weight room, the underpowered athlete should receive careful instruction on the use of free weights. Weight machines can be used, but free weights are a better choice. Weight machines may seem easier and friendlier, especially to someone unfamiliar with weight training, but a true athlete will not make significant gains in functional strength in a seated position in a weight machine. The backrest doesn't allow the trunk to control the power generated by the arms and legs.

As the underpowered athlete adds strength, power, speed, and agility, he should test to ensure that the gains don't disrupt sport skill. An athlete who notices diminished sport skill shouldn't worry. Many elite athletes who add strength in the offseason return to find that sport skills have diminished. Extra sport-specific work may be needed to refine the sport skills with the new gains in strength.

An underpowered athlete may benefit from training with a partner who will push him, watch for poor technique, and note any fatigue. A spotter is needed for strength and power exercises. Dumbbell exercises, work with medicine balls, and intervals of hill sprints and rope jumping should be the foundation of the program. Make sure the weakest link is getting the bulk of the training. Train for about eight weeks, then retest.

Underskilled Performance Pyramid

The underskilled performance pyramid (figure 3.4) reveals an optimal functional movement level, an optimal functional performance level, and a below-average skill level. This athlete, either naturally or through hard work, has appropriate functional movement patterns and good power production but does not have effective mastery of sport skills. This athlete would benefit from technique training to refine or improve mechanics or to develop a greater awareness of the movement needed to perform skills at a higher level.

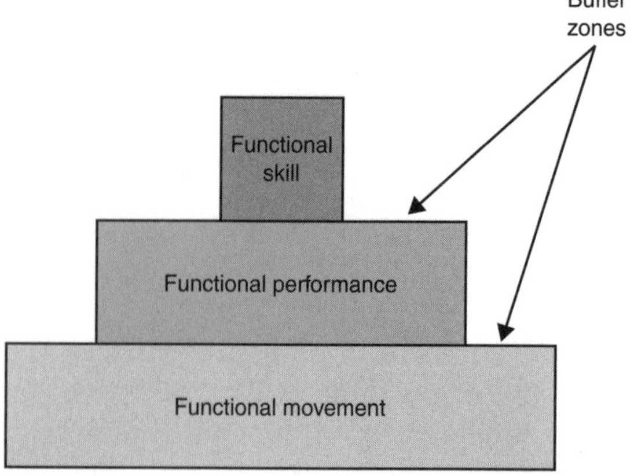

Figure 3.4 The underskilled performance pyramid.

Often underskilled athletes are in better physical shape than many of the people they play with and compete against. They may have less body fat, greater flexibility, and better weight-room stats than others, but other players consistently perform better on the field or court.

Often the key to developing an underskilled athlete is consistent and methodical practice. An athlete who isn't committed to shooting multiple free throws, hitting countless putts, or spending long hours in the batting cage shouldn't expect time in the weight room or a nutrition plan to make a difference in sport performance. Skill can be improved with the right training approach.

The underskilled athlete needs to find out what her skill weak links are. With the help of a coach or video analysis, the athlete should review good and bad performances and identify factors that contributed to the performance. Anxiety may be a factor. Creating a relaxation routine may help the athlete overcome anxiety. Sometimes taking up a new sport or activity, such as tennis, martial arts, racquetball, or golf, may help. Each of these sports isn't won through sheer athleticism alone. Control and proper technique are needed. Learning to develop skill in a new area, even if only a recreational pursuit, may help the athlete recognize fundamental flaws in her chosen sport or activity.

For some athletes, the performance pyramid will change during competition or training over a season. For others, the pyramid will remain the same. Some athletes will naturally have the ability to generate power but will consistently have to work on functional movement patterns to maintain optimal freedom of movement. Others will have excellent freedom of movement and movement patterns but will need to use supplementary training to maintain a level of gross athleticism and power production. Some athletes will find that they need to consistently work on fundamentals and sport skills, while some are naturally gifted with sport skills and should invest their time in conditioning.

Nothing good comes in life or athletics unless a lot of hard work has preceded the effort. Only temporary success is achieved by taking shortcuts.

—Roger Staubach

The performance pyramid demonstrates why simply replicating the program of another athlete will not consistently yield the desired results. Many coaches and athletes intuitively have used this approach to expose the area of greatest weakness and then work on that area. The testing in this book will provide the information needed to construct a simple performance pyramid. The testing will help target areas of focus. The performance pyramid is a simple and effective way to keep body balance in check.

4

Developing Resistance to Injury

It is impossible to discuss movement, fitness, sports, training, and conditioning without discussing pain and injury. Almost every athlete will experience a difficult injury at some point. Attitude has a lot to do with how well the athlete adjusts to the injury and comes back from it.

Take Walter Payton, for example. When faced with the decision to run out of bounds or make contact with a defender, Payton would lower his shoulder and press on. Yet he missed only one game during his career, caused by an ankle sprain during his rookie year. Payton didn't want to miss that game; it was the coach's decision. Payton felt he could have played on the ankle. When he had arthroscopic surgery on both knees following his 1983 season, he flippantly referred to it as his 11,000-yard checkup.

Payton's ability to resist injury came from his body knowledge and awareness, functional conditioning, core strength, and natural talent. Everyone can use at least three of these qualities.

To become different from what we are, we must have some awareness of what we are.

—Zen saying

Understanding Pain

The old saying "No pain, no gain" is often misinterpreted by young athletes. They think it means that any uncomfortable sensation, from the severe pain of injury to mild discomfort, can be worked through. If the saying is applied to pushing through fatigue in an endurance situation or clipping out that extra repetition, then it's probably helpful. Soreness is often the by-product of hard work and training. Pain, however, indicates a problem that needs to be examined and corrected to prevent further damage. But many athletes and fitness enthusiasts continuously push, compete, and train into pain and use ice and anti-inflammatory medications for long periods to mask pain.

Most people don't see pain for what it is. The body is smart—pain is a warning that something is wrong. In the age of medical miracles and quick fixes, we consider pain a distraction and an annoyance, but it is a signal that something is not right.

Imagine that while driving your car, you notice a red light on your dashboard. You would not take a towel from your gym bag and lay it across the dashboard so that the light would not annoy you. Rather, you would probably try to identify the nature of the problem. Most likely you would stop the vehicle as soon as you could and examine the problem in greater detail, then either fix it yourself or find help. If you continued driving with the warning light on you could damage the vehicle and compromise your own safety.

With a car, stopping to evaluate a warning sign seems quite logical. But consider that the next day while out jogging you experience knee pain. Instead of stopping, you continue to run, pushing through the knee pain. The pain persists through two or three runs. Eventually you purchase anti-inflammatory medications and various other products such as neoprene sleeves, muscle rubs, magnets, and ice packs to cover up the pain for the next run. You are throwing a towel over the dash rather than addressing the cause of the pain. The knee pain could simply be a muscle imbalance that has produced unnecessary stress in the joint or tendons. Covering up the symptom (pain) and pushing the joint further and further into activity can cause a significant amount of damage. You want the pain to go away so that you can get on with things, but by denying it you are ignoring one of the keys to refining your training.

Poor posture and body alignment can rob energy from movement. Coaches often refer to this as *wasted energy,* but it is better called *misdirected energy* because energy that is lost has to go somewhere. Misdirected energy can result from poor body mechanics, poor posture, poor technique, or an unfortunate collision with an opponent, object, or the ground, and it often injures the body and creates unnecessary fatigue.

Even though muscles are supposed to be sore when worked, they are not supposed to *stay* sore (beyond 48 hours). With normal training and conditioning, joints are not supposed to hurt. Naturally, after a competitive sporting event or a hard race, one will likely experience some joint stiffness and maybe even some pain. However, the human body was designed to have most of its mechanical stress taken in the muscles and diverted away from the joints. Therefore, in most cases soreness should be in the muscles, only temporarily, after hard work.

The joints create the framework for movement and the muscles and tendons create tension and absorb stress to move and protect the body. The muscles are strategically aligned, crossing and attaching to joints at every necessary angle to help create efficient movement and dissipate the stress sustained through movement. In other words, they were made to deal with stress. Their ample blood flow allows them to recover quickly even when they have been pushed to their limit. Blood flow brings nutrients and carries away waste. Joints, however, do not have the same circulation network, nor can they handle inflammation with the same efficiency as muscle.

Pain distorts proprioception, which creates the ability to feel when moving from turf to dirt (without looking down) or to stop on a dime and make a cutting move. Training and conditioning require body awareness. This body awareness allows each workout session to be more than just an opportunity to sweat. Each workout session can improve motor learning, coordination, and movement patterns. If body awareness is distorted by pain, then chances are the athlete will compensate or use awkward or unnatural movements to avoid the pain. These movements can create more problems. Compensation creates stress in other parts of the body as other areas work harder to achieve the same level of performance. New problems arise when normal body parts must work in abnormal situations or the athlete pushes into the pain, risking even greater injury with more complications.

It is extremely important to get to the bottom of the causes of pain. If the pain is caused by a single episode or injury, it is easy to discern the cause. However, if a nagging pain comes on slowly and lingers, it is important to find out what caused it, where the pain is coming from, and what can be done to correct it.

Pain Is NOT the Enemy

Both enemies and obstacles need to be overcome. Although you are perfectly justified in wanting to be rid of pain, it is not an enemy or an obstacle. You will not overcome pain until you understand it. Pain is simply a signal alerting you to a problem or a potential problem.

The body is intuitive and intelligent, and it knows when things are wrong. It is completely sensitive to the most minute stress, misalignment, and unnecessary strain. The same system of sensitivity that allows a golfer to create a shot with pinpoint accuracy and a quarterback to thread a needle with a football keeps you in touch with your body. The system uses pain to say something's not right or that something's going to be wrong if you persist. Sure, you can cover it up, but are you dealing with the cause or the symptom?

Today's science and technology can mask pain and allow you to push on. That's a decision that only you can make, but it's important to know that the pain is trying to tell you something, such as the following:

- You have poor form.
- You have poor technique.
- You didn't warm up.
- You didn't stretch.
- You have a small muscle imbalance.
- The right and left sides of your body aren't working together.
- The energy that you are producing for this activity is not going to this activity. It's going into stress (energy leaks).

Use pain to your advantage. If you are working out, lifting weights, jogging, or practicing, change your technique or your stance or some other aspect of movement. Look at form and the way you shift weight or the way you move. Consider your posture. Are you sticking with fundamentals? Are you moving the way a coach would like you to move? Or are you trying to clip out an extra few repetitions or push on in the presence of fatigue? Many of these little changes can give you insight into your problem. If you have already created inflammation, swelling, and irritation there is little you can do from a technique standpoint. Any activity, even high-quality activity (doing everything perfectly), will cause problems.

If you have inflamed tendons, joints, ligaments, and muscles, you can't beat the old RICE treatment. RICE stands for *rest, ice, compression,* and *elevation.* Once you've done rest, ice, compression, and elevation, don't forget to ask the question, "Why?" If you weren't injured from a fall or some sort of trauma, then chances are you have microtrauma. You have an energy leak, a weak link, a point of stress or strain. If you listen to your body, it will pay off in the long run. It is amazing how many athletes are reluctant to miss one or two workouts while seeking an answer to this question when, with a little rest and education, they could come back in a week or two with a new understanding of a weak link and maybe even better movement patterns as well.

Awareness is everything. If you know what your opponent is going to do, if you know what's around the next bend, if you know how the ball is going to bounce, then you've got an edge. Your body is looking for the same edge. It doesn't want tightness or weakness anywhere. Tight and weak muscles can lead to poor joint alignment, and when joints are stiff and not aligned they are not supportive or efficient and do not communicate effectively.

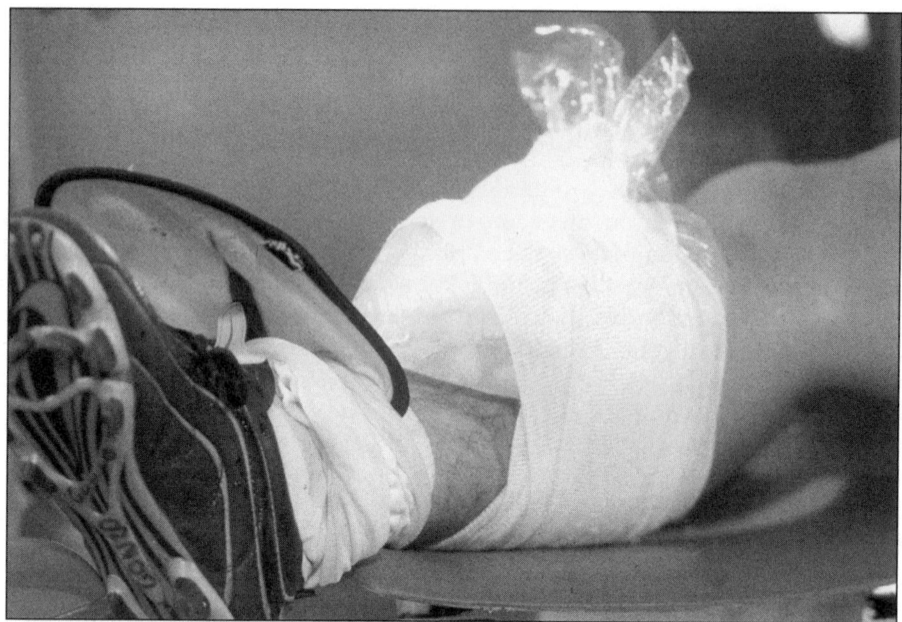

Use RICE—rest, ice, compression, and elevation—to treat pain, but also try to identify the cause.

Yes, joints talk. They talk to the brain. Muscles also talk to the brain, and joints and muscles talk to each other. When joints and muscles are not working effectively together, the brain does not have the information it needs to act and react with proper movement sequences. So it misses important information like "Don't cut so sharply—you're going to slip" or "Stop on your left foot, not your right—otherwise you'll be off balance." Many athletes think that the mind-body connection or communication is only one way. Of course the brain talks to the body, but the body also talks to the brain. There is a constant two-way conversation between the body and the brain.

Joints and muscles indicate everything that the eyes do not. The eyes can only be in one place as you perform and play. The body tells you the rest. Equilibrium helps balance. The joints tell you where your body is by their position and movement. Muscles, by their tension, indicate how you are moving and what your intensity level is. The brain sorts all of this and blends it with what you hear and see and makes you aware of what you are doing. This awareness is important, and you don't even have to think about it. Thinking takes too long and signals that you don't trust your instincts. Proper training and repetition develop instincts and allow you to become relaxed and comfortable with skilled movement during competition. Any experienced athlete would prefer to play instinctively. This is not to say that planning and preparation are not necessary. In fact, the planning and preparation are what make relaxed and instinctive play possible. Therefore, stay relaxed, focused, and aware so that you can act and react instinctively. Training is no different. Don't just practice—practice being aware.

The awareness philosophy can be applied to pain. If you have pain, be aware of it. Don't treat it as an obstacle; treat it as a puzzle. It should be your job to figure it out. Doctors, athletic trainers, and physical therapists can help you, but it's still your problem. If you can't figure it out, get help and keep seeking help until somebody can provide you with a logical explanation and a possible solution. Quick fixes and cover-ups will cost you dearly in the long run.

Remember, when you cover up pain you are covering up a weak link or an energy leak and missing an opportunity to refine the way you move and become more aware of your body. When a medical professional helps you with pain you must also find out what caused the problem. Let the medical professional know you are not interested in a cover-up. Ask whether an underlying weak link may have caused the problem. Ask what you can do to prevent the problem in the future. Be a smart consumer.

An athlete with a nagging injury or an unresolved problem should not try to lay training on top of that faulty base. Injuries and medical problems in athletics are often classified in such categories as tendinitis, bursitis, instability, dislocation, strain, and sprain. Every problem is unique, and rarely is just one thing wrong. An athlete may be aware only of the area of symptoms, but other mechanical problems may exist.

Some players with a lot of athletic ability just go out and play. Then after four or five years you don't hear about them anymore. The smart guys figure it out, and they play ten, twelve years. They do it mentally more than they do it physically.

—Ahmad Rashad

This book takes a simple approach to expose some of the major mechanical limitations that cause problems. Movement patterns reveal limitations, and the exercises in this book will break them down and try to correct them so they can be rechecked. This is a simple approach that works.

But if it does not work, do not continue to train blindly, thinking that the problem will go away. Most likely, it will not. Actively and intelligently pursue the problem. Be wary of quick fixes and suspicious when people cannot explain why the problem occurred or demonstrate how to regain control of the problem. Sports medicine clinicians are just like coaches. They are opinionated and have their own way of doing things. Be an educated consumer and make sure that the explanation and remedy make sense. If they don't, have them explained again or have them explained by someone else.

Trigger Points

If you have ever had massage or physical therapy, you may have heard the term *trigger point.* A trigger point is thought to be a small area or section of muscle that acts differently from the rest of the muscle. Many different stresses can contribute to the formation of a trigger point, but the muscle does not need and should not have trigger points. A trigger point is a section of muscle that is unusually sensitive to pressure, resulting in a pinching or burning sensation when the area is compressed. This increases tension throughout the entire muscle and also can cause pain in another area of the body (called *referred pain*). Trigger points can also cause pain within the same muscle, in muscles close to the area, or in joints close to the trigger point. Trigger points can be found in extremely tight or bulky muscles or in muscles that are overstretched and generally weak and therefore overworked.

Trigger points are thought to be associated with areas of previous trauma within the muscle. This could be a microscopic tear or a contusion that injured muscle fibers, causing them to have abnormal activity. Inappropriate use of a muscle can also cause trigger points. If you use a muscle to compensate or substitute for other muscles because of tightness or weakness elsewhere in the body, that muscle will be overstressed. It will have to work overtime during certain activities. The increased tension and trauma to the muscle sometimes can irritate the muscle. Constant irritation in a muscle can cause abnormal responses, such as the development of trigger points.

It is not uncommon to see trigger points develop in muscle after injuries that required immobilization in a brace or cast. Too much activity, not enough activity, or traumatic activity can cause trigger points. During a sport massage, trigger points become obvious. If you don't stretch, strengthen, and train after the trigger point has been relaxed, it will come back. It's simple. Get the muscle to an appropriate state, train it in that state, and then recheck it before training again.

An objective way to identify and treat trigger points is by using a roller device called a *stick*. It is a simple tool that is rolled over a muscle belly to identify areas of increased sensitivity. In many cases, these areas will be trigger points. However, not all sensitivity is a trigger point. Areas with obvious scar tissue and bruising should be evaluated by a sports medicine professional.

If the area is a trigger point, it may be treated with the stick. Gently roll the stick back and forth over the sensitive area. By rolling the stick over only the sensitive area of the muscle, you distort and stretch the fibers directly under the stick but leave the rest of the muscle alone. If you stretch or massage the entire muscle, it is unlikely that you will affect the trigger point, because it is more resistant to change than the rest of the muscle. By focusing only on the area of increased sensitivity, you isolate treatment and create an area of more normal behavior within the muscle only where that behavior was initially abnormal. This approach is more specific than stretching to reduce chronic trigger point activity.

As sensitivity in the area fades, consider the trigger point managed. If you identified the muscle with the trigger point to be a short one, then use stretching to improve the length of the muscle once the trigger point has been treated. If you try to stretch a muscle without addressing a trigger point, the muscle will lengthen but will quickly return to its original length, not because the stretching was inappropriate but because the trigger point overrides the work you just did.

You may have a muscle that feels tight but actually is not tight at all. Judge the tightness of the muscle not by the way it feels but by whether you have full range of motion. For instance, if you scored perfectly on a straight leg raise (page 36) then the hamstrings have appropriate length. Even if you feel you have tight hamstrings, if you scored perfectly on the test it is highly unlikely that this is your greatest problem. Tightness or tension in a muscle could indicate an inadequate warm-up or an attempt to compensate for a muscle that is extremely tight. Many athletes will think that they have tight hamstrings when their lower backs are tight. If a muscle has an area of sensitivity, treat the area and recheck it. Trigger points can also make muscles weak or less efficient, and it is equally appropriate to do stick work on a muscle before you train for strength, endurance, speed, agility, and quickness.

If the trigger point does not go away with treatment, seek help from a trained sports medicine professional. An athletic trainer, physical therapist, or physician with a sports background is the most appropriate choice. If the area does not change quickly with treatment, stretching, and appropriate strengthening, chances are there is some other contributing factor, or you aren't dealing with a trigger point. Areas that have recently been bruised or strained are not trigger points. Sensitivity there is due to inflammation. Most elite athletes consistently use sport massage, but this can become extremely expensive. It is best to get in touch with your own body.

Understanding Injury and Recovery

Injuries can have underlying factors and are sometimes not as simple as they might appear to be on the surface. Statistics have shown that the chance of injury increases toward the end of competition when fatigue is higher. Sometimes this fatigue could have been prevented through training. Fatigue, like pain, also reduces body awareness, affecting reaction time and coordination and causing compensations, which are usually much less efficient and place significantly greater stress on the body.

In part II, we will discuss mobility and stability testing that will help identify potential problems quickly. Undetected stiffness and weakness can cause many problems that could have been prevented. It is helpful to have a personal baseline of test results before an injury. These results can be used to chart rehabilitation and recovery and compare preinjury flexibility, speed, stamina, power, quickness, and strength to postinjury performance.

Sometimes athletes overdo training and conditioning. They compete or train beyond their limits, causing pain, soreness, and maybe even injury. If the injury is a simple strain or general muscle soreness or if the athlete has been sick or ill and is going to return to training, there are some simple low-stress forms of exercise called *active recovery* that will help the body alleviate soreness and tension and prepare for harder work in the future.

Active recovery can save time in the recovery process, but it is not a substitute for rest. If the athlete is not getting enough rest, then no amount of exercise or high-grade nutritional supplement can help. Low-level aerobic exercise increases circulation, elevates body temperature, and increases sweating and respiration.

The natural healing process can't be accelerated, but many things can inhibit or slow recovery. Too much rest does not allow an adequate amount of circulation to flush a muscle of the waste products generated in high-stress activity. Insufficient activity inhibits or slows the healing process. On the other hand, too much activity can irritate sore muscles and stiff joints or stress metabolism and create unnecessary strain. Medicine and therapy remove some of the factors that slow or delay the normal healing process, but magic does not exist in medicine. Managing symptoms and creating a cure are two different things.

Here are four forms of active recovery that you can incorporate into your program. They also work well in conjunction with a rehabilitation program if you have been injured. Remember, time is the important factor here. The longer and easier, the better.

The Stationary Bike

Almost everyone has seen a major league pitcher after a game with ice on his shoulder, arms crossed, riding a stationary bike. He increases circulation as he pedals the bike while managing inflammation and swelling in his shoulder by using the ice.

The stationary bike is a simple way to improve circulation, but it isn't a workout. Try to pedal for a long time, and keep water handy. It's best if you don't hold onto the handlebars the majority of the time you ride, so change body position often by sitting up straight, crossing your arms, and twisting your upper body left and right, stretching your arms overhead and keeping your spine in an erect but comfortable position. Keeping the spine erect will help you breathe better. Take a 10-minute break in the middle of the cycling workout and use the stretches that are most beneficial to your movement type (see chapter 5). Pedal at a comfortable rate so that your breathing is more rapid but you can still carry on a conversation.

Treading Water

Most athletes cannot spend enough time in the pool to have appropriate swimming mechanics. Swimming is sometimes too strenuous for athletes with high muscle mass, low body fat, and poor technique. However, most people can tread water. If you can't, learn.

Use a small flotation device around your waist or wear a lifejacket if you have difficulty staying afloat. The flotation device should barely hold you up so that a little bit of leg and arm action is necessary to keep you afloat. Use less and less flotation as you become more proficient at treading water. You want to be able to carry on a conversation as you tread. Set a goal to be able to tread water for at least a half-hour with periodic breaks and stretching as necessary.

Treading water is overlooked in most training programs, but it incorporates the arms, legs, and spine in natural movement patterns. It has another significant benefit: Most of us expend too much energy when we first start to tread water. This is an opportunity to learn to relax and do as little as possible but still remain afloat. Deep breathing and slower, more controlled movements of the arms and legs will allow you to conserve energy and still exercise at a low level. Flippers can emphasize leg action, and hand paddles can emphasize arm action in the event that you can use only your arms or legs. If you have access to a pool, treading water is one of the most natural and productive forms of active rest.

Hiking

Simple walking is not usually enough for an active person who is trying to recover. You need a little more activity but want to avoid impact and fatigue. Therefore, hiking, which is really just walking on uneven terrain with as many hills as possible, is an excellent alternative. Hiking with one or two walking sticks can also incorporate upper-body movement and assist you in practicing erect posture. Use this as an opportunity to tune your breathing. You easily can get out of breath when hiking, but use slow, deep, relaxed breathing when you feel like taking a break. Learn to emphasize exhaling. Make it slow and long, twice as long as your inhaling time.

Hiking can be the most strenuous form of active recovery, so know the route you are taking and be familiar with the terrain you are walking. Hiking requires slightly greater range of motion from the lower body than walking. For this simple reason, it is an excellent form of active stretching that also develops postural awareness and cardiovascular conditioning. It is safest to hike with a partner, take plenty of water and a light snack, and dress appropriately.

The Sauna

The sauna (dry heat) should not to be confused with a steam room (wet heat). The use of a sauna can elevate your metabolism almost to the same degree as low-level aerobic exercise. A hot tub or a steam room will elevate your temperature somewhat, but will not induce the intense perspiration that dry heat does.

Dry heat causes all of the blood vessels close to the surface of the skin to grow larger (dilate), moving heat away from the center of your body (your vital organs) to the surface of your body. That heat then leaves the body through evaporation into the dry atmosphere of the sauna. To move this blood and produce sweating, your heart has to work as hard as it would in response to low-level exercise. Your heart rate will often get as high in a sauna as it does when you are leisurely riding a stationary bike. Most saunas also have enough room so that you can perform a simple stretching routine.

If you are not familiar with saunas, then you probably will make a common mistake and try to endure a temperature that is too high. It is necessary to take periodic breaks from the sauna. Shower to remove the sweat from your body and then return to the sauna and continue. It would be optimal to stay in the sauna 30 to 60 minutes with as many shower breaks as necessary at a level of heat that is comfortable but produces sweating.

The benefits of sauna and dry heat have been used for centuries by many different cultures as a form of active recovery, a way to manage stress, and a way to increase metabolism. Educate yourself on the correct use of a sauna and get started.

Most champions who stay on top use a personal system to manage stress, rehabilitate injuries, perform active rest, and constantly uncover weak links. Follow their lead and educate yourself. Don't wait for someone to do it for you.

PART II

MOBILITY AND STABILITY

5

Mobility and Stability Testing

As a physical therapist and strength coach, I have pursued better ways to incorporate functional exercise into both rehabilitation and conditioning. Eventually I realized the best way to show a need for functional exercise was to develop some sort of functional assessment that would not only demonstrate the need for functional exercise but provide feedback regarding the effectiveness of a particular exercise on functional performance.

My intuition was telling me that something basic was missing in many of my previous assessments. With the help of friends and colleagues, I developed and refined a screening tool called the *functional movement screen* as a way to document and communicate what I was seeing in my orthopedic assessment of athletes. As I evaluated athletes with difficult problems and unexplained injuries, instead of focusing specifically on their injuries I took a step back so I would not miss the forest for the trees.

Then it hit me. Although I had been trained to look at both the parts and the whole, I was focusing too much on the part and not enough on the whole. Actually, it was a problem of sequence. For example, if an athlete complained of a chronic knee problem that had not been successfully managed, I would observe, evaluate, and test the knee in many different positions. Then I might ask the athlete to perform a few general movements, such as balancing on one leg, turning, twisting, or maybe even lunging. But the sequence was wrong. By looking at the knee first, I missed an opportunity to watch the body move—and because I didn't watch the body move first, I lost perspective. I was evaluating the athlete in front of me as a knee problem and not as an athlete who was experiencing symptoms in the knee but who may have multiple problems.

So I reversed the sequence. Regardless of the complaint or injury, I looked first at the whole before initiating a functional exercise or sports rehabilitation program. I made notes on the athlete's history, the type of injury, and the previous care. Then I had the athlete perform a few basic movements as I watched. Sometimes these movements provoked symptoms in the problem area. Sometimes they provoked symptoms in other areas. This gave me the opportunity to observe movement patterns. Once I had established a map of movements the athlete could and could not perform, and those that produced pain, I focused on the injury. This sequence provided a much clearer picture of the athlete's problem.

As my observation and evaluation skills improved, I wanted to communicate what I was seeing in clear and concise language to other sports medicine professionals. The functional movement screen I devised is made up of seven tests that look at fundamental movements. I use the word *fundamental* because these movements are not simply the foundation for sports movements, they are the foundation for *human* movement. These movements relate closely to the movements infants and toddlers use to train themselves to move and turn and twist and walk and climb and crawl and reach. The functional movement screen is simply a way to demonstrate how athletes who have elite strength, power, speed, agility, and sport skills may have fundamental flaws that do not show up on a stat sheet.

The movements that make up the functional movement screen look simple but require good flexibility and control. An athlete who is unable to perform a movement correctly, shows a major limitation within one of the movement patterns, or demonstrates an obvious difference between the function of the left and right side of the body has uncovered a significant piece of information that may be the key to reducing the risk of chronic injuries, improving overall sport performance, and developing a training or rehabilitation program that helps the athlete advance to a higher level of competition. Fundamental movements should not be sacrificed when the athlete seeks to perform at a higher level through advanced conditioning and skill training.

I use the movement patterns of the functional movement screen as object lessons to demonstrate how athletes who are strong, powerful, and seemingly coordinated sometimes have extreme difficulty getting into the most basic positions. Most athletes migrate toward their strengths and spend a majority of their time training their strengths. But the movement screen pushes each athlete into all movement extremes, rather than simply the preferred ones, and thus demonstrates how athletes who appear flexible and under control within their given sports can have significant restrictions and asymmetries between left and right in basic movement patterns. Their skill and speed and quickness allow them to compensate for and mask fundamental flaws in movement. These flaws rob the athlete of efficiency and may cause unnecessary stress on the body. They may either directly break down an area of the body or cause problems when the athlete is trying to rehab a traumatic injury caused by a collision or fall.

Imagine two highly skilled, highly trained athletes recovering from knee surgery. Both are dealing with the swelling, inflammation, and weakness caused by the surgery and immobilization, but one athlete also has very poor ankle flexibility and a significant amount of stiffness in the hip. To this point, this athlete's knee has been compensating for the lack of mobility in the hip and ankle. But because the knee can no longer compensate, the rehabilitation process will be delayed unless the weaknesses in the hip and ankle are addressed.

The functional movement screen is made up of seven movements:

- Squat
- Step
- Lunge
- Reach
- Leg raise
- Push-up for trunk control
- Rotational stability

The tester follows strict criteria to grade each movement. The athlete has three opportunities to successfully complete the movement pattern. Perfect execution of the movement pattern earns 3 points; execution that demonstrates compensation and less-than-perfect form receives 2 points; inability to complete the movement pattern because of stiffness, loss of balance, or another difficulty is worth 1 point; and pain during a particular movement pattern earns a score of 0 regardless of how well the athlete performed the movement.

Initially when I proposed the functional movement screen, the word *functional* created confusion because some expected to see drills and movements that closely resembled sport-specific movement. They wanted to see a more dynamic collection of vigorous movements that looked and felt like athletics, and they were puzzled by the simple positions. What they failed to realize (or I failed to communicate effectively) is that functional movement for all sport is built on the foundation of the ability to simply move without restriction or limitation. The problem with the current perspective is that it is a two-block pyramid instead of a three-block pyramid. Often athletes are assessed in terms of how they perform in their sports and in fitness, agility, power, strength, and endurance tests. But simply looking at skill and performance, the two-block pyramid doesn't recognize that the ability to perform is not separate from the ability to move free of limitation or restriction. This method looks at only the top two blocks of the performance pyramid. Adding the third block (functional movement) makes it much easier to effectively assess the problems athletes experience.

I do not see these seven movements as the bricks that make up the foundation of functional movement in sport; rather, they are the clay that makes up each brick. These movements tie all sports together because they are fundamental and representative of human movement. The biggest mistake made in sports medicine and sports conditioning today is moving to sport-specific movements too quickly.

The movement screen is not a law or an absolute. It is simply one way to demonstrate the most fundamental aspect of human performance—the ability to move freely. If you refer back to the performance pyramid described in chapter 3 (page 13), you'll see that the first block of the pyramid represents the ability to move freely; the second is the ability to move with a certain degree of raw athleticism or gross performance; and the third is the ability to take that raw athleticism and gross performance and turn it into a specific skill. The functional movement screen makes the performance pyramid possible.

For the purposes of this book, I've created a modified version of the functional movement screen. It is less specific but more user friendly, and the tests can be self-administered. The self-screens that follow, if used correctly, can still provide a great deal of information about movement. For more information about the seven-point movement screen, see chapter 2 in *High-Performance Sports Conditioning* (Bill Foran, editor; Human Kinetics, 2001), or go to my Web site at www.functionalmovement.com.

Understanding Mobility and Stability

The fundamental concepts of *mobility* and *stability* are not hard to understand. Mobility and stability must coexist to create efficient movement in the human body.

While flexibility is the ability to elongate a muscle, such as when the hamstrings are stretched during a forward bend, mobility is a broader concept and involves the muscle and joint. Mobility is also more inclusive when describing freedom of movement. A good example of mobility is the ability to keep the heels flat while squatting past the point where thighs are parallel to the floor. Note that the squat involves multiple joints and muscles.

While strength can be defined as the ability to *produce* force or movement, stability is the ability to *control* force or movement. In most cases, stability is a precursor to strength.

The movement system in the human body is similar to a system of levers. Tendons connect muscles to bones and pull the bones into different positions to create movement. Consider the example of moving one arm above the head. First the arm must have adequate mobility within the joints and muscles to go above the head. Next the muscles of the shoulder blade must anchor the shoulder to the body and hold it in a relatively stable position so that the muscles of the arm can contract and raise the arm over the head. The first muscles to contract are those that do not produce a large amount of movement: they stabilize the shoulder blade. Actually there is movement at the shoulder blade, but it is at a much slower rate than the arm and therefore less obvious. The first muscles to contract are the stabilizers and the second are the movers.

Mobility and stability usually occur naturally. For example, think about the way a child learns to move. Children do not usually have mobility or flexibility problems. They do, however, lack stability. They don't just lack strength; they lack control. This is the optimal situation for learning to move. As children move, they develop control through trial and error and by feel. Infants naturally roll or crawl or try to take steps. If they do it correctly by stabilizing certain body parts and moving other body parts, they move in the direction they want to go. If they make a mistake or have faulty balance or coordination, they do not move in the direction they want to go. Usually they do not repeat the activity that did not produce the result they wanted. Only the *correct* motor programs will be reinforced as the child slowly learns body control. The child doesn't need to compensate, because his mobility is not restricted or limited. Therefore, children develop efficient motor programs through trial and error.

An adolescent, teenager, or adult learning a movement pattern or skill for the first time creates a motor program. The body's current level of mobility and stability influences the motor program. If a movement problem exists because of reduced mobility (muscle tightness or joint stiffness) or reduced stability (poor strength, coordination, or control), then the movement pattern is altered to compensate, creating a suboptimal motor program. This can become a problem, especially when another motor program and another movement pattern interacts with it. It is like continually adding to a house that is built on a shaky foundation.

Movement patterns result from habits, activities, hand or leg dominance, and previous injuries. Habits are forms of behavior that are consistently repeated. Activities develop certain movement patterns, just as lack of activity allows some movement patterns to deteriorate. Previous injuries may not have fully rehabilitated and therefore present a limitation in mobility or stability.

Even if an injury is completely rehabilitated, a temporary compensation during recovery may still be present. Consider a knee injury that requires surgery. Before and immediately after surgery, the athlete may have to walk on crutches. Even after rehabilitation, the athlete may limp temporarily because of pain or stiffness in the injured leg. Walking for a period of time with the limp requires the ankle and hip to function differently. This can result in a hardware change by allowing the ankle or hip to become stiffened or weakened, or a software change by using a different sequence of coordination of muscles in the hip and ankle.

Bruce Lee once said, "Training for strength and flexibility is a must. You must use it to support your techniques. Techniques alone are no good if you don't support them with strength and flexibility." His words remain profound and timeless, demonstrating how fundamental movement supports specific movement. Mobility and stability are the fundamental building blocks of strength, endurance, speed, power, and agility.

When these building blocks are not in place, the athlete compensates, developing bad biomechanical habits that allow her to continue performing a skill. Compensations increase the chances of poor performance as well as injury.

Incorrect body mechanics caused by inadequate mobility and stability can produce poor efficiency, requiring more energy and more effort to execute skills. It is easy to see how this could affect sports skills. Great athletes develop efficiency through mobility, stability, and motor programs that use the least amount of energy with the greatest possible result. This allows the athlete to stay relaxed while functioning at an extremely high level. Poor biomechanics not only affect performance, they also can create unnecessary stress, resulting in injury. Playing and training without appropriate mobility and stability will create faulty motor programs, which can create frustration, greatly hinder gains in performance, and increase the risk of injury.

Before Core Training

Testing mobility and stability is the starting point for a balanced training and conditioning program. Since the advent of weight training, most exercise approaches have been targeted at specific muscles and muscle groups. This is called *isolation training,* and it does produce muscular development. But physical performance is about movement development, which is not the same as muscular development. Physical performance is about integration, everything working together. In the case of human movement, the whole is greater than the sum of its parts. Simply speaking, if you train the muscle you may not completely develop the movement, but if you train the movement the muscle will develop appropriately.

It is nearly impossible to gain any valuable movement information by doing tests that isolate specific muscles or muscle groups. It is more appropriate to test and train movements than to test and train muscles. As you learn to understand the basic movements that demonstrate mobility and stability, you will develop greater awareness and learn to refine your training.

Mobility and stability training is the fundamental key to creating freedom of movement and control of motion. Training for mobility and stability must start at the spine. The spine must be flexible enough to adapt to many different situations and movements and stable enough to support the body and transfer power. Most forceful movements producing power, speed, agility, and quickness require the extremities (the arms and legs) to move freely while the spine is maintained in a tall, erect posture.

Even the best athletes do not always maintain perfect posture. In most cases, when you see the athletic spine bend or twist to an extreme, it is in the follow-through movement or after the explosive movement has occurred. When the spine remains stable, the arms and legs are simply pulled toward or away from the trunk to create movement. For efficient movement to occur, it is important that the spine remain stable.

Many athletes think that abdominal training, such as crunches and sit-ups, will improve spine stability. It is true that a strong midsection is a fundamental building block of spine stability, but spine stability cannot be trained when the spine is moving, as it is during crunches and sit-ups. Spine stability is trained by keeping the spine stable in the presence of movement around it (in the arms and legs). The brain and muscles can remember only the way they were trained, so they must consistently be trained the way they will be used in the sport or activity.

When the abdominal muscles work in isolation, they bend the spine forward and flex it or twist it to one side. But they work in conjunction with the powerful hips and extensor muscles of the back to create spine stability. When the muscles in the hip and trunk work together, they form a functional segment called the *core.*

Core training is an attempt to centralize the strength, flexibility, coordination, and power of the body into the most powerful region of the body—the hips and torso. The center of mass is located in this area, and it is the point of stability. In football, when a defender is guarding a receiver, he often is instructed not to take the head fake but to focus on the receiver's midsection because the receiver cannot go anywhere without it. The midsection is the center of mass, so when it is off balance the body is off balance. If this area is strong and stable, the body has a platform from which to drive. Don't get caught up in focusing only on the abdominals—focus on the core. The hips must be flexible and the torso must be strong, and they must work together to generate power.

Optimal core performance relies first on a mobile and stable body. If mobility and stability are inadequate, then the core will compensate in some way. You *think* about moving your arms and legs, but your core functions on reflex (automatic) reactions based on your movement, your balance, and your task. These reflexes cannot function normally if your core must compensate for left hip tightness, poor abdominal strength, poor balance on your right leg, or tightness with left torso rotation. The reflexes that automatically control your core are altered and delayed when you don't take time to balance your body. An abdominal routine that makes your abs burn does not necessarily train your core: it just helps you get really good at an exercise while lying on your back. The strength and endurance you gain while lying down will not completely transfer into a standing position, because that's where your imbalances come into play. Consider movement screening a way to clean up your movements so you can truly train your core.

Self-Movement Screen

The self-movement screen is a simplified and modified version of the functional movement screen. It will give you a quick reference to gauge your ability to perform basic movement patterns. If you want a more in-depth appraisal of your movement patterns, reference the functional movement screen at www.functionalmovement.com or locate a professional currently using the screen. Remember that the self-movement screen and functional movement screen are only screens and not medical evaluations. If you are recovering from an injury or currently have pain, the screen is not for you; you need a complete musculoskeletal evaluation to identify and explain your problem. If you do not have pain or a preexisting problem but experience pain during either movement screen, you also should have a complete musculoskeletal evaluation before initiating a training program.

The self-movement screen can be performed with minimal warm-up. A few jumping jacks (no more than 20) should do the trick. You will need a doorway 32 or 36 inches wide, tape (masking tape works well), and a dowel that is approximately 4 feet long. The best time to perform a movement screen is when you are fresh (before strenuous activity) and not sore from a previous workout.

The scoring system is simple. Completion of the movement is considered a *pass* if all criteria are met. If you are unable to complete the movement within the criteria provided you receive a *fail* for the movement. If you have pain, do not exercise until you receive a complete assessment and appropriate treatment of the problem responsible for the pain. The self-movement screen includes the following tests.

1. **Deep squat:** Examines the symmetrical movement of squatting—the left and right sides of the body do the same movement. To pass this screen, you need optimal mobility at the ankles, knees, hips, and shoulders, and optimal stability throughout the spine.
2. **Hurdle step:** Examines the asymmetrical movement of stepping—the left and right sides of the body perform opposite movements. To pass this screen, you need optimal mobility of one ankle, knee, and hip while demonstrating optimal stability and balance of the other ankle, knee, and hip, as well as the spine. The test is performed on the left and right sides.
3. **In-line lunge:** Examines the asymmetrical movement of lunging. To pass this screen, you need optimal mobility, stability, and balance of both legs in the opposing positions of hip flexion and hip extension. Lunging also requires optimal spine stability. The test is performed on the left and right sides.
4. **Active straight leg raise:** Examines the asymmetrical movement of a straight leg raise. To pass this screen, you need optimal mobility of the legs and optimal core stability in a supine position (on your back). The test is performed on the left and right sides.
5. **Seated rotation:** Examines the ability to rotate the upper torso left and right in a seated cross-legged position. To pass this screen, you need optimal upper-torso mobility as well as optimal hip mobility. The test is performed on the left and right sides.

DEEP SQUAT

In a doorway, place a strip of tape on the floor so that the tape is your foot length away from the doorjamb. Stand in the doorway with your feet shoulder-width apart with half of your body on each side of the door and your toes touching the tape. The feet should be parallel and not turned inward or outward. Hold a dowel overhead to create a 90-degree angle of the elbows and shoulders with the dowel. Press the dowel upward and extend the elbows to a straight position (figure 5.1a). If you hit the top of the door with the dowel, finish extending your elbows as you descend into the squat position.

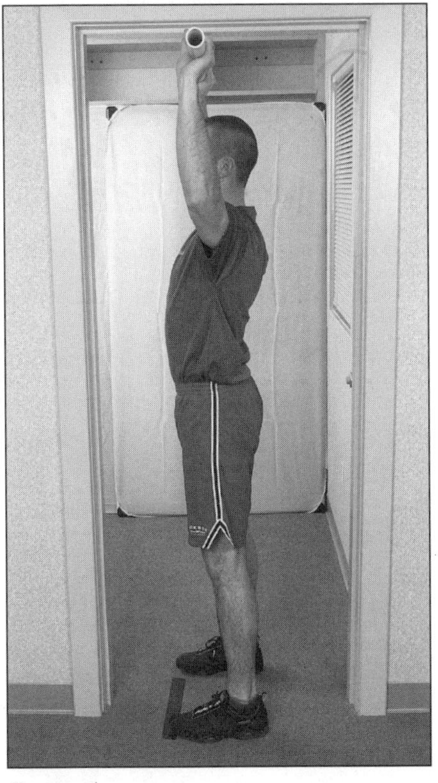

a

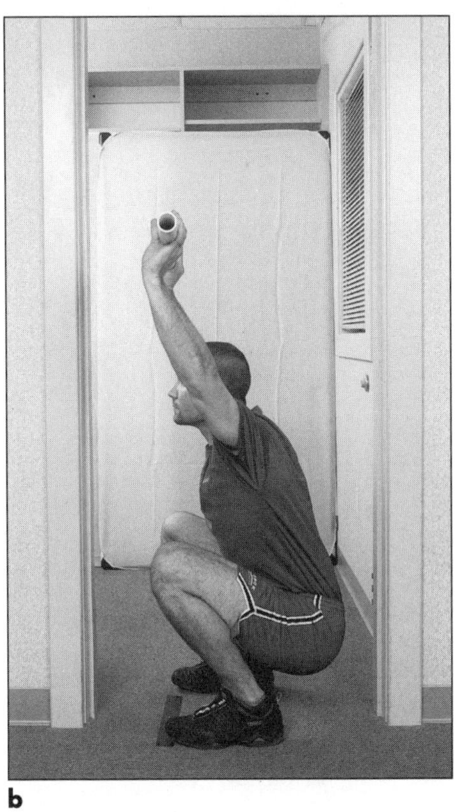

b

Figure 5.1 Deep squat: *(a)* hold the dowel overhead; *(b)* lower into a full squat position.

Once you are in the proper position, descend slowly into a full squat position as deep as you can go (figure 5.1b). Your heels should be flat and your feet should not turn outward or slide as you descend or achieve the full depth of your squat. The dowel should remain overhead at all times and the dowel, your face, or your head cannot touch the doorjamb. To successfully complete the squat, heels must remain on the floor, the head and chest must face forward, and the dowel must be maximally pressed overhead. You have up to three chances to complete the squat, but it is not necessary to perform the squat again if it is achieved on the first attempt.

You pass if the heels stay down, the feet do not slide or rotate, the hips are below the knees, the knees are aligned over the feet, and the dowel does not touch the wall. You fail if any of the five elements is not presently possible. If the movement causes pain, no score is given. It is recommended that a medical professional perform a thorough evaluation of the painful area.

HURDLE STEP

Fasten a strip of tape across a doorway to create a hurdle. The tape should be placed on the outside of the door where you plan to stand when you perform the test. Adjust the tape to the height of the bump on the upper shin just below the kneecap *(tibial tuberosity)*. Assume the starting position by placing the feet together. Position the dowel across your shoulders, not on the neck. The dowel should be just behind the door face as you stand erect with it across your shoulders. Align the front edge of the toes directly beneath the tape (figure 5.2a).

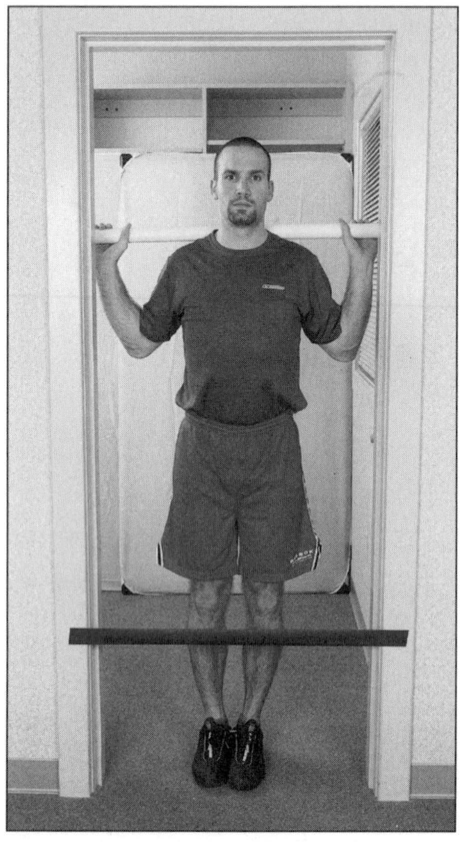

a

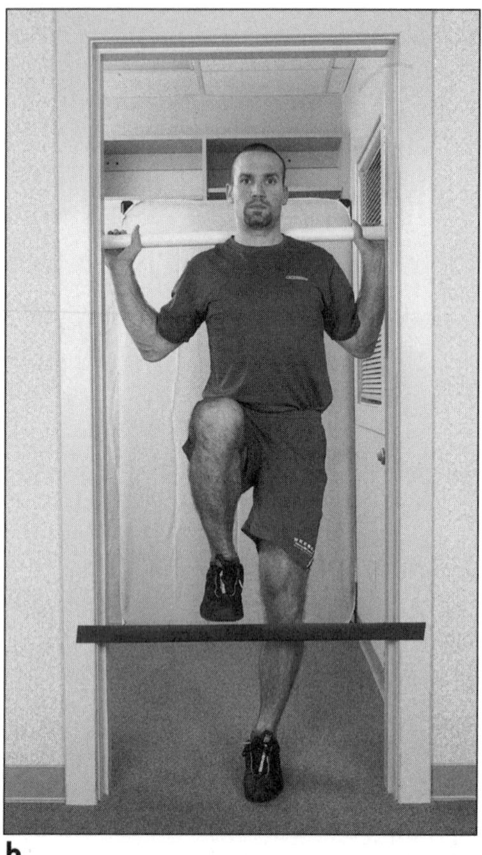

b

Figure 5.2 Hurdle step: *(a)* stand with feet together in front of tape; *(b)* lift foot over tape.

Step over the tape and touch the heel to the floor while maintaining balance (figure 5.2b). Do not put your weight on your heel. Only touch the floor lightly and return to the starting position. Try not to touch the tape as you move the foot over and back. The hurdle step should be performed slowly, as many as three times per foot if needed.

Perform the hurdle step on each side and give a passing grade if the hips, knees, and ankles remain aligned forward, the dowel and hurdle remain parallel (the dowel cannot dip to the left or the right), the dowel does not touch the wall (this would happen if you leaned forward), and balance is maintained. You should have no movement above the waist. The goal is not just to clear the tape. Score yourself hard here. If you get over the tape but have to contort your body and compensate to do so, then you have identified a problem that should be corrected. Give a failing grade if any of the four elements is not presently possible on either side. If the movement causes pain, no grade is given for the test. Have a medical professional perform a thorough evaluation of the painful area.

IN-LINE LUNGE

Cut a strip of tape that equals the length of the lower leg from the bump below the kneecap to the floor, the same measurement used for the hurdle step. Place the tape on the floor through the center of the doorway, with the doorway marking the halfway point of the tape (half the tape on one side of the door and half on the other side). Stand over the tape with the toes of the rear foot touching the back end of the tape and the heel of the front foot touching the front end of the tape. The dowel should be placed in the same position used in the hurdle step screen (across the shoulders; see figure 5.3a).

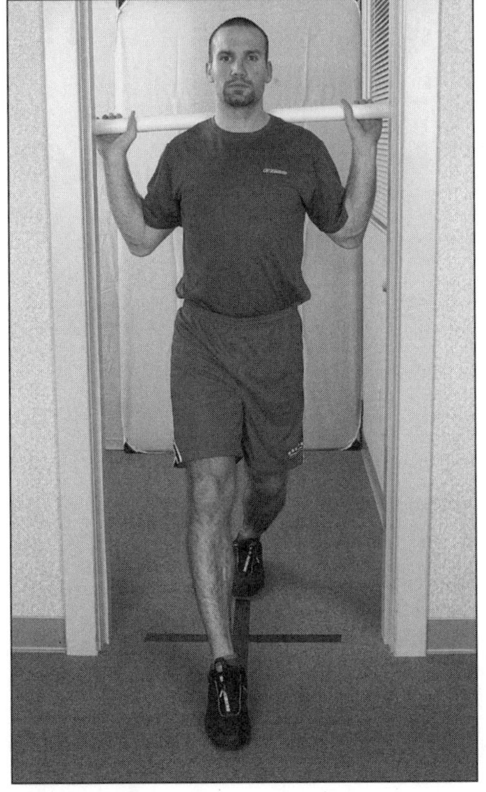

a

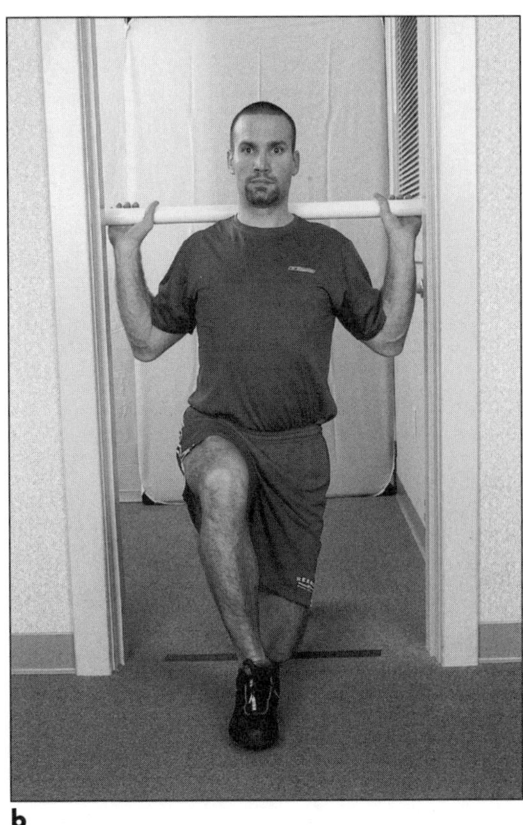

b

Figure 5.3 In-line lunge: *(a)* stand with feet on the tape, dowel across the shoulders; *(b)* descend so the back knee touches the tape.

Lower your back knee enough to touch the tape behind the front foot (figure 5.3b). The heel of your front foot should remain flat on the floor. Your feet should be on the same line and pointing straight throughout the movement. Perform the lunge up to three times on each side in a slow, controlled fashion.

Give a passing grade if there is minimal to no upper-body movement, the feet remain on the tape, the back knee touches the tape behind the heel of the front foot, the dowel does not touch the wall, and balance is maintained (the dowel must not tip left or right). Give a failing grade if any of the five elements is not presently possible. If the movement causes pain, no grade is given for the test. Have a medical professional perform a thorough evaluation of the painful area.

ACTIVE STRAIGHT LEG RAISE

Assume the starting position by lying on your back perpendicular to (through) the doorway with your arms at your sides, palms up, and head flat on the floor (figure 5.4a). The midpoint between the hip and the top of the bend of the knee is in line with the door frame.

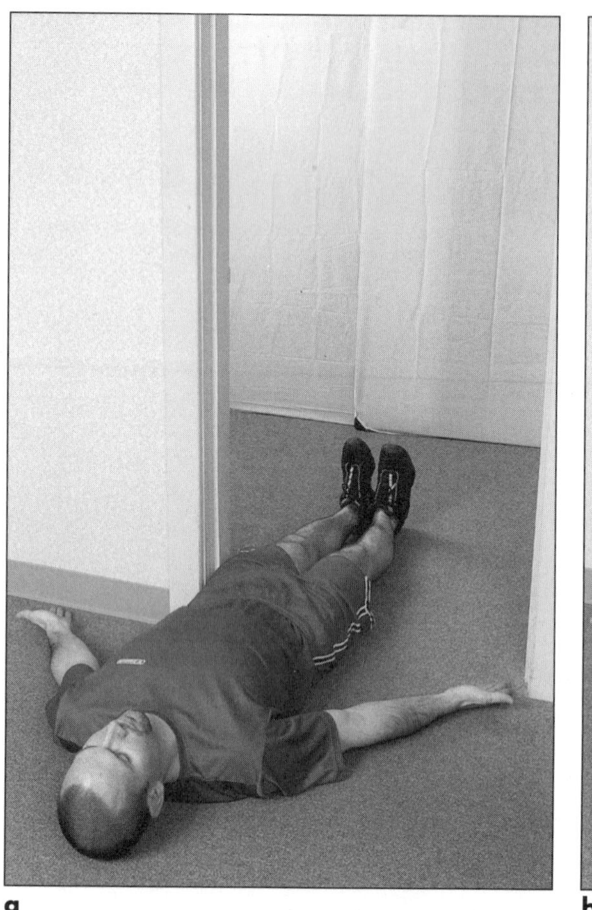

a

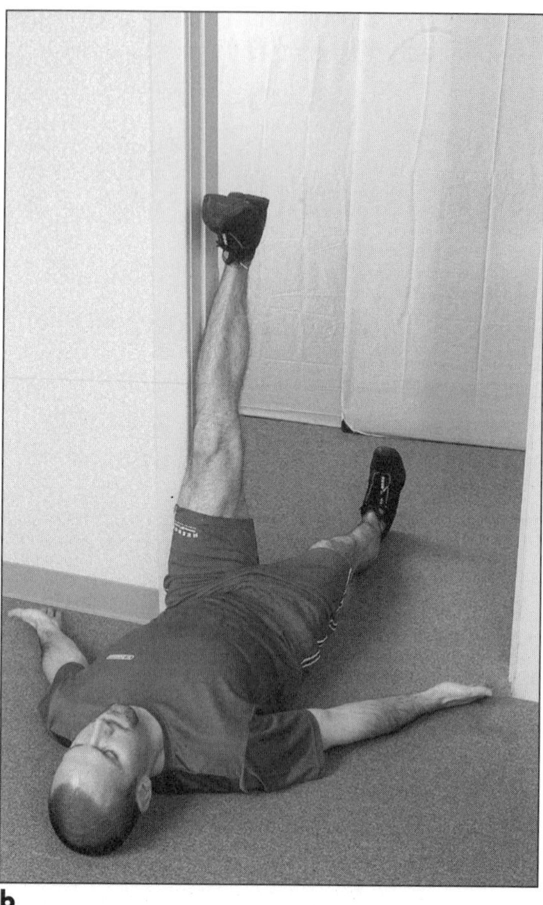

b

Figure 5.4 Active straight leg raise: *(a)* lie on your back in the doorway; *(b)* raise your leg.

Lift the leg that is closer to the door frame while keeping the foot flexed and knee extended (figure 5.4b). During the test, the other leg should remain in contact with the floor and not move. The head should remain flat on the floor, and the arms should not move. The test may be performed as many as three times on each side.

Give a passing grade if the ankle bone *(lateral malleolus)* of the lifted leg clears the doorjamb and the floor-bound leg does not move. The foot of the floor-bound leg should point straight upward for the entire test. The knee of the floor-bound leg should remain extended without the slightest degree of flexion. Give a failing grade if any of these elements is not presently possible on either side. If the movement causes pain, no grade is given for the test. Have a medical professional perform a thorough evaluation of the painful area.

SEATED ROTATION

Sit upright on the floor, back straight, with legs crossed. One foot should be on each side of the doorjamb. Hold the dowel above your chest in front of your shoulders (figure 5.5a). It should touch your collarbone and the front of both shoulders at all times.

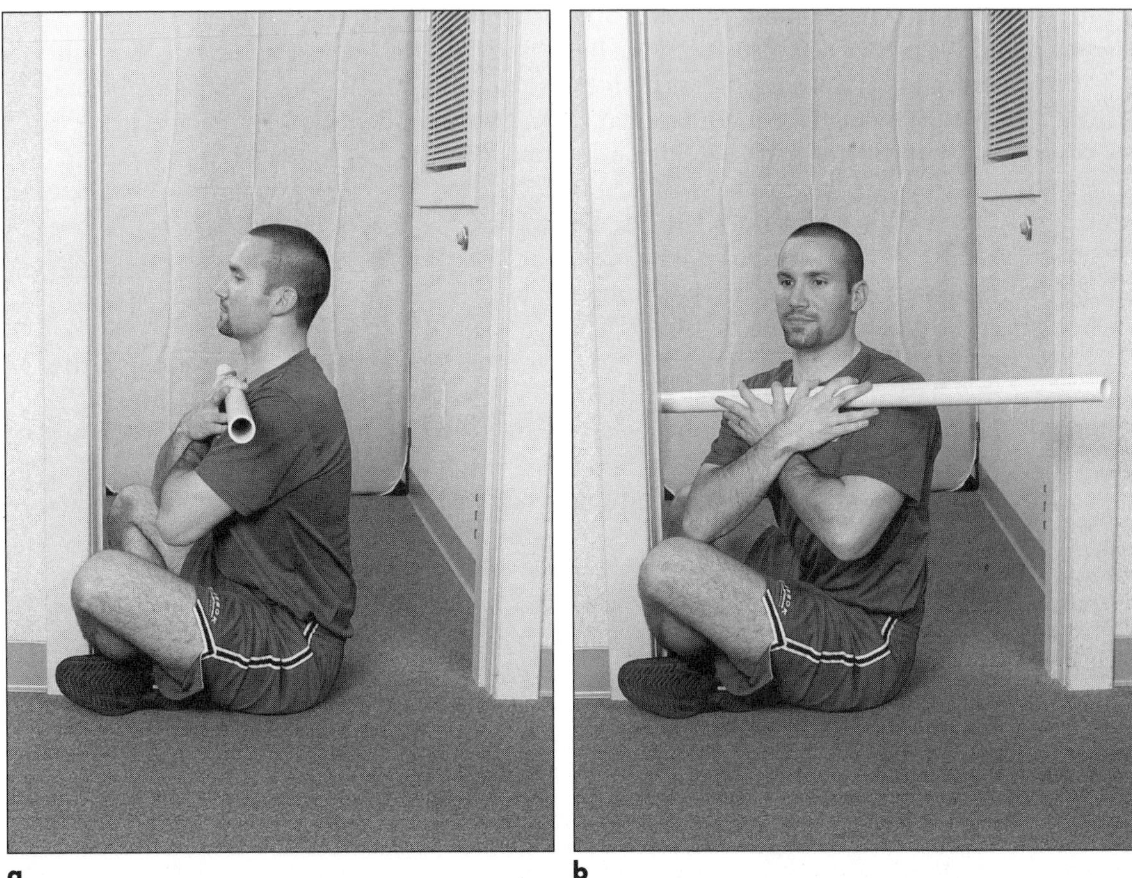

a b

Figure 5.5 Seated rotation: *(a)* sit in doorway with legs crossed; *(b)* rotate to the side.

With your back straight, rotate to each side (figure 5.5b). Attempt to touch the dowel to the door frame. During the test, maintain an upright position and limit leaning toward the door or bending the spine in any direction.

Give a passing grade if the dowel touches the wall, the dowel remains level and in contact with the chest, and the spine remains straight and upright. Give a failing grade if any of the three elements is not presently possible. If the movement causes pain, no grade is given for the test. Have a medical professional perform a thorough evaluation of the painful area.

Scoring and Exercise Progressions

In chapter 6 you will find a recommended exercise progression for each of the five movements described in the self-screen. However, I recommend that you follow only one corrective exercise progression. Once you have graded the screen, look at your grades to choose the most appropriate exercise progression. You will have one grade for the squat and two grades for each of the other screens because the left and right sides are screened independently. Record your grades (pass/fail) in table 5.1.

It is best to work on the movement pattern that presents the greatest difficulty. Also, focus first on movement patterns that expose a right-left asymmetry. For instance, say you failed the squat. You also failed the hurdle step on the left but passed on the right and passed all remaining screens. Both the squat and hurdle step present problems, but it is best to focus on the hurdle step first because it identified an asymmetry. As you work on the hurdle step, you may also improve the squat by correcting the asymmetry. If further testing doesn't show an improvement in the squat, start the exercise progression for the squat once the hurdle step asymmetry no longer exists. To use another example, let's say you passed the squat. You passed the hurdle step on the left but failed on the right. You failed the lunge on both sides and passed all other screens. You should still work on the asymmetry first.

If you fail multiple screens, start with the exercise progression that presented the most difficulty and retest to check for changes. If the exercise progression is too difficult or does not yield effective results, start with the exercise progression you feel most comfortable with and progress from there.

It is not necessary to stop your current workout just to correct a movement pattern, but use the exercise progression as a warm-up or cool-down whenever possible. Also, consider that some part of your current workout may be counterproductive to correcting a movement pattern. You can expect to improve most movement patterns within two months of corrective exercise work. Many movement patterns will change quickly; others will change very little. Focus your energy on correcting movements and maintaining the best possible movement screen score. At the very least, do not allow asymmetries to go uncorrected. The corrective exercise progressions can also be used to maintain a movement pattern.

Table 5.1 Self Mobility Screen Scoring Sheet

			Final grade	
Test	**Pass**	**Fail**	**Pass**	**Fail**
Deep squat				
Hurdle step	L R	L R	L R	L R
Inline lunge	L R	L R	L R	L R
Active straight leg raise	L R	L R	L R	L R
Seated rotation	L R	L R	L R	L R

6

Balance Training

Although this chapter is titled "Balance Training," it is not about improving equilibrium. The word balance is used to describe training designed to create movement symmetry between the right and left sides of the body and to promote a balance of mobility and stability within the body. Mobility and stability should be the starting point for a training program. Although mobility and stability may sound as if they are opposites, they must exist together to form an effective foundation for movement and activity. If testing reveals poor mobility and stability, you must focus on an effective fundamental mobility and stability program before any other kind of training. This type of training, when done correctly, will greatly improve movement awareness, especially between the right and left sides of the body.

Pete Draovitch, a well-respected physical therapist, trainer, and strength and conditioning expert, has worked with athletes in many sports. He has used the functional movement screen in many situations over the past few years. One of his success stories involves a professional basketball player who underwent ankle surgery for an OCD lesion (a defect in the cartilage). Following acute rehab, he began an aggressive offseason conditioning program. The functional movement screen revealed failure on the deep squat, hurdle step, in-line lunge, and active straight leg raise. Eight weeks after receiving additional clinical care and doing an exercise routine that specifically targeted balance training (mobility and stability training) to address the imbalances in the hip and leg, the athlete was running and jumping without pain. He improved his squatting technique within two and a half weeks and was able to add weight on squats and lunges. The athlete even reported that he was jumping higher to dunk off that leg than he had in the past. If his quality of motion had been assessed earlier in his career, he might not have required surgery according to Pete. Balancing mobility and stability is a fundamental element of both rehabilitation and performance training.

It is best to work on one movement problem at a time. It is also best to work on right-left differences before working on limitations. When there is more than one imbalance, the imbalance with the greatest limitation or greatest difference between left and right sides should be addressed first. Frequent retesting will provide feedback on how much work is needed. Retesting can be done every one or two weeks. Frequent retesting can confirm improvement and redirect attention to another problem area. Testing can also be performed following rehabilitation of an injury or to determine whether adequate mobility and stability is being maintained through conditioning.

Postural Habits and Activity Habits

Postural habits and activity habits influence the way the body moves. *Postural habits* can be defined as the way the body is held or positioned during both rest and activity. The word *posture* usually is used to describe the way a person holds the spine, but the spine is not the only factor. The arms and legs also are held in certain positions. Some people stand with their knees hyperextended, whereas others do not extend their knees even to a straight position. Some people naturally hold their shoulders back, whereas others have shoulders that round forward and a head that slumps in front of the body.

Postural habits are developed in sports and activities—the way a golfer addresses the golf ball, a batter stands in the batter's box, a basketball player stands at the free throw line, or a linebacker assumes the ready position in football. The way the body is held has a lot to do with the way it moves; the starting position influences the movement that is to follow. When the body begins in a suboptimal position, the brain tries to make up for the problem by unnecessarily altering body mechanics in an attempt to catch up or to correct the movement. Simple stretching and warm-up exercises that focus on movement as well as static positions will demonstrate how postural habits can influence the way the body moves.

Activity habits are movement habits. There are many different ways the body can move. Some are efficient and some are not. Some are correct and some are not. Sometimes what feels natural is incorrect and what feels extremely awkward is correct. Do not assume that what feels natural is the best way to move. Even the world's greatest athletes can develop bad habits, get sloppy, and lose their fundamentals.

Muscles do not get tight or weak for no reason. Muscles grow tight because of the way they are used. If muscles are tight it's because the athlete has chosen to use them in a shortened range, and the activities they perform do not lengthen them to their full potential. As a result, over time the athlete develops movement patterns that rely on short muscles. The brain remembers the short muscle position; just because the muscle is stretched one day does not mean that it will stay elongated. It will return to the length that it is most familiar with and that is used most often.

The same theory applies to weak muscles. Muscles that normally are not engaged effectively, that the athlete avoids using, or that may at one time have been injured can fall into this category. Following an injury, movement patterns are altered to avoid using a muscle that may have a strain, contusion, or tendinitis. By the time the muscle recuperates, a movement pattern has been developed that neglects this particular muscle or uses it less. The body has become familiar with this movement pattern and has no reason to change back.

Every muscle is opposed by another muscle in the body, usually on alternate sides of the joint. When one muscle is extremely tight, its counterpart often becomes weak and lengthened to accommodate the tight muscle. Most of this happens not for mechanical reasons but for neurological reasons. Opposite muscles often inhibit each other in an attempt to make a movement pattern more efficient. Maintaining good movement patterns keeps the muscles strong and flexible. Remember, muscles are tight because of how they are used. Muscles are weak for the same reason.

Getting Started

The exercises in this chapter are specifically designed to work on a particular movement problem. If you experienced pain with one of the movements during the self-screen in chapter 5, these exercises are not the cure. Have the problem checked and treated by a medical professional. However, if you experienced tightness, stiffness, loss of balance, or difficulty during the testing, this is the place to begin.

The exercise program starts with a few helpful stretches to raise awareness of left-right differences as well as overall limitations. The foundation drills are exercises following the stretches designed to train the brain to use the new mobility and gain stability. The program will improve movement memory and provide quick access to the benefits stemming from the increase in functional movement.

Eventually the movement exercises can take the place of the stretches because they are actually a more dynamic form of stretching. Those who have significant flexibility problems may want to continue the passive stretching program and the movement learning exercise as well. Doing both provides extra reinforcement.

One of the movements in the screen may have seemed impossible; if so, that shows your weakest link. You may never have a perfect score. Work on the movement pattern continually because the body can use even subtle improvements to become more efficient and reduce the chance of injury.

Deep Squat

The deep squat is the first movement in the self-assessment. Ability to deep squat successfully is a fairly good indicator of overall movement quality. Failure on the deep squat generally means one of two things: generalized stiffness throughout the body, or asymmetry. In this context, the word *asymmetry* indicates an imbalance between the right and left sides of the body regarding mobility, stability, and coordination. Even though the squat does not look specifically at the right and left sides of the body (unlike the other tests), it requires maximum range of motion in both legs and both arms in the exact opposite direction of their resting or standing position.

Improving the deep squat and going deeper through the full range of motion will improve movement when shifting weight from left to right. It also will improve the ability to quickly get into the universal athletic ready position, which is somewhere between deep squatting and standing erect. If the squat is severely limited, then the ready position is not between squatting and standing—it is between standing and whatever the squatting limitation is, which may not be optimum or efficient for long periods of time or for all of the activities a sport requires.

If a restriction exists on only one side of the body (for example, the right hip), in most cases the body will learn to squat only as deeply as the restriction will allow, thus making it look like the entire squatting movement is limited instead of simply the one point of restriction. Other parts of the body will move inappropriately to try to make up for the lack of movement in the area of restriction, contorting the body in such a way that the squat will feel extremely difficult. If this is the case but the other self-assessment movements did not show a significant right-left asymmetry, the exercise progression that follows is recommended.

If the other tests revealed a significant asymmetry or earned a low score, it is recommended that the asymmetry found in the other test or tests be addressed first. Then, if a squat continues to present difficulty, progress to the recommended exercises on pages 42 to 46 to improve the deep squat movement pattern.

The following program includes some simple exercises to improve deep squatting. Most of the improvement for this particular exercise progression will be the result of enhanced body awareness and coordination. Difficulty in deep squatting is rarely a simple flexibility problem. Squatting is a complex movement that requires stability of the trunk and mobility of the extremities through constantly changing tension and position. The tension between the muscles of the trunk and limbs must coordinate perfectly—as one relaxes, the other must contract to maintain balance and an erect spine through the entire motion. If coordination is skewed, the deep squat will feel extremely awkward and limited.

TOE TOUCH PROGRESSION

The toe touch progression is a simple exercise to improve body awareness (or sensory awareness) for deep squatting. The toe touch progression is a fundamental component of the exercises needed for the deep squat and shouldn't be overlooked. It simply teaches relaxation of the tension in the lower back and how to shift weight from the heels to the toes in a smooth and consistent fashion.

Stand erect with feet side by side, heels and toes touching. The balls of both feet should be elevated onto a 1- to 2-inch platform such as a board or free-weight plate. Insert a towel roll or foam roll between the knees by flexing the knees slightly and separating them without changing foot position (figure 6.1a). The towel or foam roll should be thick enough that the knees cannot be locked backward or hyperextended. This position will feel bowlegged and extremely awkward, but do not change it. If foot position is altered in any way, the towel roll is too large; unroll a layer or two before continuing. The back should be relaxed and without tension. You should feel tension from the outside of the knee up through the outside of the hips.

Reach for the ceiling, stretching the arms as high as possible with palms facing forward. Hollow out the abdomen by pulling in as deeply as possible with the abdominal muscles. This should not alter breathing. If it does, continue practicing the movement until it can be done without significantly changing breathing.

Bend forward so that the fingertips touch the toes (figure 6.1b). If the fingertips do not make it completely to the toes, remember to keep the abdominal area pulled inward. Also, squeeze the towel roll slightly to help relax certain muscles in the outer

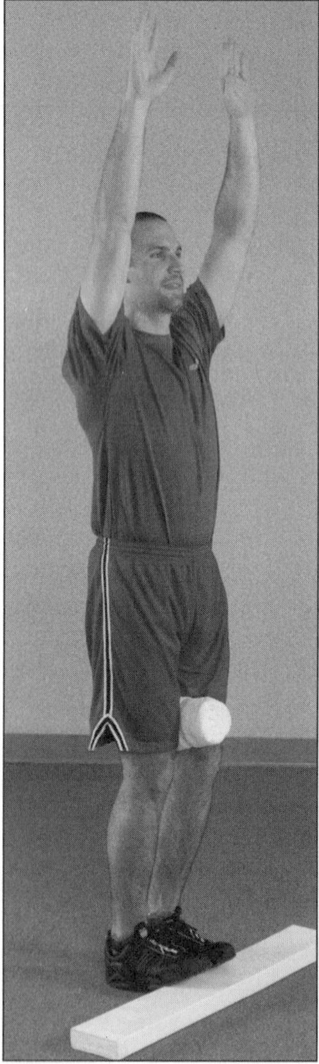

a

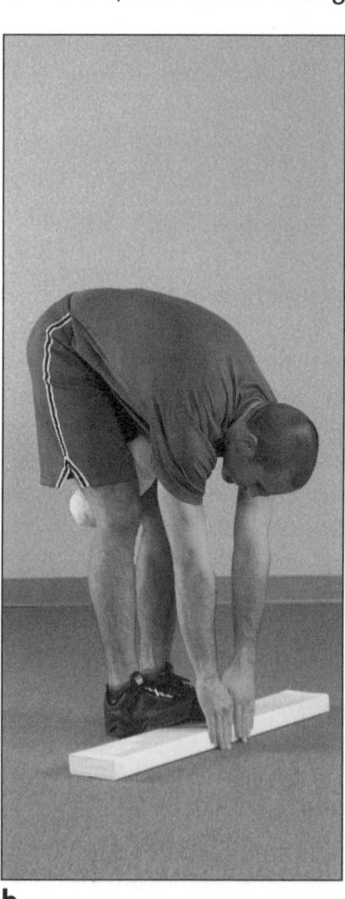

b

Figure 6.1 Toe touch progression, phase I: *(a)* stand with balls of feet elevated on a platform and a foam roll between knees; *(b)* touch the toes.

thigh and back so that the toes can be reached. If you still cannot reach the toes, bend the knees slightly to reach them for the first repetition.

Return to the starting position, keeping the heels on the ground and the hands raised as high as possible overhead with palms facing forward. Keep the abdominal region pulled inward and repeat the movement. If a slight knee bend was required for the first repetition, try to bend the knees a little less this time. Reduce the knee bend with each repetition and try to go a little farther each time. Do 10 to 12 repetitions. You will feel tension in the calf behind the knee, in the hamstrings, and possibly in the lower back.

Phase two of the toe touch progression uses the same movement but from a different position. For phase two, elevate the heels on a 1- to 2-inch platform (figure 6.2a). The toes should be on the ground. Insert the towel roll between the knees without changing the foot position. Repeat the toe touch movement, reaching up to the ceiling, pulling in the abdominals, and reaching to the toes (figure 6.2b). There may be slightly greater tension in the lower back and hamstrings and slightly less tension in the calves than in phase one. Bend the knees as little as possible to allow a toe touch, and bend the knees less and less with each repetition until they can be held in a nearly straight position. At no time during the exercise should the knee hyperextend or the foot position change. You should be closer to touching your toes or doing so more comfortably following this drill. You should be comfortable touching your toes before starting the deep squat progression.

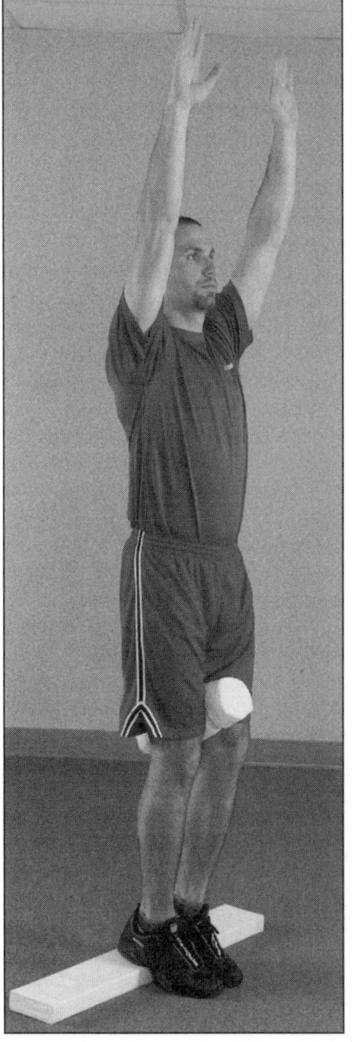

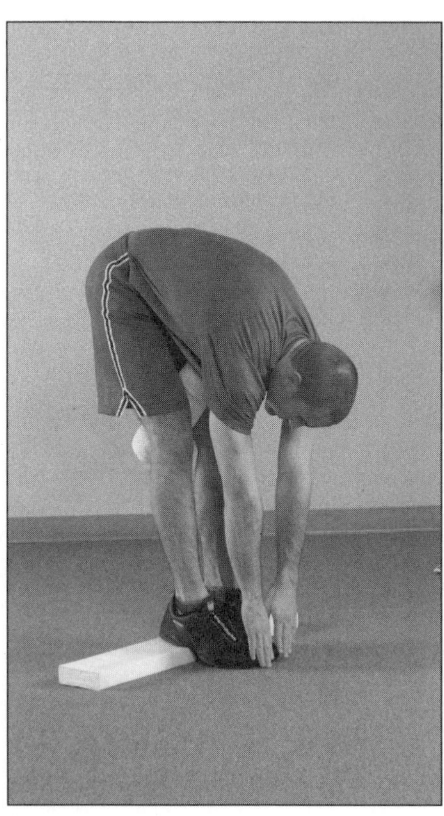

a b

Figure 6.2 Toe touch progression, phase II: *(a)* stand with heels elevated on a platform; *(b)* touch the toes.

DEEP SQUAT PROGRESSION

With the heels on a 1- to 2-inch platform, spread the feet until they are shoulder-width apart or wider. Bend forward until the entire palm can be laid flat on the floor or on a 2-, 4-, or 6-inch platform (figure 6.3a). Use only what you need and gradually reduce the platform, or get rid of the platform altogether. Free-weight plates, wooden blocks, or small bricks can be used. The entire palm must lay completely flat, so it is better to use a slightly taller brick or block than to overreach and be off balance. Heels should remain flat and the knees should be extended but not hyperextended. The head and neck should be relaxed and looking downward.

Without moving the hands off the platform, slowly bend the hips, knees, and ankles and lower the body into the squat position with the knees going to the outside of the elbows (figure 6.3b). Do not change foot position during the descent. If it is hard to control foot position during the descent, hold the knees outward or widen the feet slightly, but keep the feet pointed straight ahead at all times.

With the hands flat on the platform, keep the heels in full contact with the 1- to 2-inch platform and sit deeply into the squat. Concentrate on keeping the knees outside of the elbows and try to relax as much as possible. If this position causes a stretch, maintain the stretch for approximately 20 seconds. Try pulling in the abdominals as in the toe touch progression to make this movement easier. Use long, slow, deep breaths and exhale during the stretch.

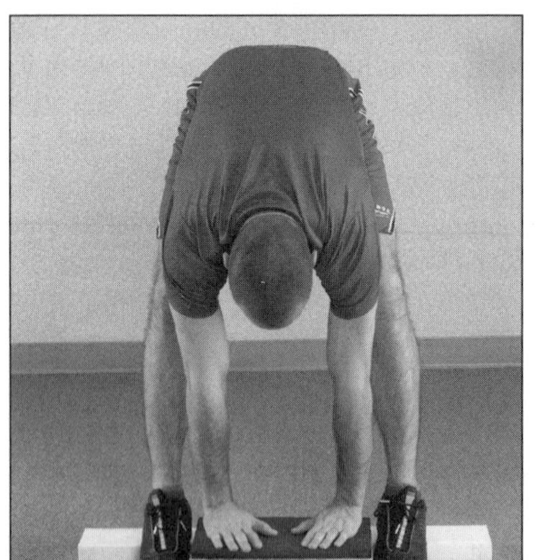

a

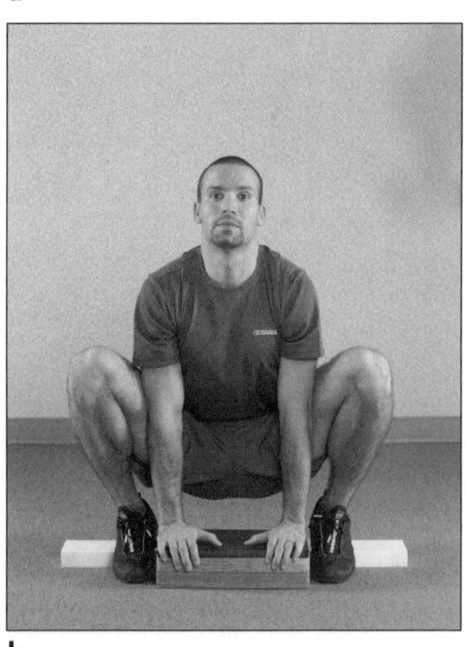

b

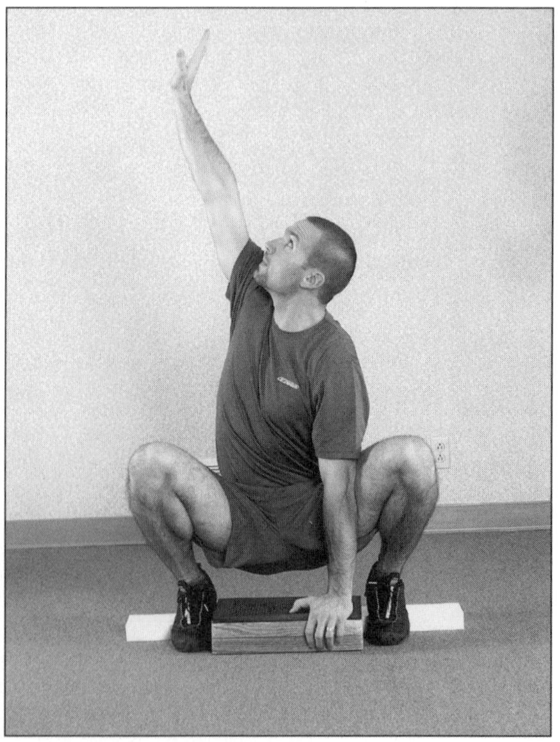

c

Figure 6.3 Deep squat progression, phase I: *(a)* bend forward and place hands on platform; *(b)* descend into a deep squat; *(c)* reach one arm toward the ceiling.

If you cannot achieve a comfortable sitting position, use a slightly greater heel lift and a slightly elevated hand platform.

Once the squat position is comfortable, elevate one arm as high as possible over the head, reaching for the ceiling without changing the hip, knee, or ankle position (figure 6.3c). Do not shift weight. Keep both feet flat and both legs in the same position. Follow the movement of the hand with the eyes. Turn the head to the side of the arm that is being raised. Do not attempt to take the arm straight backward; rather, reach overhead, keeping the spine as long and tall as possible throughout the entire movement.

This movement should take approximately 20 seconds: 8 to 9 seconds on the way up, 2 to 4 seconds to hold the stretch while reaching as tall as possible, and 8 to 9 seconds to return to the platform. Repeat on the other side. You should note which side is tighter or presents greater difficulty. Try to achieve equal movement by working the tighter side three times more than the other side.

Once the movement can be done with the lower body completely relaxed, the upper body moving freely, and the right and left sides feeling about equal, proceed to the next phase of the exercise.

Start from a deep squat position with the hands on the platform. Raise both hands into a Y position and take them as far back and up as possible, maintaining complete balance and keeping the lower body fully relaxed (figure 6.4a). There should be no change in foot, hip, or knee position. If the hands are directly above the head, reach and then stand up out of the squat (figure 6.4b). It will feel difficult at first because this move uses the most powerful muscles of the hips and thighs in a new position. Numerous repetitions of this exercise will improve motor memory and increase coordination.

Return to the start position by bending forward and touching the 2-, 4-, or 6-inch raised platform with palms flat. Drop again into the squat, then resume the Y or overhead reach with both arms.

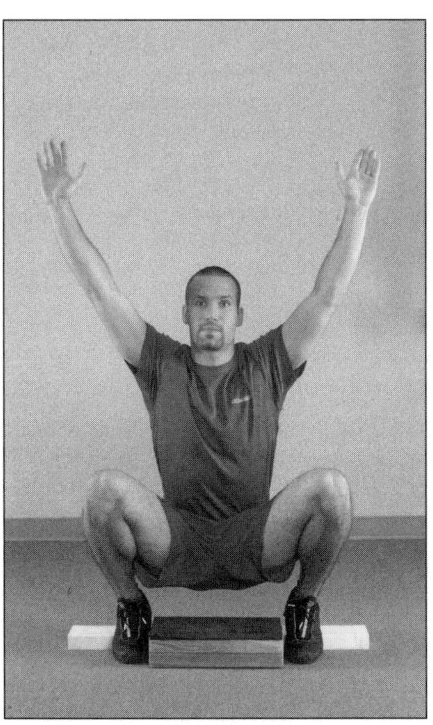

a

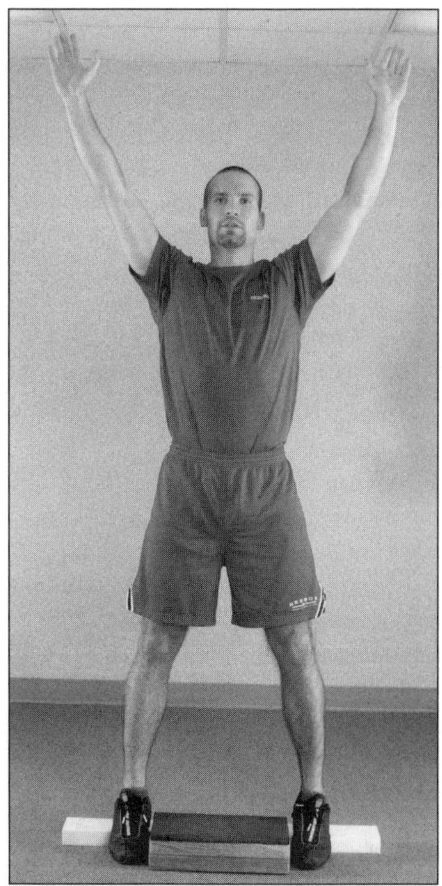

b

Figure 6.4 Deep squat progression, phase II: *(a)* raise both arms; *(b)* stand up.

Now stand slowly. Practice for 10 to 12 repetitions. Reduce the elevation of both the heel lift and hand lift until both heels and palms are on the floor. Once you can perform this comfortably in a relaxed and easy manner, attempt deep squatting with heels flat on the floor while holding a dowel as described in the self-screen (see page 33). Retest after at least 10 to 12 repetitions of practice.

This exercise progression may seem a little awkward, but it is one of the quickest ways to teach the body the proper sequence and muscle coordination for deep squatting. Conventional weight training rarely takes the hips below parallel, thereby reinforcing limited movement.

Ultimately it is a personal choice whether to use deep squatting movement patterns with weight training. Regardless of your preference, work to achieve the hip mobility needed to perform deep squatting to maintain optimum joint and muscle function as well as body awareness, balance, and control. Touching the toes first relaxes the lower back. Once the lower back is relaxed, drop into the squatting position without ever taking the hands off the floor. This maintains the relaxation in the back but also puts the abdominal muscles at a mechanical advantage. Once in the deep squat, allow the back to erect itself. Tighten the back muscles only after the abdominal muscles have been properly engaged by the flexed spine–flexed hip position.

The back squat is a popular weightlifting exercise in which a barbell is held on the upper back and shoulders. It allows one to use a large amount of weight and is great for hip and leg development. However, the back squat should not be the only form of squat training used for hip, leg, and trunk development. Before the back squat was invented as an exercise, few human beings ever squatted deeply with anything on their backs. They usually bent into the squatting position, grabbed an object, held it close to the chest, and stood up. Therefore, they went into the squatting position unloaded with a relaxed spine but came out of the squatting position with an erect trunk and protected spine. When the spine is loaded at the top of the movement the erector muscles of the spine will sometimes contract incorrectly and pull the spine into too much extension. This reduces the ability of the other core muscles to create a balance of stabilizing forces around the spine. It is impractical to start the squat in the low position; however, much of this problem can be remedied by doing a front squat instead of a back squat.

A child does not learn to squat from the top down—in other words, he does not suddenly make a conscious decision one day to squat. Actually, he is squatting one day and makes the conscious decision to stand. Squatting precedes standing in the developmental sequence. This is the way a child's brain learns to use the body as the child develops movement patterns. Therefore, a child is probably crawling, rocks back into a squatting position with the back completely relaxed and the hips completely flexed, and stands when he has enough hip strength. This approach makes a lot of sense and can be applied to relearning the deep squat movement if it is lost. Someone who doesn't perform well on the squat assessment test does not know what deep squatting feels like. It's like going on a journey without knowing the destination. By relaxing the lower back and doing the toe touch and deep squat progressions, the hips, knees, and ankles get into the squatting position and then set the spine when the hands are lifted off the raised platform. This allows the squatter to feel where she is going. She already knows what the top of the squat feels like—that's standing. Now she knows what the bottom of the squat feels like. The exercise will become an opportunity for motor learning and working out the coordination between the start and finish position.

Use three or four of the stretches and drills as a warm-up and cool-down, or make them part of a workout for one week and retest. Check all movements, not just the one being focused on, and see what has happened. Sometimes the difference will be obvious; sometimes it will not. Be persistent and consistent, and you will start to see change. Follow directions and work on the asymmetries (left-right differences) first and limitations (general stiffness noted on both the left and right sides) second.

Once you improve your ability to deep squat and pass the deep squat screen, you can proceed to the supplementary work to reinforce deep squatting. (See part III on strength and endurance.)

Hurdle Step

When performing the hurdle step test, it is important to note whether an asymmetry exists between the right and left side. If an asymmetry does exist, you will need to do approximately three times more work on the weaker side. It is important to do at least some work on the more proficient side simply to feel the more refined activity, improved coordination, better stability, and better mobility present on that side compared to the other.

For example, if the right leg down and left leg over the hurdle presents difficulty but the left leg down and right leg over the hurdle is normal, start training in the left leg down and right leg over position to improve awareness of what is normal. Then do the majority of work in the other position (right leg down and left leg over) to reduce the asymmetrical difference between the left and right sides of the body. Do not try to simply isolate this test to a single muscle weakness, muscle tightness, or joint stiffness. Work the pattern.

The hurdle step involves many muscles and joints working together in unison to create a balanced and stable body while one leg moves through a nearly full range of motion. Difficulty could be due to inappropriate balance on the down leg or inappropriate mobility in the up leg. Unless there is pain or a history of injury, the location of the problem is not as important as the understanding of the difference between the left and right side while performing the hurdle step. With practice, the problem can be resolved. Knowing which muscle is tight or weak or which joint is stiff will simply distract from the problem at hand—a movement problem, not a structural problem.

Advanced Stretches

Although these may look like stretches, this group of movements require more than simple stretching. You must hold a stable position with your spine. Unlike most stretches, focus should be on not only the area being stretched but also the area that is holding you stable. You will be required to hold your spine and one leg stable while you relax and stretch the other leg. You will soon learn to focus on the parts of your body that are stable.

TABLETOP STRIDE

Stand next to a table or a bench that comes to mid-thigh level. Place one foot on top of the table or bench, leaving the other foot on the floor with the heel flat. Slightly bend the knee of the leg on the floor and maximally bend the knee of the elevated leg. Feet should be in line and pointing forward at different elevations. Keep the spine erect, allowing the body to sink down by bending the knee of the lower leg, elongating the stride between the left and right leg. Remain tall and elongated through the spine and pull in the abdominal muscles to reduce stress on the back. Pulling in the abdominal muscles should not affect breathing. If it does, practice pulling in the abdomen and breathing normally before continuing the stretch. Hold the stretch for 30 seconds and then return to the start position with both feet on the floor. Repeat the stretch three times. Staying balanced and relaxed are the keys to performing the stretch well.

For a more advanced stretch, add a torso twist. With the spine erect and tall, put the arms out to the side at 90 degrees from the shoulders with palms up and rotate the torso toward the elevated leg. Shift weight when rotating the torso, making subtle changes to maintain balance. Let these changes occur naturally; do not force them. Hold the stretch for 20 seconds, return to the start position, and repeat the stretch two times. This stretch places equal emphasis on both legs. It also emphasizes relaxation and balance, not simply forced muscle stretching. Learn to relax the muscles and let them lengthen. Remember, don't contract the muscle you are trying to stretch.

TABLETOP HIP STRETCH

This drill isolates the elevated leg. Use the same table or bench as in the tabletop stride. Place one leg on the table. Rotate the hip outward and lay the leg flat on the table. To protect the elevated knee, place a towel between the lower leg and knee and the table. Keep the ankle in a neutral position or flex the foot as much as possible. If the knee does not lie flat comfortably, use a larger towel until the towel roll supports the leg so that equal weight is on the knee and ankle. Adjust the position of the hip so that all the tension is in the buttocks and lower back. The thigh should be moved inward so that it is in line with the foot on the floor. Twist the torso toward the elevated hip using the arm on the same side as the elevated hip to hold the stretch. Hold for 20 seconds, then return to the start position. Repeat two times.

STANDING QUAD STRETCH WITH HIP EXTENSION

Stand erect on one leg and grab the opposite ankle with the knee maximally flexed and pointed forward. Slowly extend the hip back and hold for 30 seconds. As you extend the hip the knee should point downward. Maintain balance for the entire stretch. Learn to relax the thigh during the stretch. Hold for 30 seconds and repeat with the opposite leg.

STANDING GLUTE STRETCH WITH HIP FLEXION

Stand erect on one leg and pull the other knee to the chest. Hug the knee with both hands and squeeze the thigh toward the chest. Hold for 30 seconds, balancing the entire time. Do not let the spine bend or round when the hip is flexed. Perform two to three times per leg. Work toward symmetry. Perform more repetitions on one side if necessary.

Foundation Drills

Perform 8 to 10 repetitions of each exercise on each side, working one leg at a time. If you have a right-left imbalance, do two more sets of 8 to 10 repetitions on the problem side. If not, do two sets on each side.

ELEVATED MOUNTAIN CLIMBER CYCLE

Using a step, low bench, or table, assume a push-up position with arms directly under shoulders. To decrease difficulty, increase bench height; to increase difficulty, reduce bench height. The back and legs must be completely straight. Keeping the spine as long as possible with no observable movement, draw one knee toward the chest by bending

a

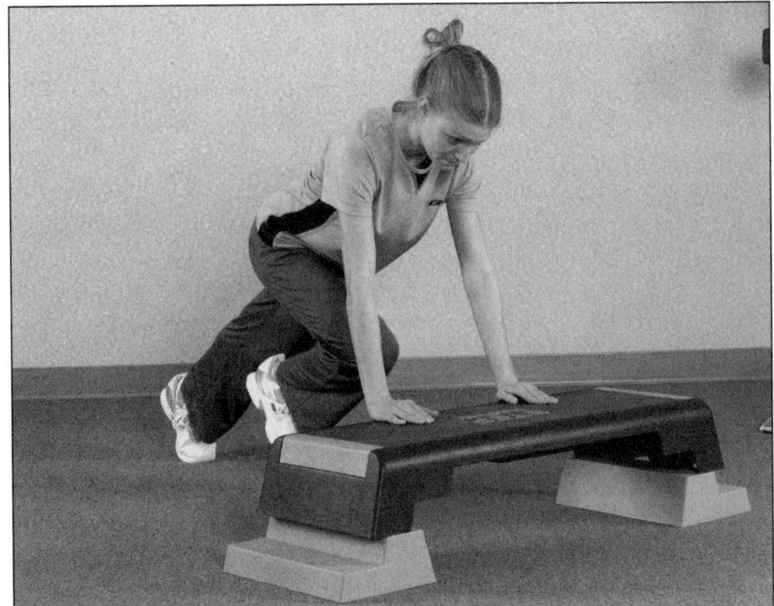

b

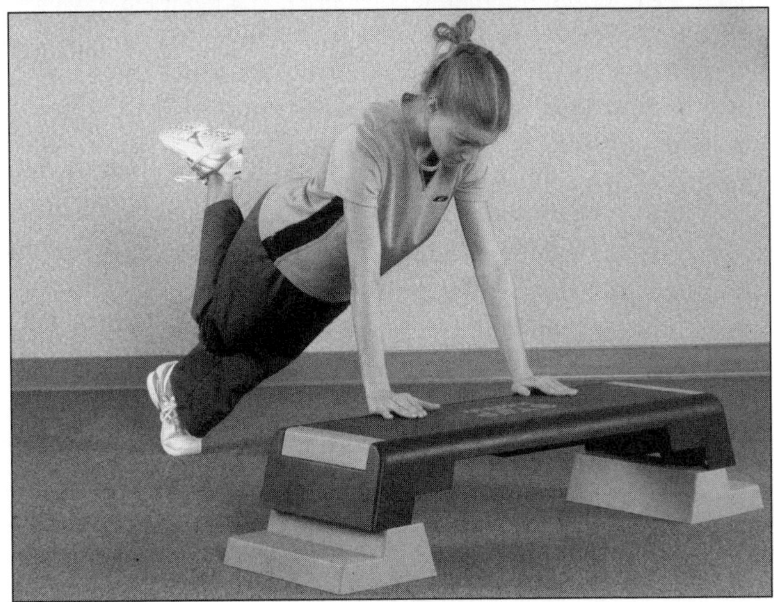

Figure 6.5 Elevated mountain climber cycle: *(a)* bring one knee to the chest; *(a)* move leg back and bend the knee.

both the knee and the hip (figure 6.5a). Bring the knee as close to the chest as possible and then straighten the leg. Make the leg as long as possible and only lightly touch the toe to the ground. Now bend the knee to greater than 90 degrees (figure 6.5b). Do not allow this position to change the spine position. The spine and nonmoving leg should look like a straight line. If this causes a great stretch on the thigh, you're doing it correctly. If the move is difficult, continue to work between the two movements. If it is not too difficult, add a third movement—extend the hip without changing the back or other leg position.

To increase the level of difficulty, get rid of the bench. Assume a push-up position on the floor. Hands should be directly below the chest and collarbone. Follow the same movement pattern. Or try a narrow stance to increase the difficulty of the movement: move the hands closer together under the face. Moving the hands forward on the floor will increase difficulty. Move the hands inward to narrow the stance and increase difficulty again. Follow the same movement pattern.

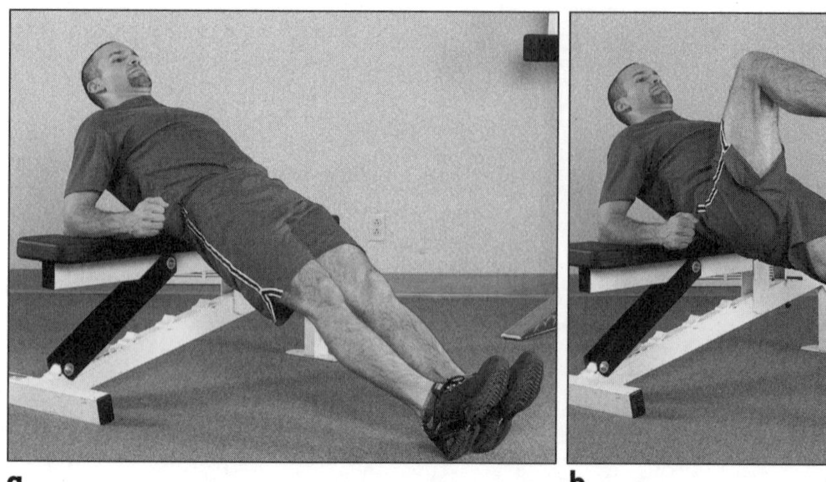

Figure 6.6 Elevated dip cycle: *(a)* lean back on bench; *(a)* bring knee toward chest.

ELEVATED DIP CYCLE

The elevated dip is a reverse of the mountain climber. The leg movement is the same but the body position is reversed. With the back to the step, low bench, or low table, bend the elbows and rest the forearms on the step, bench, or table (figure 6.6a). To decrease difficulty, increase bench height; to increase difficulty, reduce bench height. Extend the legs. The spine should remain straight at all times. Draw one hip and knee toward the chest, keeping the other leg extended and the spine straight (figure 6.6b). Return the leg to the extended position to complete the repetition.

To increase the level of difficulty, remove the bench and extend the elbows. Rest the hands on the floor, fingers forward. Perform the same movement pattern.

Pick three or four of the stretches and foundation drills to serve as a warm-up and cool-down, or make them part of a workout for one week and retest. Check all movements, not just the one being focused on, and see what has happened. Sometimes the difference will be obvious; sometimes it will not. Be persistent and consistent and you will start to see change. Follow directions and work on the asymmetries (left-right differences) first and limitations (general stiffness noted on both left and right sides) second.

Lunge

The lunge is an extremely important movement pattern for athletics. Some degree of a lunge movement pattern is adopted for both deceleration and cutting movements. The ability to lunge effectively with good technique demonstrates how the upper and lower body can move in an independent fashion and yet complement each other with balance and weight shifting.

The lunge movement pattern is difficult. To improve this pattern, you must improve what you feel when attempting the pattern. In the discussion about the squat, an exercise program was introduced that allowed the participant to learn to squat from the bottom up. This allows the participant to get into a squatting position with a little help and gain a better feel of what deep squatting requires of the body. In the same way, because the lunge is a complicated pattern, it is best to start at the bottom of the lunge and work up.

Foundation drills are designed to use mobility gained from stretching and create stability through motor learning. The drills create coordination because they are dynamic. Coordination is necessary if you are going to incorporate a more complete lunging pattern into your current athletic movements.

You may want to place a line of tape on the floor the same length as the one used in testing. The tape will help with foot placement and force you to have a narrow base. The narrow base is important because mechanics must be nearly perfect. Use mobility and stability to perform the drill. Even though no lunge in sport will be this narrow, you should develop this movement skill under extreme conditions (very narrow base). This forces the body and brain to work together. You create a little stress and overcome that stress. With the narrow base you will wobble—everyone does. Work on not wobbling. That is mobility and stability in action. If you take these drills as seriously as you do weight training or speed and agility work, you will be rewarded.

HALF-KNEELING DOWEL TWIST

Get into a half-kneeling position, keeping the spine as tall as possible (figure 6.7a). Do not hyperextend the hip. Hold the body erect in line over the down knee. Bring the foot of the front leg to within four inches of the end of the tape line if you use a tape line. The down knee should be on the back end of the tape line. The front heel must be equal with the front end of the tape line, but it can be up to four inches to the side to widen the base and reduce the difficulty when you start this exercise. The front of the down thigh, the back of the front thigh, and the calf of the front leg should form a box. Maintain this box throughout the entire exercise.

Hold a dowel or stick across the shoulders (not the neck) and twist in the direction of the front leg (figure 6.7b). Keep the spine as tall as possible and do not lean. Twist only as far as possible without losing posture or original leg position. Don't fight the stretch. Relax and hold the position for at least 30 seconds.

Now twist toward the down leg. This move will be easier to do, but the position will be harder to hold. The hips will want to rotate, but don't let them. Stay tall and twist. Hold the position for at least 30 seconds.

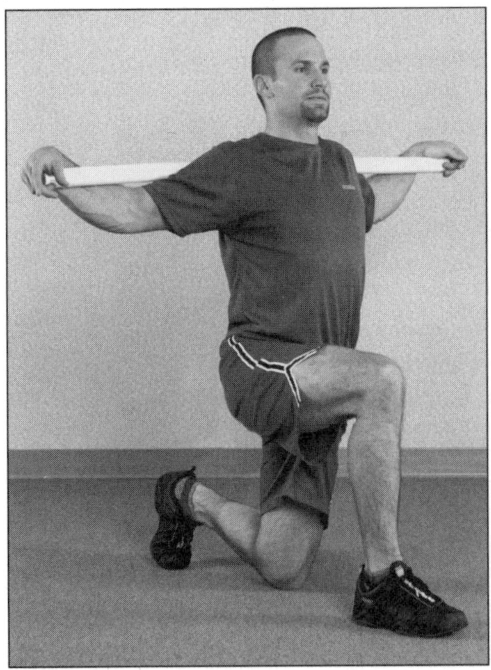

a

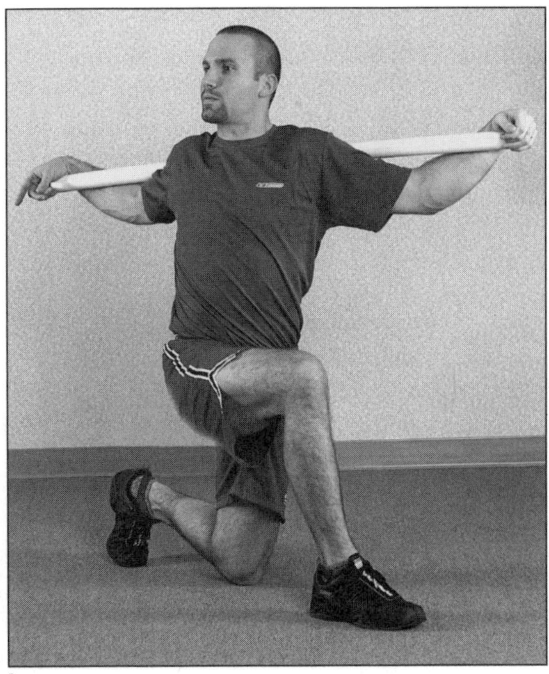

b

Figure 6.7 Half-kneeling dowel twist: *(a)* start in a half-kneeling position with the dowel across your shoulder blades; *(b)* twist to one side.

Compare the twists to each side and note the differences. Use this simple active stretch to eliminate the differences. Don't just twist harder. Hold your spine taller, breathe, and relax. Grade the difficulty to help you understand the problem. There are four positions: rotate right with right knee down; rotate left with right knee down; rotate right with left knee down; and rotate left with left knee down. One or two positions may be more difficult than the others, so work them more, even two to three times more. If all movements are equal but stiff, slowly work on holding the position and relaxing, not straining or forcing the movement. Stretching and movement training are more productive when the motion is not forced. You will notice greater gains in shorter time by simply doing more reps, not just trying harder. As you progress, move the front foot toward the tape line. This will narrow the base and improve your stability and coordination.

IN-LINE LUNGE

Stand over the tape with one heel touching the back end of the tape and the other foot touching the front end of the tape. Place the dowel behind your back so that it touches the head, upper back, and buttocks (figure 6.8a). The hand on the same side as the back foot should grasp the top of the dowel at neck level; the other hand grasps the bottom part of the dowel at the lower back. (Note: These are the only two points at which the dowel is not in contact with the body.) Lower your back knee enough to touch the tape behind the front foot (figure 6.8b). Your feet should be on the same line and pointing straight throughout the movement.

Perform the lunge 10 to 15 times on each side in a slow, controlled fashion. Restart the drill if you lose your balance. If one side presents difficulty, perform an extra set on

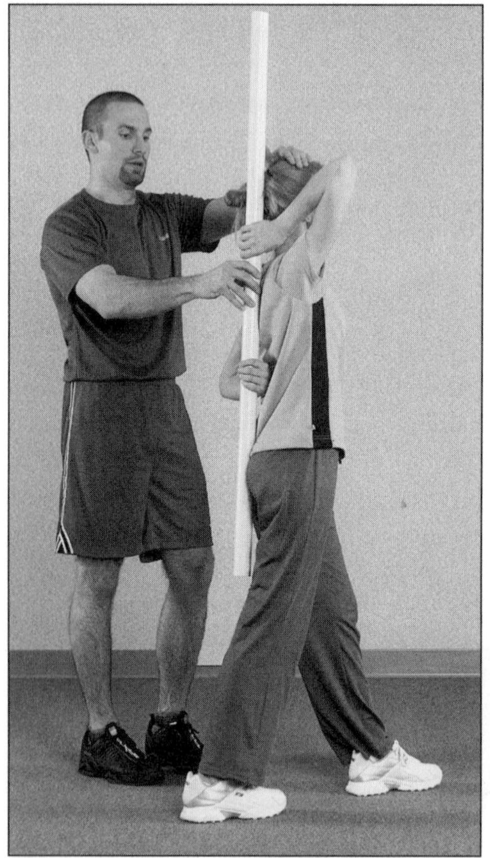

a

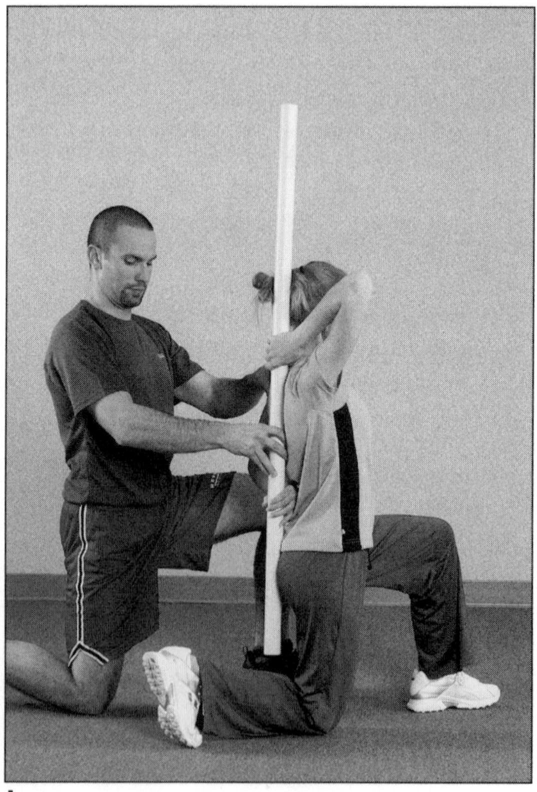

b

Figure 6.8 In-line lunge: *(a)* stand with dowel behind your back; *(b)* descend so that the back knee touches the tape.

that side. The dowel should remain vertical from a front and side view through the entire lunge movement. The dowel should also remain in contact with the three points previously mentioned.

Like the squat and hurdle step, the lunge is a fundamental movement pattern. But remember, it is not designed to simulate a particular exercise or sport movement. It is designed to demonstrate the athlete's ability to go through a left and right movement pattern by subjecting the body to a few extremes. The special hand placement for the lunge movement pattern uses specific range of motion in the upper back and shoulders and requires the athlete to stabilize the lower back and demonstrate an extreme striding motion without losing balance. Many who have participated in the lunge assessment have said, "I'm all wound up," or, "My body feels as if it's locked up and can't go any farther." Typically, it is not simply a flexibility or a strength problem, as is often initially assumed. It is just a pattern that places the athlete in an unfamiliar position. The athlete does not adequately contract and relax the muscles in a coordinated fashion to allow for movement. You may be tempted to blame a poor test score on tightness or weakness in a single muscle, but this is rarely the case. Habits, activities, hand and foot dominance, and level of fitness all come into play. But being aware of a movement pattern limitation allows the athlete to do the necessary work to regain that pattern and, it is hoped, some movement efficiency.

Use three to four of the stretches and foundation drills as a warm-up and cool-down, or make them part of a workout for one week and retest. Check all movements, not just the one being focused on, and see what has happened. Sometimes the difference will be obvious; sometimes it will not. Be persistent and consistent and you will start to see change. Follow directions and work on the asymmetries (left-right differences) first and limitations (general stiffness noted on both left and right sides) second.

Active Straight Leg Raise

At first glance, the active straight leg raise may appear to be less functional than the deep squat, hurdle step, and lunge. The active straight leg raise was not chosen as an assessment because of its similarity to sport movement, but rather because it is a simple movement that creates an appreciation of left-right differences or unobserved limitations. It combines leg flexibility with trunk strength. Difficulty with this test usually is caused by a combination of strength and flexibility imbalances or timing problems. Someone who can easily touch her toes but has difficulty with the active straight leg raise may be performing the toe touch by overstretching the spine to compensate for a flexibility problem in the lower body. She also may have poor coordination throughout the abdominal muscles, resulting in limited leg-lifting ability.

The core, the midsection of the body, should be the first group of muscles to fire. In nearly any activity, they stabilize the spine so that the extremities can be moved. The lack of this coordination sequence can really be seen in the active straight leg raise because the hip flexor muscles often will fire first, tilting the pelvis forward and pulling the low back off the floor into an arched position. This position reduces the effectiveness of the abdominal muscles as well as the other muscles that stabilize the trunk. When the core is functioning effectively the trunk and pelvis stabilizers fire before the hip flexors. The hip is effectively flexed without changing the position of the trunk. This is a true example of core stability.

One of the greatest conditioning mistakes is to assume that ab strength and endurance developed in one exercise will carry over into all movement patterns. Most people train their abs with crunches. However, crunches do not create the stress on the lower back that forces the abs to be completely reactive and coordinated. The scissors movement of the legs in the active straight leg raise does. Another problem in conventional conditioning is abdominal function symmetry. There are few ways to check for left and right differences in abdominal strength and function. The active straight leg raise may give some insight into the asymmetry. Simple crunches or sit-ups may demonstrate ab strength or endurance but do not reveal significant left-right differences when it comes to functional movement.

The active straight leg raise does require leg flexibility. It would be easy to assume that hamstring flexibility is the most important factor. It is not. If you are concerned only with the lifted leg, you will forget the leg on the floor. The leg on the floor must be flexible in the direction of extension; the leg being lifted needs flexibility in the direction of flexion. The striding motion used is not dependent on just one muscle but on groups of muscles on each side of the body, allowing for a full and unrestricted stride in either direction.

The final and most often overlooked attribute of this simple test is core stability. Stability implies control of motion, not the production of motion or the strength of the core. Stability means the core doesn't move when the extremities do.

If you want the core to move more, then do crunches, sit-ups, and roman chair extensions. If you want the core to be stable, do tests and exercises that demonstrate stability, such as the active straight leg raise. Move the limbs and note whether the core moves, too. If it does, it's not stable. Don't dismiss this simple test. Practice the following exercises to improve your score.

LEG-LOWERING PROGRESSION

Lie on your back and lift your legs to as close to a right angle as possible (figure 6.9a). Relax the feet or point the toes. Arms should be in a T or Y position to help balance the weight as you lower the leg. Lower one leg while keeping the other leg straight (figure 6.9b).

At first, use a 6- to 8-inch block or step. The important thing is not how much you lower the leg but how still you keep the upright leg. Keep the spine and legs as long as possible.

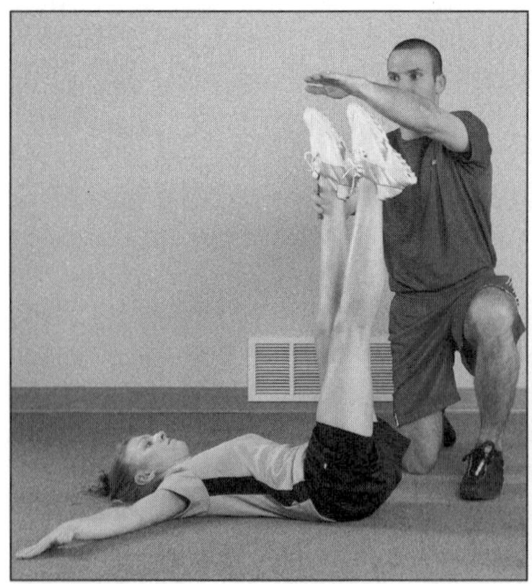

a

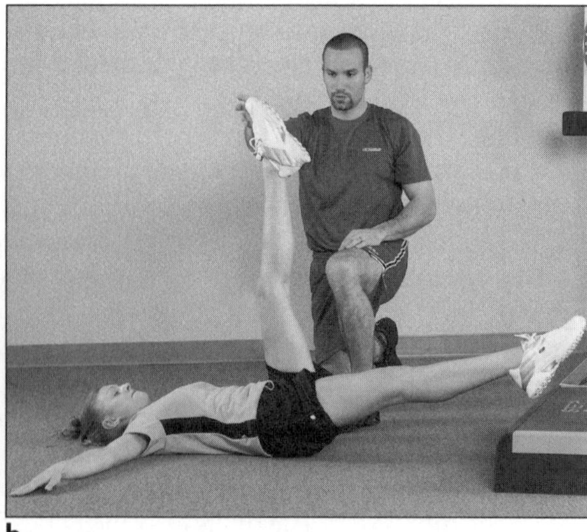

b

Figure 6.9 Leg-lowering progression: *(a)* lie on the floor with feet lifted; *(b)* lower one leg.

Relax and don't strain. If you are straining, make it easier (increase box, chair, or bench height) and do more reps.

Make sure the left and right sides are symmetrical in ability and control. Once you feel equal between the left and right sides, move to symmetrical activities that will help reinforce strength in this new pattern, such as the curl-up.

CURL-UPS TO MODIFIED CURL-UPS

This exercise should be used only as a supplement to the leg-lowering progression. It will help maintain leg flexibility and improve motor learning, leg relaxation, and trunk control. The stability program with leg lowering is more functional and should always come first. This exercise is only a complement.

Lie flat on your back with your arms over your head and toes pointed at the ceiling (figure 6.10a). Bring the arms toward the legs. Keep the shoulder blades flat on the floor. Slowly lift the head so that the chin comes into contact with the chest (figure 6.10b). Leave the shoulders back and curl up the spine one segment at a time, hands reaching for the toes. Squeeze the knees and feet together. Perform a smooth curl-up with no jerking. The legs should not come up.

If you experience difficulty with the movement, try pointing the toes to the sides and squeezing the legs together before initiating movement. This simple move will keep the legs out of the curl-up. Hollow out the abdomen by drawing the abs back. Try to flatten the back and attempt the curl-up again. If this still presents difficulty, use a slight incline under the back until you can complete 12 repetitions.

The curl-up prepares the abdominal muscles for the next activity. Begin by lying on your back in a doorway with the right leg on a wall and the left leg through the doorway. Move into the wall until you feel an adequate hamstring stretch. Pull in the abs. The left leg should be bent at the knee with the foot flat on the floor. Slowly lift and straighten the left leg so that it is beside the right leg. Flatten the back and relax the shoulders. Place hands above your head and slowly lower the left leg until it touches the ground. Relax, take a breath, and slowly lift it back.

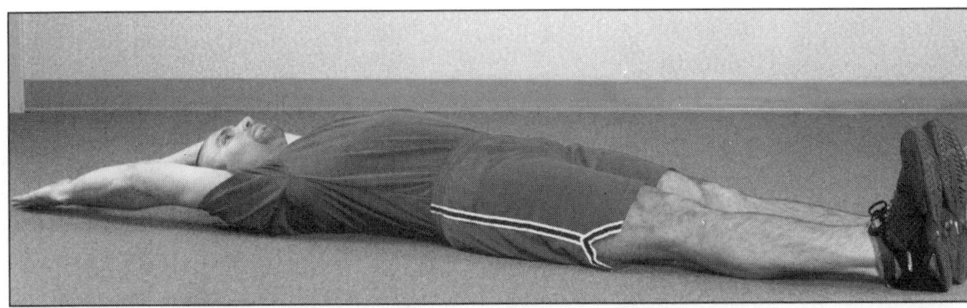
a

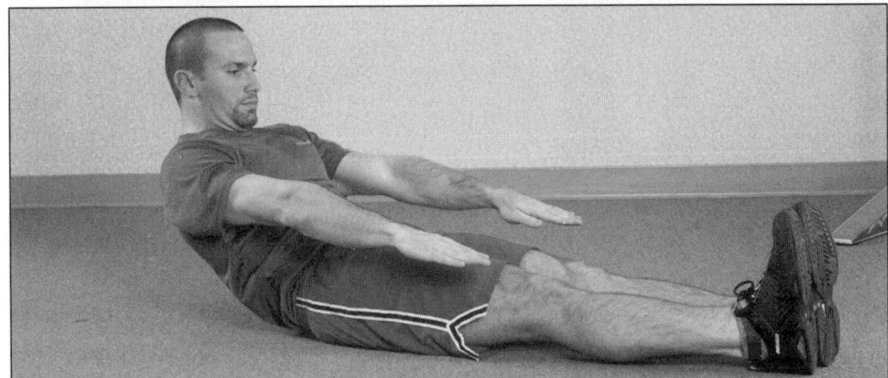
b

Figure 6.10 Curl-ups: *(a)* lie on the floor with arms overhead; *(b)* reach for your toes.

If the low back comes off the ground during the movement or the hamstring stretch intensifies, you are not staying stable through the core. The quickest remedy is to put a small rolled towel under the left knee so that it does not have to go into full extension on the floor. Reduce the bulk of the knee roll each day until you no longer need it. This activity will prepare you for a new way to train abdominal muscles and will help resolve significant left-right differences in coordination and body awareness.

LEG-LOWERING PROGRESSION WITH SUPPORT

Lie on your back near a doorjamb, corner, or another narrow stable surface. Extend both legs and prop them against the support. Slide toward the support until you are close to a right angle. Go as far as you can. Relax with your arms by your side and keep your spine as long as possible. Legs should be as long as possible. Relax the feet or point the toes.

Lower one leg while keeping the other on the wall (figure 6.11a). Rest your heel on a small 6- to 8-inch block when you lower your leg. You may use a larger block if you need to. Reduce the height of the block as you gain flexibility and control. Touch the block and raise the leg back to the original position. Do 10 to 12 repetitions, then switch legs.

Once you have equal ability and control on each side, try to go to the floor (figure 6.11b). If originally you were not at a right angle, move closer to the wall before going lower with the leg. This will ensure that you get the maximum benefit from the exercise and can observe left-right differences.

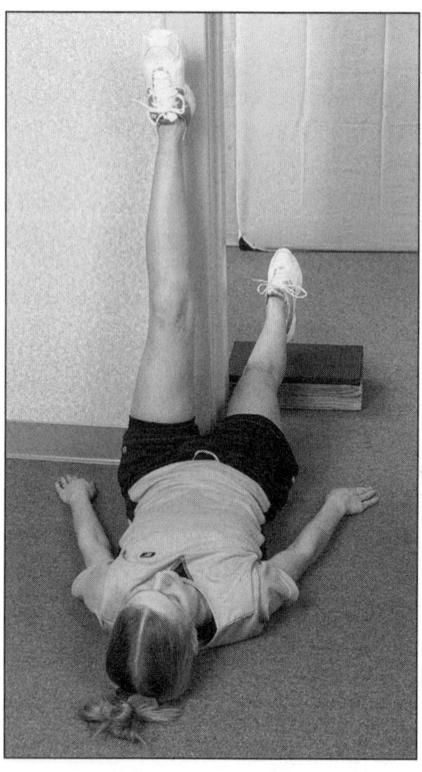

a

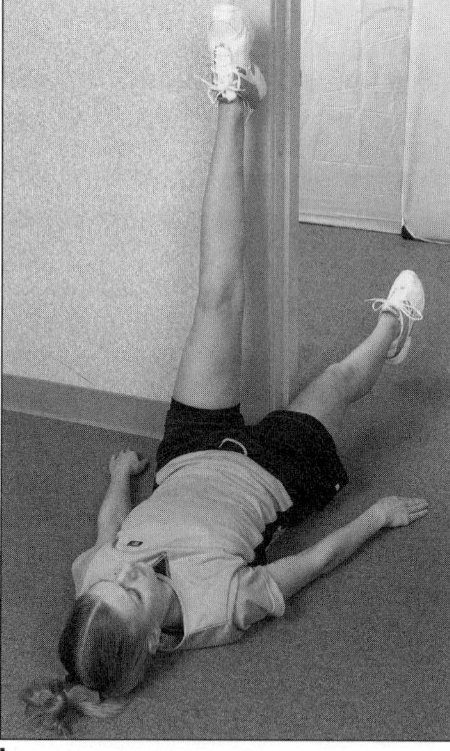

b

Figure 6.11 Leg-lowering progression with support: *(a)* lower your ankle to the elevated platform; *(b)* lower your ankle to the floor.

Use these stretches and foundation drills as a warm-up and cool-down, or make them part of a workout for one week and retest. Check all movements, not just the one being focused on, and see what has happened. Sometimes the difference will be obvious; sometimes it will not. Be persistent and consistent and you will start to see change. Follow directions and work on the asymmetries (left-right differences) first and limitations (general stiffness noted on both left and right sides) second.

Seated Rotation

The seated rotation assessment shows how tightness in one area of the body can significantly affect the movement of another. Someone who is slightly stiff even getting into a cross-legged position will unknowingly flex and contort the spine to take stress off the hips. Doing this reduces the spine's ability to effectively rotate left and right. If hip tightness isn't the problem but the seated rotation is still difficult, then it is probably safe to say that most limited movement is in the spine, represented by general stiffness rotating right and left.

The secret to performing the seated rotation adequately is to keep an erect and elongated spine, pull in the abdomen, and keep the shoulders back. It is best to go through the movement screen before moving into this section because it is important to know what you naturally do, not what you are willing to do with appropriate cues. The body naturally has good mechanics. It is through bad habits, unnecessary tension, sedentary activities, and unbalanced exercise that natural efficiency is lost and bodies try to compensate. Improving ability in the seated rotation will reduce stress on the spine and improve overall posture.

SIDE-LYING ROTATION

Lie on your right side. Flex the left knee and hip slightly greater than 90 degrees. Place the right knee on top of the left ankle to lock into a rotated position. If necessary, use a ball or towel under the left knee for support. Rotate the shoulders to the left. Do not break contact between the left knee and the towel roll, ball, or floor. Maintain consistent pressure.

Reach up and out with the left arm (figure 6.12a). Do not force the movement into a backward rotation as if trying to lay the shoulders flat on the floor. Pick up the right arm and reach toward the ceiling (figure 6.12b). This will engage the abs. Do not move the lower body. Use the abs while reaching the right arm toward the ceiling to help rotate farther to the left. Maintain pressure on the ball or towel throughout the movement.

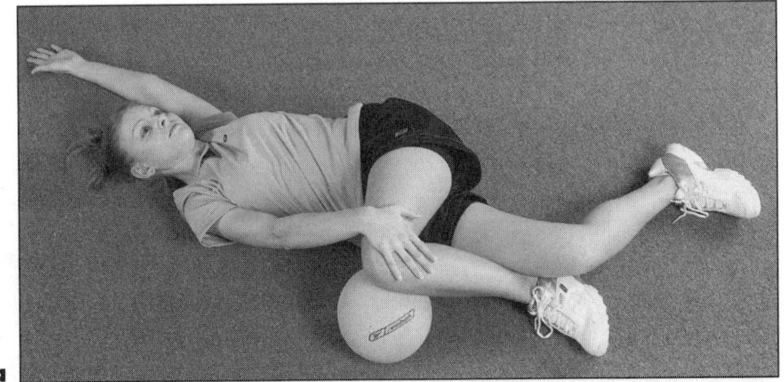

a

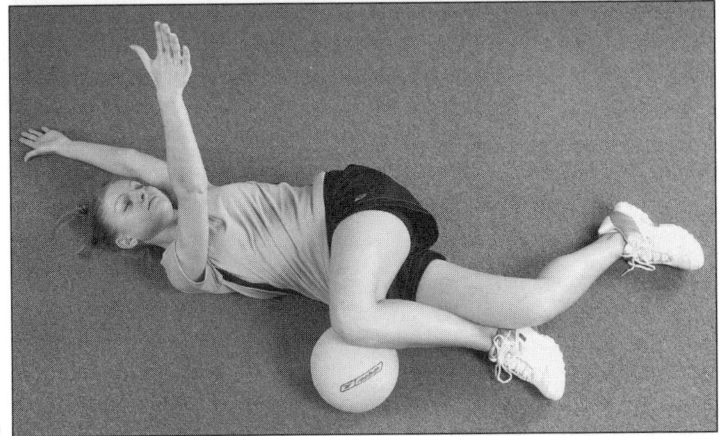

b

Figure 6.12 Side-lying rotation: *(a)* reach with the left arm; *(b)* reach with the right arm.

SHOULDER ROTATION

Lie on your left side. Flex the right knee and hip slightly greater than 90 degrees. Place the left knee on top of the right ankle to lock into a rotated position. If necessary, use a ball or towel under the right knee for support. Rotate the shoulders to the right. Do not break contact between the right knee and the towel roll, ball, or floor. Maintain consistent pressure.

Reach up and out with the right arm (figure 6.13a). Do not force the movement into a backward rotation as if trying to lay the shoulders flat on the floor. Rotate the right forearm, palm toward the floor, hand just above the buttocks. Keep the forearm flat on the floor and slide the hand up toward the mid-back while maintaining a retracted position with the scapula and rotated position with the spine (figure 6.13b).

a

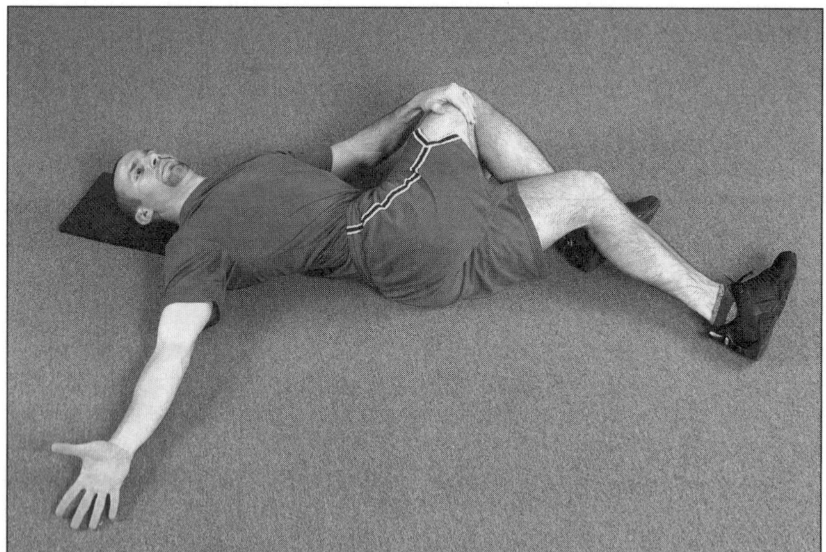

b

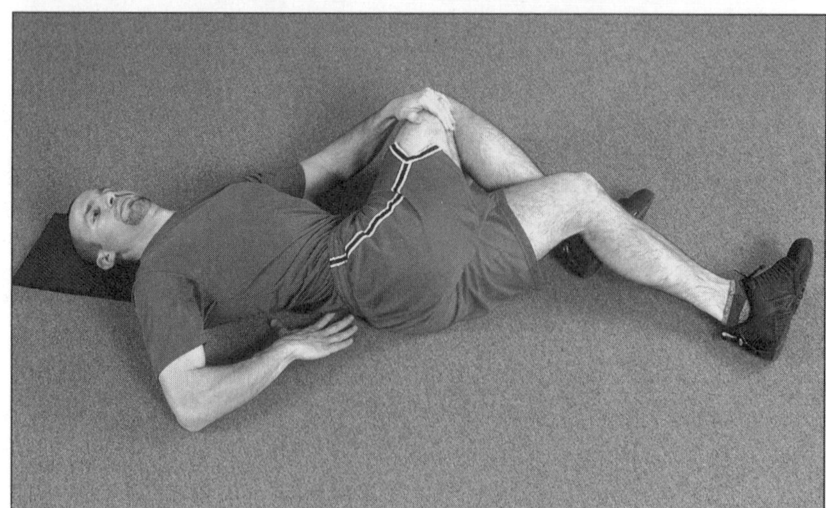

Figure 6.13 Shoulder rotation: *(a)* reach with the right arm; *(b)* slide the hand to the mid-back.

TRUNK ROTATION

Lie on the floor with arms to the side and palms turned up (figure 6.14a). Shoulders should be retracted and abs should be pulled in. Hips and knees should be flexed to 90 degrees. Place a small bolster, foam roll, or medicine ball between the knees. Support the head with a towel if necessary.

Rotate the knees to one side while keeping the arms out (figure 6.14b). Keep the knees and hips flexed; make sure hips are flexed slightly more than 90 degrees. Keep the shoulders flat and retracted; keep the neck relaxed. Reaching each arm out will help maintain position. Maintain contact between the floor and the low back. The trunk should remain relaxed during the movement. Take specific note of left and right differences and work through those by relaxation and core stability. Return to the center and repeat.

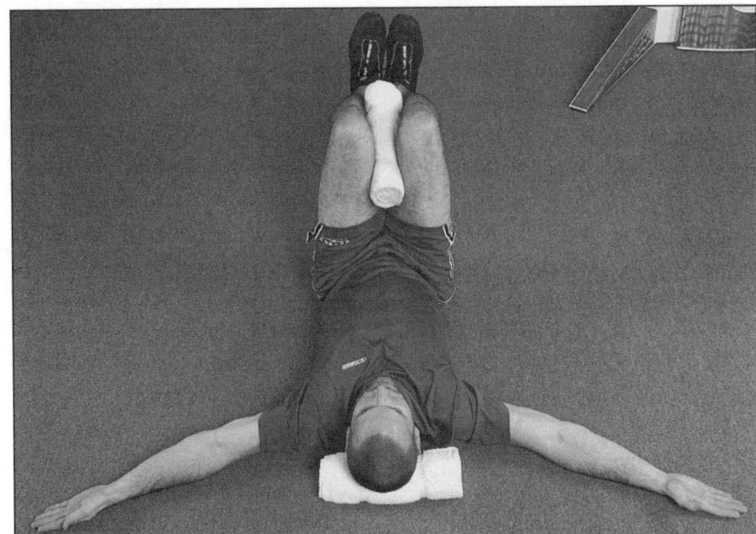

a

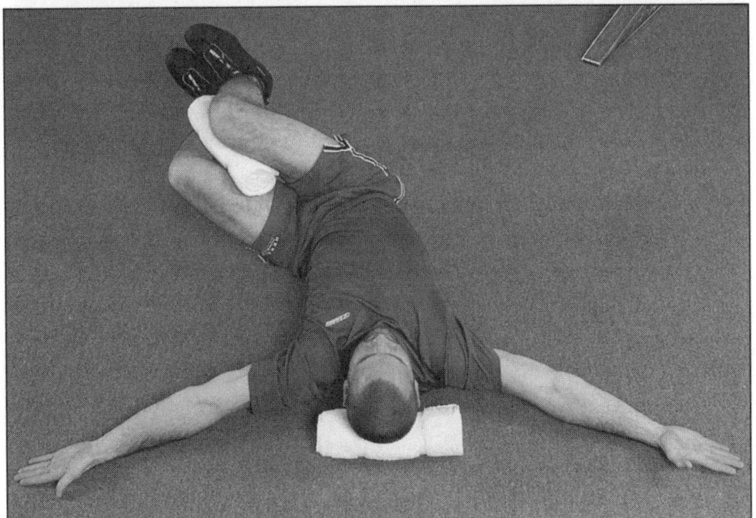

b

Figure 6.14 Trunk rotation: *(a)* lie with arms at the sides, palms up; *(b)* rotate the knees to the side.

TRUNK STABILITY

This movement will reinforce developing mobility and create awareness if the trunk is weaker in one direction. Lie on the floor with the arms to the sides slightly flexed more than 90 degrees (figure 6.15a). One palm should be turned down; the other palm should be turned up. Shoulders should be retracted and abs should be pulled in. To increase shoulder mobility, rotate the right palm down as far as it will go while rotating the left palm as high as it will go. Keep the arms reaching out as far as possible, widening the distance between the fingertips of the hands.

Rotate the knees toward the palm that is turned down (figure 6.15b). Keep shoulders flat and retracted. Keep the neck relaxed, supporting the head with a towel if necessary. Keep arms spread as wide as possible, maximizing the distance between fingertips. Reach the toes toward the ceiling and elongate the legs as much as possible. The spine should be flat and the abs should be pulled in. Remember, this is not a mobility move; it is a stability move. Therefore, the buttocks should remain flat the entire time. Rotating the knees left and right should be done through adduction and abduction of the hips. The shoulders remain flat, with the scapula retracted and the neck relaxed.

This exercise reduces the motion from the previous exercise, which targeted mobility. This is to reinforce stability and improve spine stability motor programming. If it is difficult to maintain a perfect vertical orientation of the legs, use a small folded towel under the tailbone to help flatten the back. As you progress, slowly reduce the bulk of the towel until you no longer need it.

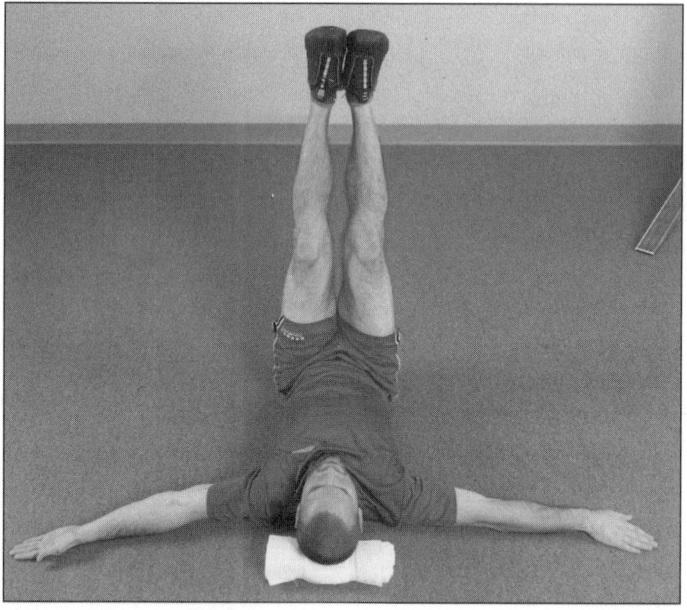

a

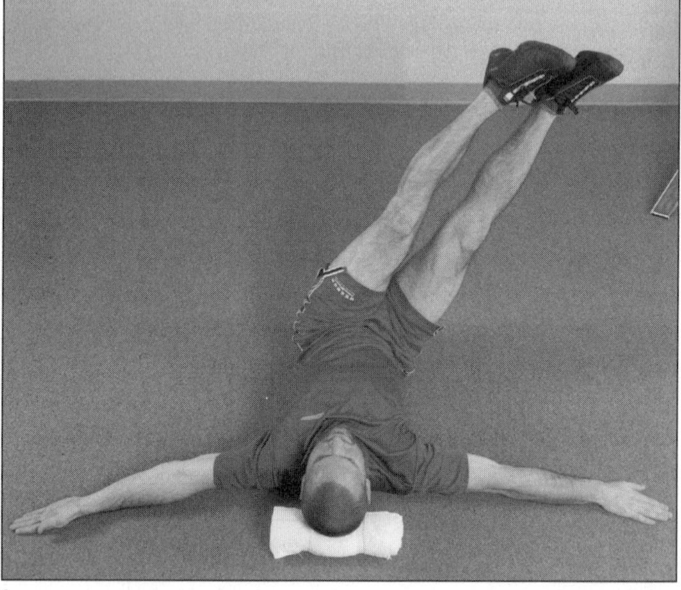

b

Figure 6.15 Trunk stability: *(a)* lie with arms to the sides, one palm down, one palm up; *(b)* rotate the knees.

Use three to four stretches or foundation drills as a warm-up and cool-down, or make them part of a workout for one week and retest. Check all movements, not just the one being focused on, and see what has happened. Sometimes the difference will be obvious; sometimes it will not. Be persistent and consistent and you will start to see change. Follow directions and work on the asymmetries (left-right differences) first and limitations (general stiffness noted on both the left and right sides) second.

7

Core Training

Core training has become a hot topic in the field of sport and fitness training. Many fitness gurus teach that getting stronger requires heavy weights, more repetitions, and more sets. But the deep muscles of the back and the deepest layers of the abdominal muscles run at the reflex level. This means they cannot just be called into play and isolated to develop strength as the biceps or quads can. Motor programs control these muscles. These muscles kick in automatically as a result of movement and resistance. If poor flexibility, muscle imbalances, inappropriate training, or one-dimensional conditioning habits have altered movement, then they may also alter the way these core muscles react and stabilize.

The functional movement screen is an excellent way to determine weaknesses in core strength and balance. Al Biancani, the strength coach for the Sacramento Kings, uses the functional movement screen on many athletes who enter the program to determine which areas need to be worked on for the benefit of the athlete and the team. When the screen revealed imbalances for Rondell White, Al was able to use the core board and core training to help White attain better body balance. Chris Webber also used the core board and core training to strengthen his ankle. "I feel using the screen core training and the core board is a must," Al says, "if we are going to attain proper body balance and subsequently improve the skills of our athletes."

My strength comes from my abdomen.
It's the center of gravity and the source of real power.

—Bruce Lee

Although many strength coaches and fitness professionals talk about core training, natural core training actually occurs during early childhood development without any coaching. It is a natural phenomenon. Most babies spend about six months doing aggressive core training before taking their first steps, mostly by practicing moving their spines and hips. Only after mastering movement of the spine and hips do they develop greater levels of control. They roll, push up onto their elbows, then eventually push up onto all fours. They crawl and attempt to stand, only to fall and try again. All of these simple little movements build and develop the core. Babies do not perform multiple repetitions trying to build strength because core training is not about strength. It's about stability and coordination. Strength is the ability to produce force, whereas stability is the act of controlling force. This is an extremely important distinction.

The word *core* represents the central part of the body, the torso and hips. The core is the powerhouse of the body. Even though the abdominal muscles are an important part of the core, core training is not about abdominal conditioning. The abdominals should never be totally isolated in training because they are never totally isolated in movement. Abdominal muscles work in coordination with hip muscles and back muscles during activity.

Two excellent examples of core training are basic yoga and the mat work developed by Joseph Pilates. Both forms of exercise are popular because they are basic, no-nonsense approaches that demand more strength from the core than the extremities (if done correctly). Many athletes who demonstrate excellent power-to-weight ratios in the weight room (meaning that they are able to move large amounts of weight relative to their body weight) have a very hard time getting through some of the basic core movements in yoga or Pilates. It may appear that this happens because of a lack of flexibility, but core stability is the other factor. These people are not weak and they have been successful in the weight room, but they are unsuccessful in balancing the body and developing the core. The strength of the extremities is not supposed to exceed the strength of the core. The core is the foundation of power and strength.

Imagine a martial artist. The only way he can put power behind his punch is to transfer the energy generated by his leg through the trunk and into the shoulder turn, resulting in powerful movements of the shoulder, arm, and fist. This translates to other sport movements as well. Almost every movement in sport requires a transfer of energy—from arm to arm, from arm to leg, from leg to arm, or from leg to leg—and the core is the common denominator.

Core stability can become automatic. Consider a runner. She doesn't have to think about her abdominal muscles or back muscles while she is running. These muscles automatically do their job if her movements are correct. The muscles are driven by reflex behavior, but the reflex behavior can be altered by poor movement patterns, poor flexibility, muscle imbalances, poor posture, or a poor warm-up.

Core training will lay the foundation for strength, power, speed, and agility training. However, it is very important to successfully complete the flexibility program and foundation drills in chapter 6 before beginning core training. This will reduce left-right differences in flexibility or movement and minimize any unnecessary tightness. You do not need to have a perfect score on the movement screen, but you do need to focus on the areas identified by the screen as limited and asymmetrical as long as they exist. In short, try to eliminate major asymmetries or restrictions before moving into core training; but if you decide to start core training with limitations and restrictions, use stretching and foundation drills to complement the core training. The core is the body's gyroscope. It tries to balance the network of forces acting on it and redistribute those forces appropriately. The core will try to compensate for differences between right and left shoulder flexibility, right and left hip flexibility, or poor flexibility in the spine. Without proper flexibility, the core ends up absorbing some of those forces. This can cause injury and a loss of power. Serious athletes cannot afford either.

Before proceeding with core training, you need an adequate understanding of your goals and needs. You also need movement screen information and an understanding of the need for functional movement patterns. Note individual scores on the movement screen and any problems, asymmetries, or difficulties. Many problems can be fixed with a targeted flexibility program. The movement screen should have increased your awareness of limited movement or tightness on one or both sides of your body. The greater your balance as you begin core training, the more quickly the core will stabilize and the sooner you will be able to move on with the program. If flexibility and functional movement haven't received adequate attention, the core program will be difficult. Even if the athlete can perform the routine and exercises, he will not get the maximum benefit from the exercises because he will compensate without realizing it.

Rid yourself of all preconceived ideas about core training. The biggest mistake is thinking that multiple sets and reps or the isolation of a certain muscle group are needed. Core training is training for movement patterns and stability. If the spine moves, as it does during crunches, sit-ups, or roman chair exercises, the core muscles are strengthened but the core is being made mobile, not stable. Remember, the definition of stability is the ability to control movement and force, not the production of movement or the generation of force. Therefore, the best core training programs require the spine to be held in a natural or neutral position while breathing and while moving the arms and legs in motions that mimic the functional ways the core will be stressed in a given sport or activity.

The following core program can be the turning point of a conditioning program. It doesn't require running, jumping, or throwing a medicine ball. A spotter isn't needed, and you don't need to put chalk on your hands. You don't need mirrors or weights. With patience, you will tap into what every martial artist, gymnast, wrestler, and acrobat knows—the core is the source of power, and creating greater stability in the core can accelerate performance.

It's what you learn after you know it all that counts.

—John Wooden

Core Program Progressions

The following program builds on the information already covered in this book. Instead of arbitrarily doing the entire core program presented in this chapter, I recommend doing the core routine that directly addresses the greatest problem revealed in your movement screen. Attend to any obvious flexibility problems and balance any specific asymmetries identified by the movement screen before beginning core training. If minor flexibility problems, asymmetries, or imbalances still exist, it is OK to start the core training program. But continue to do several stretching exercises between core training exercises. If flexibility problems persist, alter the program so that you do two stretching sessions for every one core training session. If the movement screen shows no serious flexibility problems or asymmetries, start with the core exercises that address the movement pattern that presented the greatest amount of difficulty according to scores or notes.

The core training exercises for each movement pattern are presented in a particular order called a *progression.* They should be performed in that order because one exercise builds on the other. The circuit can be completed more than once, but watch for fatigue. Fatigue may cause a loss of stabilization, making it more difficult to execute with proper technique. Remember, the brain will remember improper technique as well as proper technique. Improper technique is usually noted with greater frequency at the end of a workout, which makes it the last thing remembered. Don't let this happen. It's better to do 10 good repetitions than to do 25 bad repetitions.

After one week of performing the chosen core routine, recheck the movement screen to see whether the score has changed. If the movement pattern being worked on still presents difficulty, continue working on that sequence of exercise. If the movement screen has changed and now another movement pattern presents greater difficulty, switch and start performing that core routine.

These core routines are excellent warm-up activities and can precede conditioning, weight training, or competition if performed in moderation to activate (not fatigue) core muscles or to reinforce core stability. They also can be used at the end of a workout for a cool-down and to show whether any core stability is left at the end of a workout or training session. This will demonstrate the presence of a reserve of stability. This reserve of stability will kick in during fatigue to push the body to the limit. If core exercise technique is extremely poor after a workout or seems to be declining, you might be overtraining (which requires time off to give the body a chance to repair and rest) or have major efficiency problems. It could also indicate poor core endurance and efficiency. Efficiency problems can be fixed by continuing to improve flexibility or by increasing the frequency and volume of core training. However, temporarily cut back on other forms of training to make sure that fatigue isn't causing poor form.

Another way to add core training is to do it in the morning, beginning the day by focusing on the core. Later in the day, run through a few exercises to warm up for the normal workout. The movements resemble yoga by design, not so much as a workout but as a tuneup or rebalancing. Starting the day with core training activates the basic motor programs that build the correct foundation for all activities. These movements were designed to show left-right differences and stabilization flaws. Rushing will prevent learning. As proficiency increases, use the exercises as a warm-up to a workout only, or continue a morning routine. Don't be surprised if the best days start with a focus on the core.

Before beginning core training, warm up by stretching and jogging in place, jumping rope, or performing jumping jacks. Use the stretches and foundation drills to address the problem areas indicated by your movement screen. Dedicate 5 to 10 minutes to your warm-up each workout.

Core Board Squat Progression

The core board is the preferred piece of equipment for this program, but the exercises also can be performed on the floor or, preferably, on a step or slightly elevated surface. The core board provides resisted tilting and twisting for added feedback. However, a small amount of force can be exerted into the step or floor to produce similar results. You will not feel movement as you do with the core board, but you should feel tension develop. This tension will help core stability.

TOE TOUCH SQUAT

Stand about a foot in front of the core board with feet slightly wider than shoulder-width apart. If needed, place towel rolls under the heels to assist with the squat. Reach to the ceiling, trying to make your body as tall as possible while pulling in the abdominals (figure 7.1a). Pull the abdominals inward but don't let this alter your breathing.

Bend forward, placing the hands on the edge of the core board, keeping the knees as straight as possible without hyperextending. Let the spine comfortably round and press on the core board hard enough to make it tilt in your direction (figure 7.1b).

While maintaining consistent pressure (enough to keep the board tilted forward), go into the squat position as deep as possible, splitting the knees wide enough so that they do not touch the elbows (figure 7.1c). Make the spine as tall as possible while keeping the feet flat and the weight on the heels. Keep the board tilted forward the entire time.

Remove the hands from the board, reach overhead as high as possible without changing weight on the heels, and maintain a tall spine (figure 7.1d). Return to the standing position and relax the arms. Perform 10 to 15 repetitions.

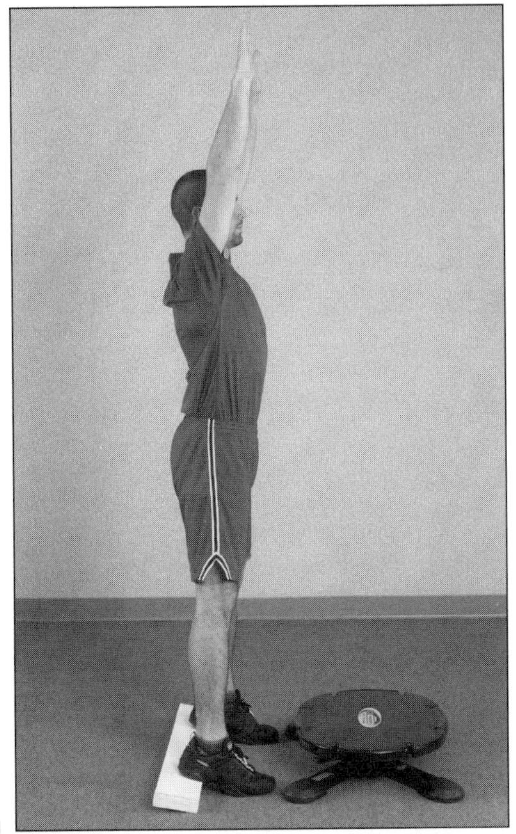

a

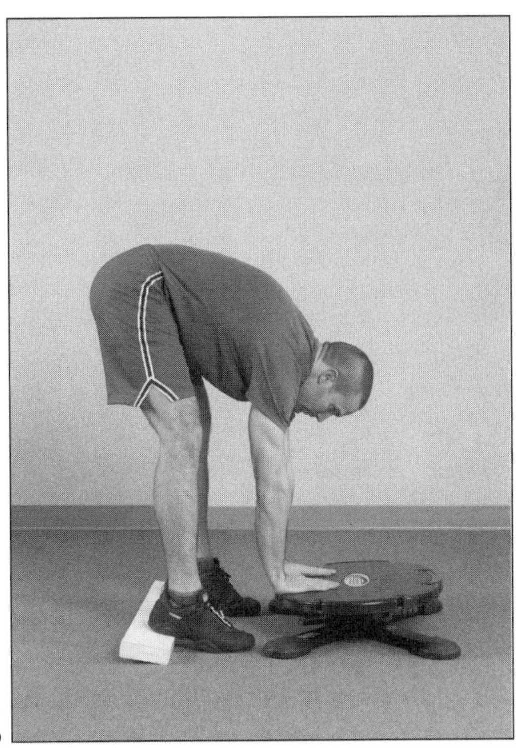

b

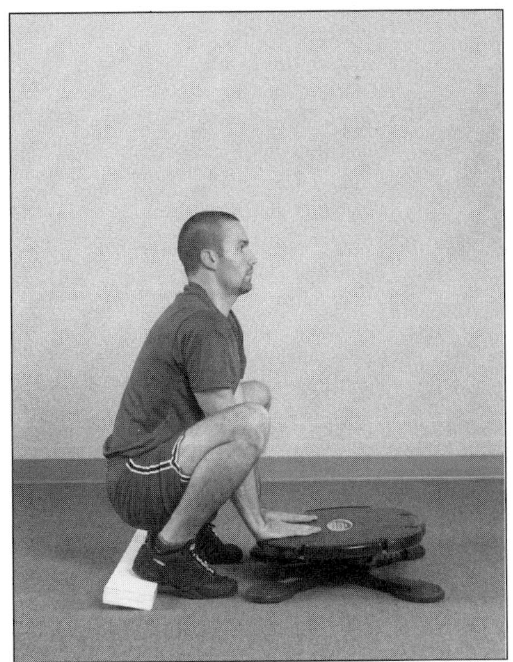

c

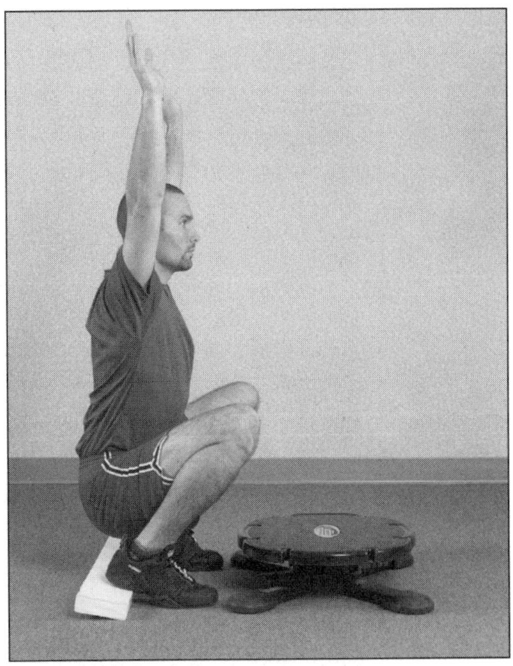

d

Figure 7.1 Toe touch squat: *(a)* reach to the ceiling; *(b)* bend forward and press on the core board; *(c)* go into a deep squat; *(d)* reach overhead.

SQUAT REACH

Once you are proficient with the deep squat progression, add a one-arm reach to the movement. Use the same start position as the deep squat progression. Bend forward and then drop into squat position. Maintain pressure on the board. Instead of lifting both arms into the air, place the hands on the outer edges of the board and twist and rotate the board by pressing down and turning it to the left (figure 7.2a). Keep weight on the heels, pressing into the board by using the abdominals and not by shifting body weight forward.

Lift the right hand back and up, looking over the right shoulder and rotating the shoulders as far as possible without losing the twist produced onto the board (figure 7.2b). This means you must at all times maintain a downward rotating pressure in the opposite arm.

The squat reach can be performed on the last repetition of the deep squat progression. You can alternate from the left to the right hand or perform 10 repetitions on the left and repeat on the right.

a

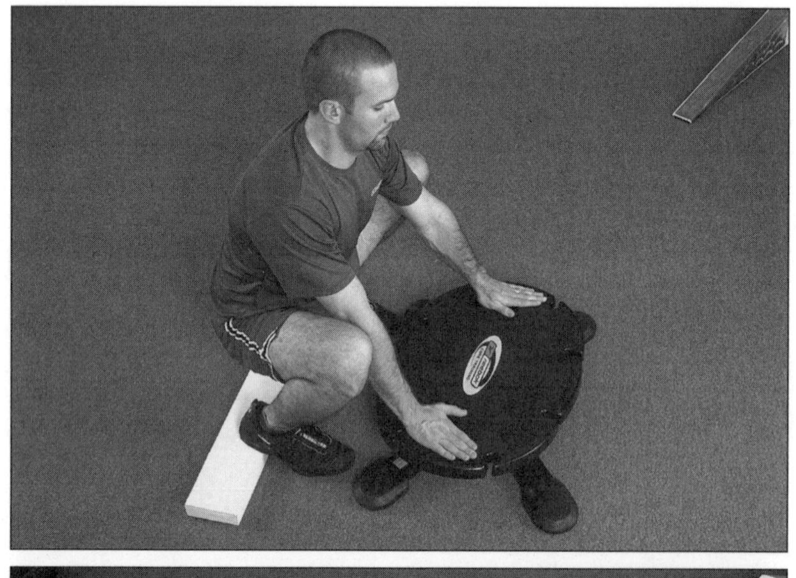

b

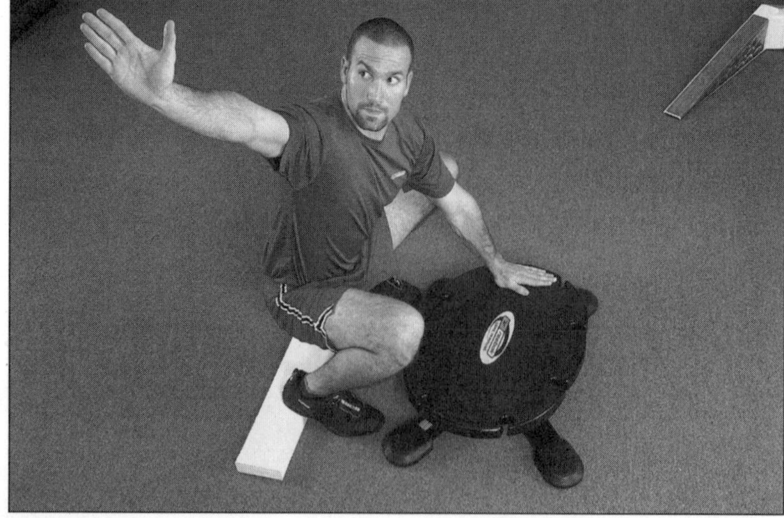

Figure 7.2 Squat reach: *(a)* rotate the board; *(b)* lift the right hand and look over the right shoulder.

DEEP SQUAT ON SLIDE BOARD

Deep squatting on a slide board may seem a little crazy, but it's not. When you deep squat, you mostly are concerned with the downward motion of the body, but often the squat motion places torque on the hips, knees, and ankles. Because your shoes or feet grip the floor, this torque is not always obvious. When you stand on a slide board, the traction component is gone and if the toes turn outward relative to heel position you will be aware of it immediately. On the slide board you will have a continual balance of the muscles of the hip, knee, and ankle, keeping the joints aligned as you descend into the squat.

Do not do the deep squat exercise on a slide board if you can't do a full comfortable deep squat. If you notice that the feet turn out even slightly, stop. Your feet must be parallel. If necessary, use a towel roll under the heels, slowly reducing the bulk of the roll as you become proficient as long as you can demonstrate the same quality of movement.

Hold a dowel vertically in front of you on the ground to help you balance for your first rep. Stand on the slide board and place towel rolls under your heels, if necessary. Descend into a squat, keeping the knees aligned over the feet (figure 7.3a). (You can use pieces of tape on the slide board to make sure your feet do not turn outward or slide relative to knee or heel position.) Return to standing with no foot movement or turning.

Now hold the dowel over your head. Descend into the squat with no foot movement or sliding (figure 7.3b). Perform 10 to 15 repetitions.

The deep squat exercise on a slide board is excellent for training stability while squatting. It also is a good exercise to include with a superset of front and back squats with weight or for leg presses, hang cleans, and jump training because it incorporates both flexibility and stability as well as body control and balance. Slide boards have been used for many years to simulate skating, but in most sports the object is *not* to slide. This drill provides an excellent tool to increase awareness of unnecessary torsion, and therefore unnecessary energy expenditure, within squatting movement patterns.

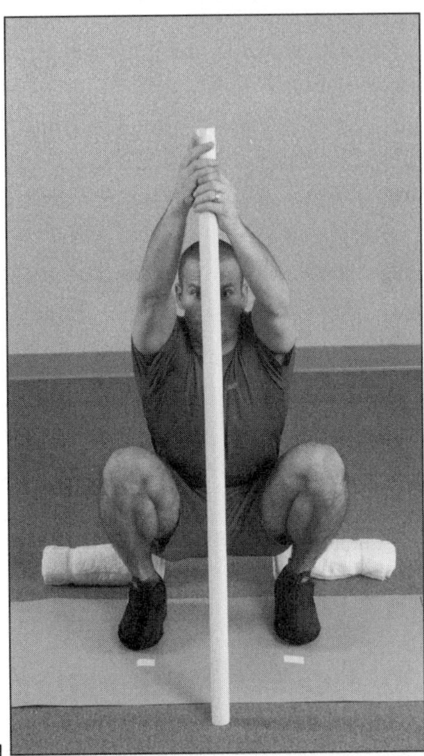
a

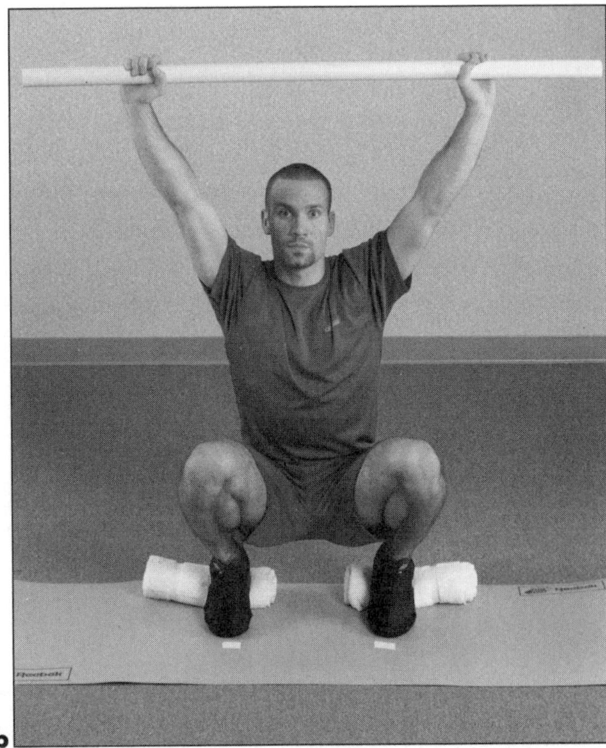
b

Figure 7.3 Deep squat on slide board: *(a)* with dowel vertical, lower into squat, then stand up; *(b)* hold the dowel overhead and lower into squat.

Core Board Hurdle Step Progression

Core training for the hurdle step will help you learn how to become more stable as you transfer power from one leg to the other. The push-up position is used to get the trunk muscles to fire and stabilize the spine and pelvis. This will reduce compensation at the core and help you focus on the hurdle or stride position of the hips.

DOUBLE-LEG STRETCH

Begin in a push-up position, hands about shoulder-width apart, weight supported by your toes and hands (figure 7.4a).

Walk the feet forward to a position at which the heels can maintain contact with the floor (figure 7.4b). The feet should be slightly wider than shoulder-width apart. With your hands at the widest position possible, maintain pressure into the core board, creating a slight tilt toward you and thus engaging the abdominals. Feel a slight stretch throughout the back of the legs and buttocks. Relax and repeat.

Perform 10 to 15 repetitions.

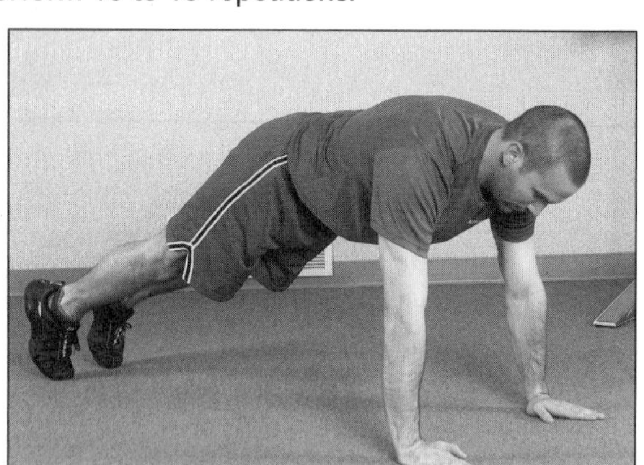
a

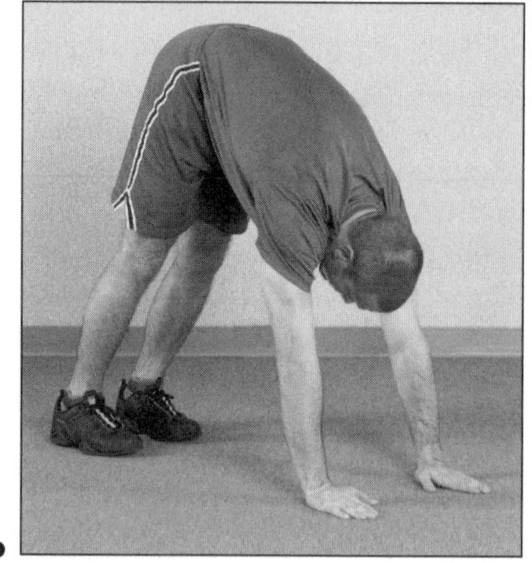
b

Figure 7.4 Double-leg stretch: *(a)* push-up position; *(b)* bring feet forward.

SLOW-MOTION MOUNTAIN CLIMBER

Begin in a push-up position, hands about shoulder-width apart, weight supported by your toes and hands, hands on the core board at the widest part (figure 7.5a). Allow no movement or twisting to occur with the core board.

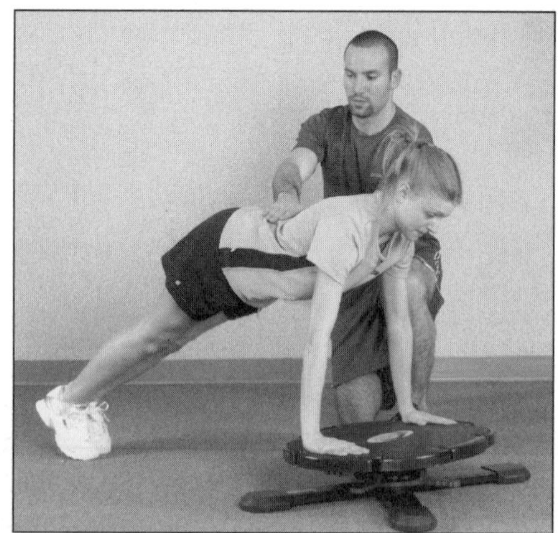
a

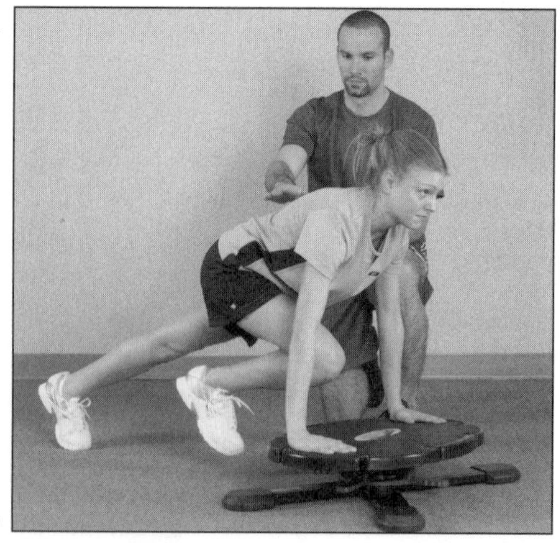
b

Figure 7.5 Slow-motion mountain climber: *(a)* push-up position with hands on the core board; *(b)* bring knee toward chest.

Flex the right hip and knee but do not make contact with the floor (figure 7.5b). Keep the foot flexed while maintaining a flat spine and tilt with the board. Flex the right knee as much as possible while maintaining maximal hip extension. Maintain a tall spine. Straighten the right leg and return to the pushup position, pointing the right toes. Do not sway or hyperextend the lower back. Repeat on the left side. Perform 10 to 15 repetitions on each side.

MOUNTAIN CLIMBER SLIDE AND STRIDE

The motion in this exercise is similar to that used in the elevated mountain climber cycle exercise in chapter 6 (page 48). Place your hands off one end of the slide board and wear socks or the slick boots provided with the slide board (figure 7.6a).

Keep the spine as long as possible. Bring one knee to the chest by bending both the knee and hip (figure 7.6b). Bring the knee as close to the chest as possible and then straighten the leg. Because of the socks or slick boots, the feet will slide forward and backward in a more piston-like motion with less jarring of the low back. It should be easier to maintain the low-back position, but sometimes it's harder to stabilize the sliding foot. This adds an extra dimension to a classic exercise.

For best results, perform the exercise in intervals with repetitions counted for performance. Pick an interval of time, such as 20, 30, or 40 seconds, and perform as many repetitions as you can in that time. Rest for a set time, such as 60 or 120 seconds, and try to perform two or three more sets of the same number of repetitions (or more) in the same time interval. Make sure your technique is good. Use a water bottle and lay it across the sway in the lowest part of your spine. Keep the water bottle steady and don't let it fall. This will help you move your hips without moving your spine.

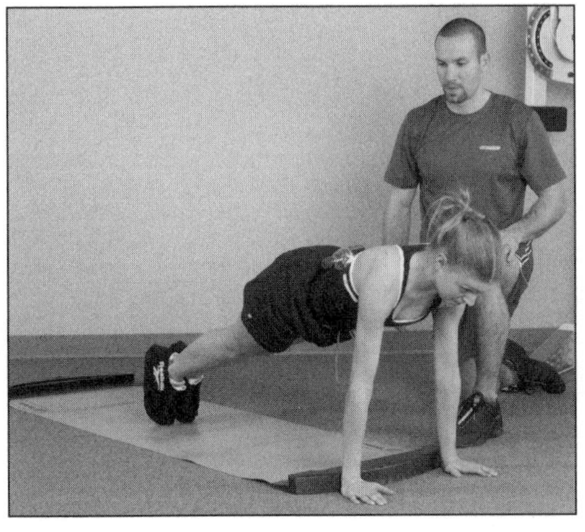

a

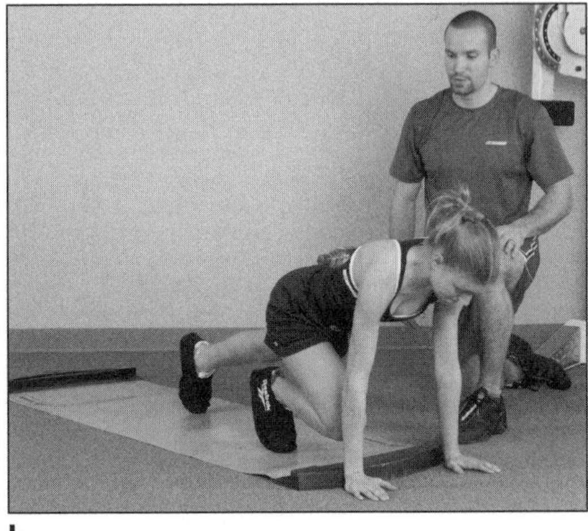

b

Figure 7.6 Mountain climber slide and stride: *(a)* pushup position over slide board; *(b)* bring knee toward chest. Prop a water bottle on your lower back to help you keep your back steady.

Core Board Lunge Progression

The importance of the lunge is disassociation of the hips and trunk. Hip tightness and poor core stability can greatly reduce lunge performance. The maximum stride required for the lunge should not cause trunk or pelvic rotation. It should be predominantly a hip movement using flexion and extension of each hip. Use these core exercises to keep mobility in the hips and legs and stability in the core.

STRIDE AND TWIST

Begin in the forward bend position (figure 7.7a). Place the hands on the edge of the core board, keeping the knees as straight as possible without hyperextending. Let the spine comfortably round and press on the core board hard enough to make it tilt in your direction. Keep abdominals pulled in.

Move into a stride position by extending the right leg, keeping the spine long, looking forward, and bending as deeply as possible through the left hip, knee, and ankle (figure 7.7b). The left heel should stay in contact with the floor. The left thigh should be under the chest.

Pull with the left arm and push with the right arm to press and turn the board while continuing in the stride position.

Maintain pressure with the right arm. Lift the left arm, rotate the spine, and turn the head (figure 7.7c). Hold the hand toward the ceiling with the arm fully extended and palm turned up. Do not rotate the pelvis. Turn only the shoulders. Maintain a stable position of the flexed left knee. Return to start position. Perform 10 to 15 repetitions. Repeat on the other side.

a

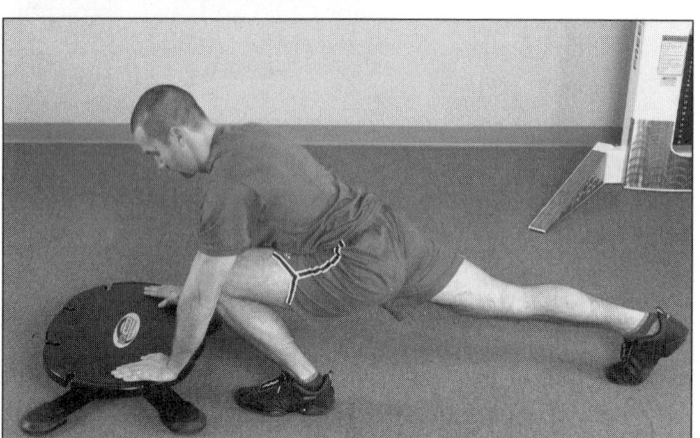

b

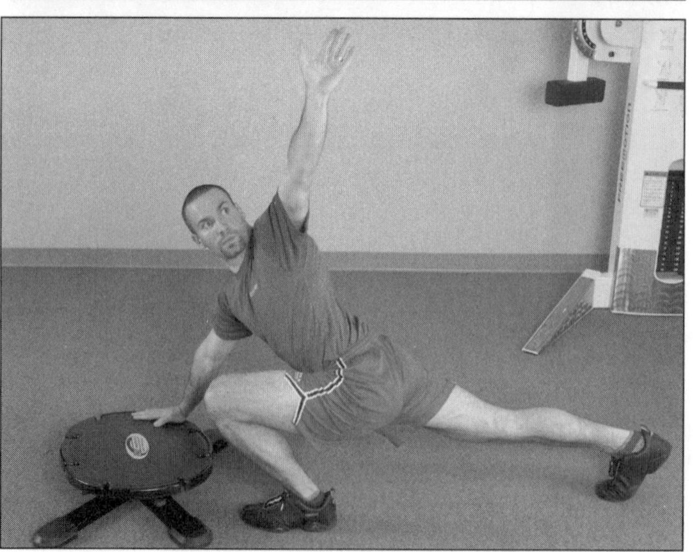

c

Figure 7.7 Stride and twist: *(a)* forward bend position; *(b)* extend the right leg; *(c)* lift the left arm.

LUNGING DOWEL TWIST (DYNAMIC LUNGE)

For this exercise you will need a dowel and a piece of tape the same length as your lower leg. Stand with feet side by side, the dowel or stick on your shoulders across your shoulder blades. Stride into a lunge position (figure 7.8a). Feet should be within the four-inch centerline. Create a box with your legs as in the half-kneeling dowel twist (page 51), except the back knee should not touch the floor. Allow it to hover about an inch off the ground. Keep the spine tall and twist toward the front leg (figure 7.8b). Return to standing and repeat the movement in a smooth and controlled fashion. Stride into the lunge and begin to twist near the lowest point of the lunge. Pretend that the dowel is a gun and that you want to shoot at a target directly in front of you. Don't lean forward or backward. Twist, shoot, and return.

Twist to the side with the forward knee, then try to twist to the other side. Note the differences. Work on the differences, trying to balance the left and right sides as much as possible to create a foundation for the more advanced moves to come.

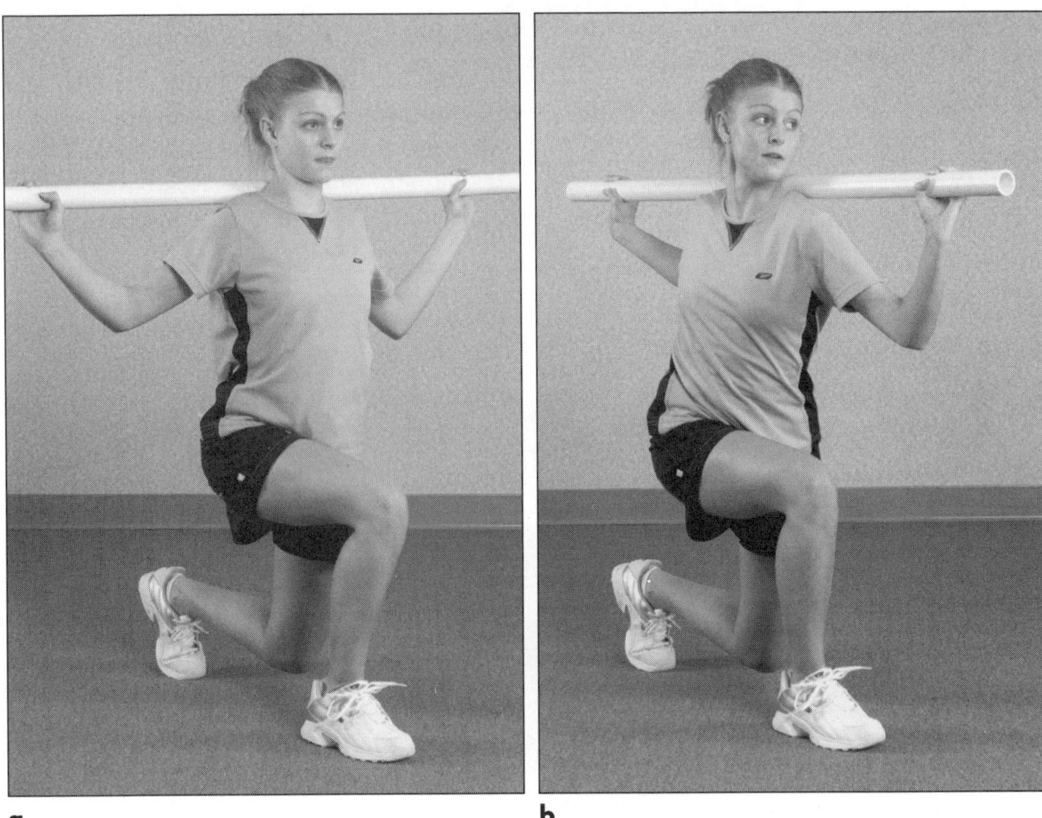

Figure 7.8 Lunging dowel twist: *(a)* lunge position with dowel across shoulder blades; *(b)* twist toward the front leg.

Core Board Active Straight Leg Raise Progression

Core training for the active straight leg raise is unique. For the squat, hurdle step, and lunge, the lower body creates the foundation for movement. The active straight leg raise is considered an *open-chain movement.* In contrast, a *closed-chain movement* is one where the upper or lower extremities are planted and stable and the body moves around the axis or point of stability created by their contact with a stable object. In an open-chain movement the body must anchor onto itself. Core training for the active straight leg raise will reinforce this type of stability.

SINGLE-LEG BRIDGE

Sit on the core board with the buttocks at one end and the feet at the other. Hands should be on the floor with arms slightly behind the shoulders.

Bridge upward by pushing down with the feet and lifting the buttocks until the hips are extended (figure 7.9a). The edge of the board nearest you will tilt upward. Maximize hip extension in order to keep the buttocks off the board. Do not hyperextend the spine. Keep abdominals pulled in during the movement.

Extend the right leg and point the right toe without changing hip position or lowering the back (figure 7.9b). Do not let the buttocks touch the edge of the board.

Perform an active straight leg raise by flexing the right hip (figure 7.9c). Do not lose hip extension or hyperextend the spine. Do not lose balance by leaning to the right or left. Keep the left knee aligned with the foot. Keep abdominals pulled in. Repeat on the left side.

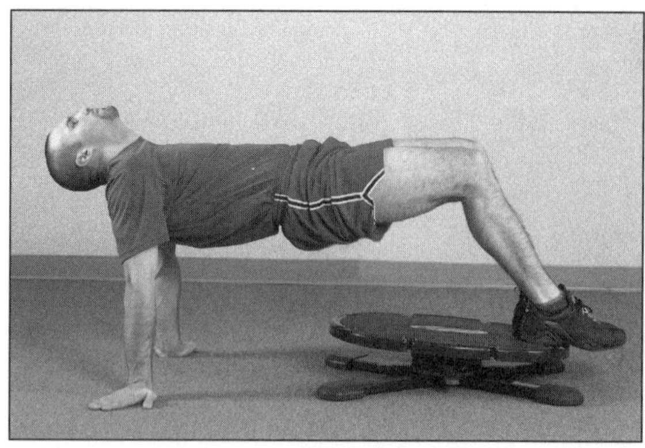

a

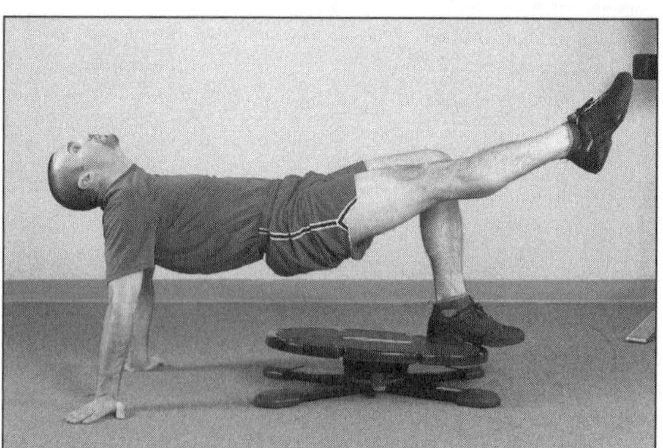

b

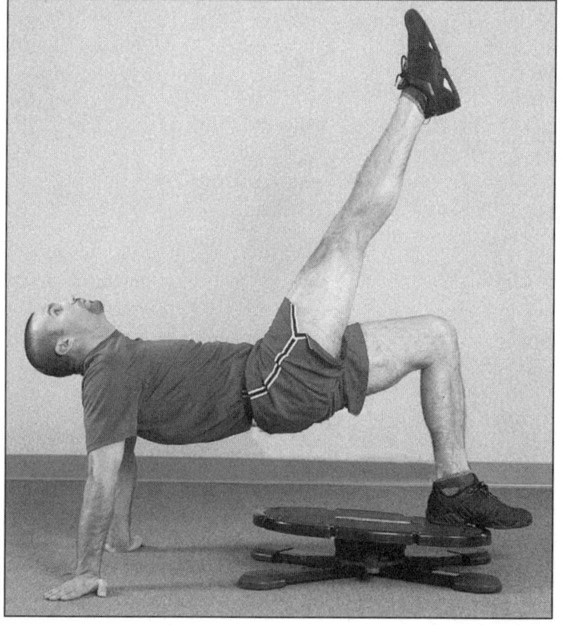

c

Figure 7.9 Single-leg bridge: *(a)* lift the buttocks to create a bridge; *(b)* extend the right leg; *(c)* lift the right leg.

DIP BRIDGE

Sit at one end of the board with feet flat on the floor and knees bent. Place the hands on the other end of the board.

Press into the core board with the hands, extend the hips, and lift the buttocks off the board, knees bent to 90 degrees (figure 7.10a). Keep the feet flat, pull in the abdominals, and extend the elbows while keeping the spine straight. The hips should be fully extended.

Extend the right leg to a horizontal position parallel to the floor and point the toes (figure 7.10b). Do not lose balance. Keep the abdominals pulled in and maintain hip and spine extension. The focal point should be maintaining the left hip extension as the right leg is lifted.

Flex the right hip, point the toes, and raise the leg as far as possible without losing spine or hip extension on the left leg (figure 7.10c). Do not flex the cervical spine. Do not allow the left knee to drift or move out of the starting position. Perform 10 to 15 repetitions. Lower the buttocks to the board and repeat on the left side.

Please note two common mistakes in this movement: (1) the neck is hyperextended and (2) the hip is *not* extended. This can be remedied by elevating the surface on which the hands are placed and moving to a more stable surface than the board. In proper technique, 7.10 b should show the model in a straight line.

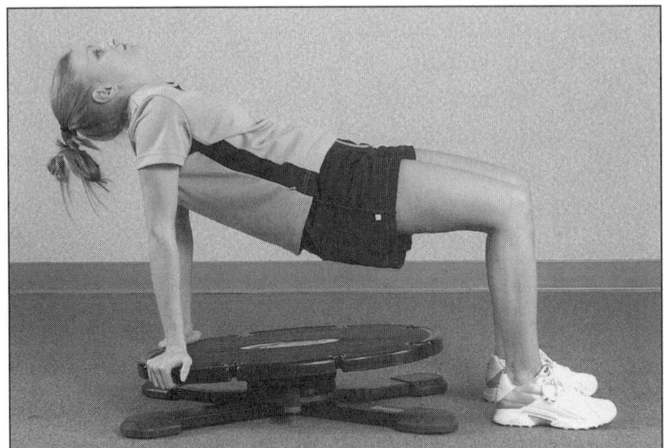

a

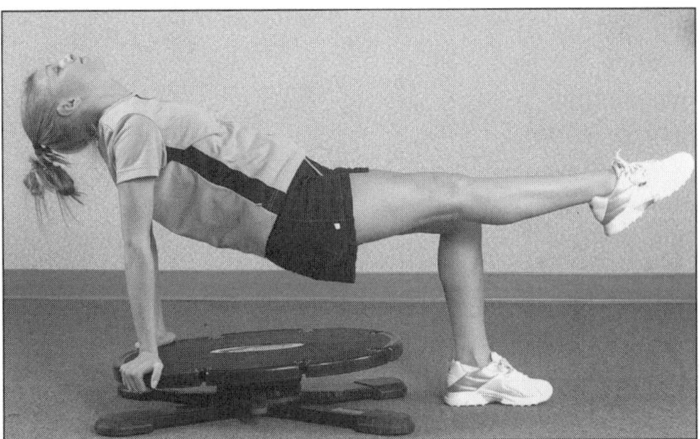

b

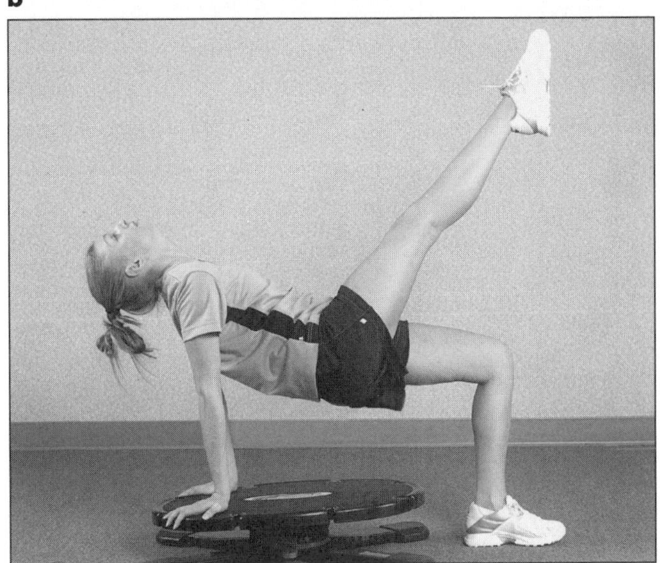

c

Figure 7.10 Dip bridge: *(a)* lift the buttocks off the board, creating a bridge; *(b)* extend the right leg; *(c)* lift the right leg.

STRAIGHT LEG RAISE

Lie on the core board with feet on the floor so that you are tilted slightly toward the head. Support the head with your hands. Maintain proper low-back alignment, pulling in the abs to keep the back flat on the board for the entire length of the spine.

Raise both legs by flexing the hips and knees, then extend the legs and point the toes at the ceiling while flexing the hips (figure 7.11a). Keep your abdominals pulled in.

Lower the left leg while maintaining position with the right leg extended and hip flexed, toes pointed toward the ceiling. Simultaneously, reach back with the right arm while supporting the head with the left hand (figure 7.11b).

Raise the left leg so both legs are in a hip-flexed position, pointing the toes at the ceiling, keeping the knees extended. Continue to keep the toes pointed throughout the movement. Perform 10 to 15 repetitions. Repeat on the left side.

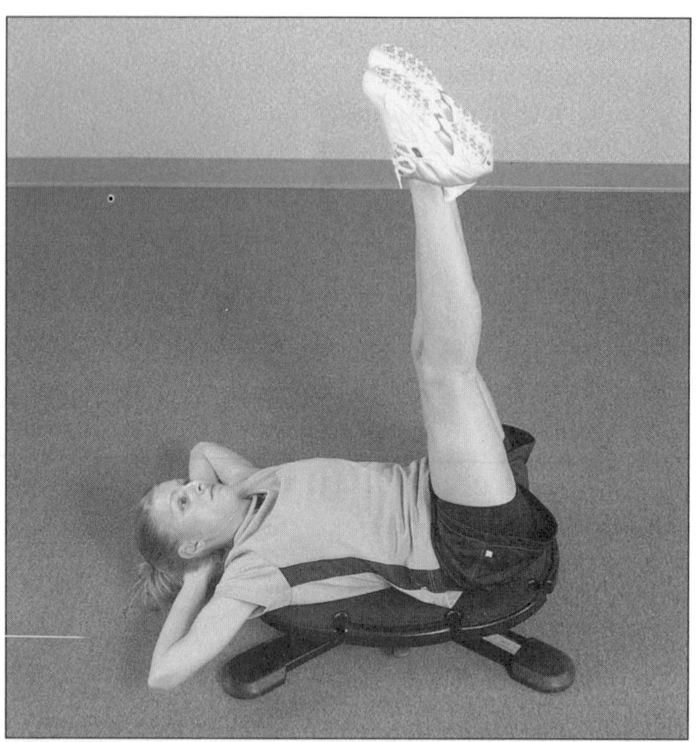

a

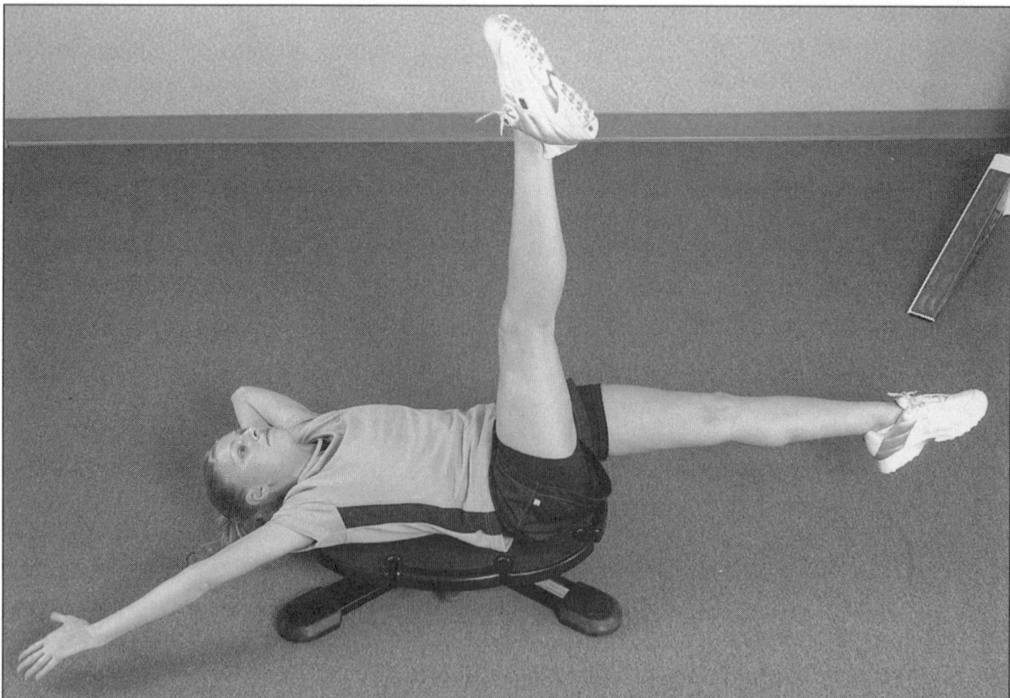

b

Figure 7.11 Straight leg raise: *(a)* raise both legs; *(b)* lower the left leg and reach back with the right arm.

Core Sequences

Core sequences represent a chain of exercises linked together in a continuous flow. Both tai chi and yoga are exercise forms in which one exercise or movement links to another. The most common form demonstrated in yoga is the sun salutation, which is simply a series of movements that require mobility and stability of the arms, legs, and spine in various functional movement patterns linked together in sequence. This is the next level of movement training. The sequence is simply the progression exercises modified and linked together in a continuous flow. The flow from one movement to another is important to motor learning. While going through a sequence, such as in tai chi or yoga, first focus on the sequence, committing it to memory, then learn to relax and focus on breathing instead of the sequence. The sequence happens automatically. The body becomes more efficient as the focus shifts from the sequence to breathing, balance, and posture as the body moves from one position to the next.

To the typical American athlete, this sequence of exercises may seem a little goofy or foreign compared to the way training has been done in the past. It's OK to think that way, but remember—most champions and elite athletes create their own stretching and exercise rituals, sometimes based on nothing more than superstition. The routines provided are based on the movement patterns that presented you with the greatest amount of difficulty.

Sometimes the ritual is actually more important than the routine because going through a familiar activity, regardless of what the activity is, sometimes has a calming effect before training and competition. This promotes focus and relaxation and helps the athlete avoid overthinking, which can sometimes distract from athletic tasks. The more ritualistic you make a routine, the more automatic it will become. Do not look at the sequence as something to master; think of it as a systems check for your most limited or difficult movement pattern.

The sequences that follow are based on the squat, hurdle step, and lunge. Perform the sequence that represents the most difficult pattern. Those who scored well on the squat, hurdle step, and lunge can create a routine of five to seven exercises based on the core exercises covered earlier. Pick five to seven movements that flow nicely so that you do not spend a lot of time changing body position, and choose exercises that move the body in different directions. A better way would be to choose the sequence that most closely represents the activities being prepared for.

SQUAT SEQUENCE

The squat sequence would most benefit swimmers, rock climbers, volleyball players, Olympic-style weightlifters, golfers, athletes in paddle sports or rowing, football linemen, snowboarders, skiers, and baseball catchers. If you don't have a core board, stand on the floor and use a step or box in place of the core board.

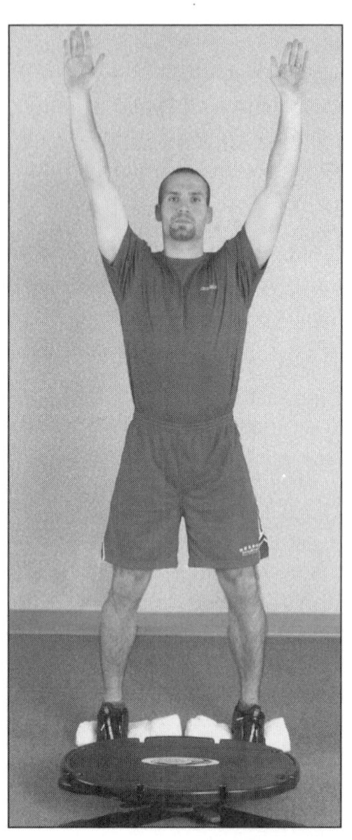
a

Stand with feet slightly more than shoulder-width apart about a foot in front of a core board. If needed, place rolled towels under your heels. Reach to the ceiling, trying to make the body as tall as possible while pulling in the abdominals (a).

Bend forward. Place the hands on the edge of the core board, keeping the knees as straight as possible without hyperextending. Let the spine comfortably round and press on the core board hard enough to make it tilt in your direction (b). This is the forward bend position.

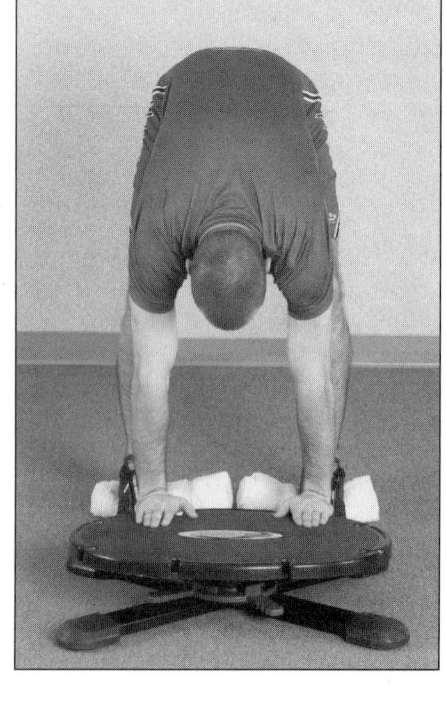
b

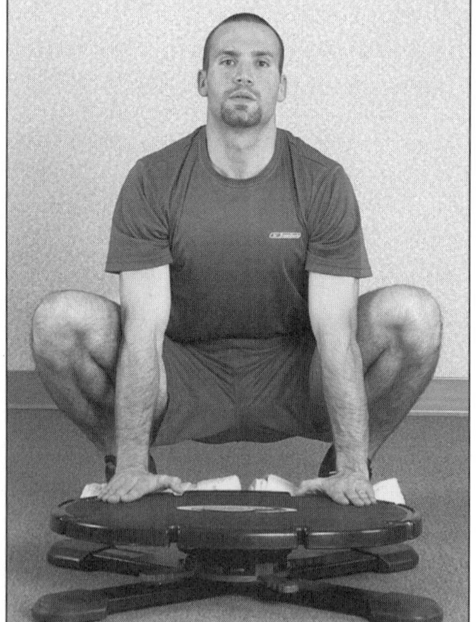
c

While maintaining consistent pressure (enough to keep the board tilted forward), go into as deep a squat as possible, splitting the knees wide enough so that they do not touch the elbows (c). Make the spine as tall as possible while keeping the feet flat and the weight on the heels. Keep the board tilted forward the entire time.

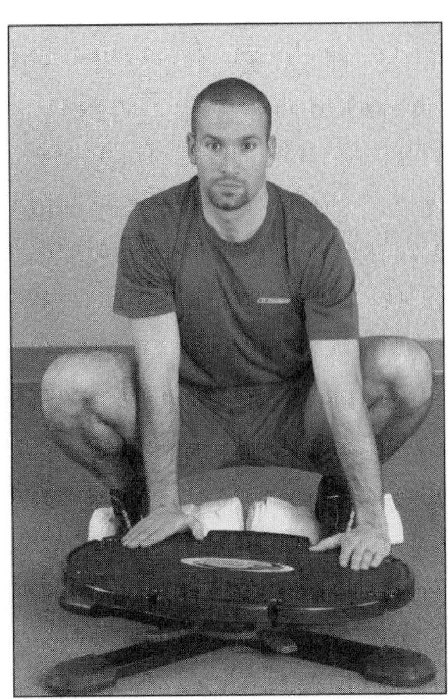

d

Move the hands to the outer edges of the board. Twist and rotate the board by pressing down and turning it to the left (d). Keep your weight on the heels. Press into the board by using the abdominals, not by shifting body weight forward.

Lift the right hand back and up, looking over the shoulder and rotating the shoulders as far as possible without losing the twist (e). Return the hand to the board.

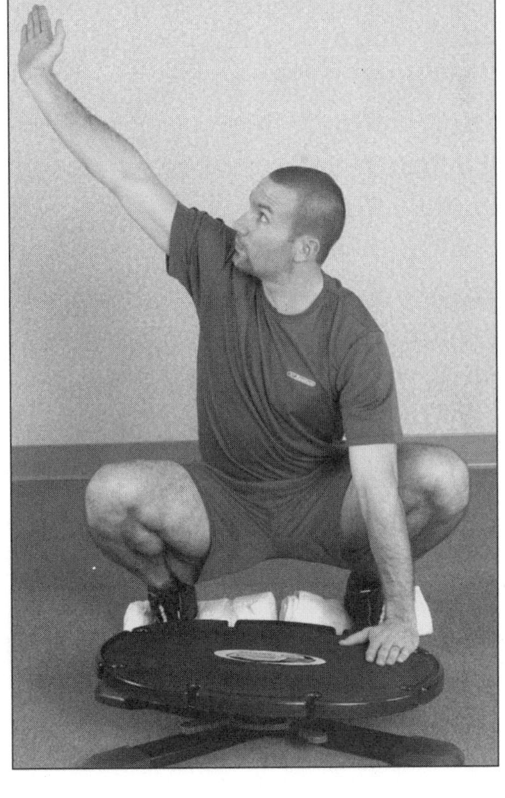

e

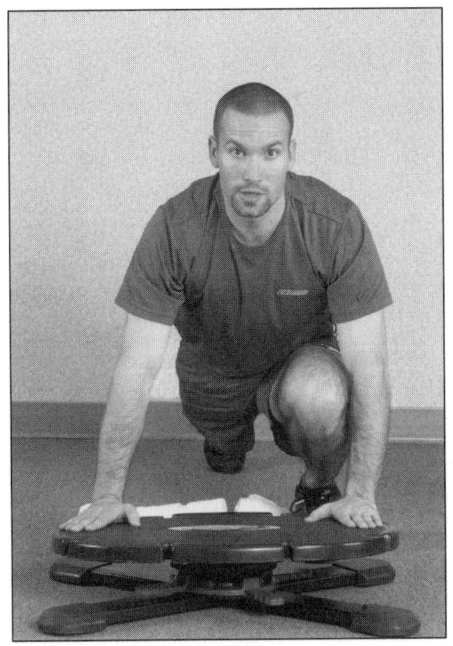

f

Step into a stride position by extending the right leg, keeping the spine extended, looking forward, and bending as deeply as possible through the left knee and ankle (f).

Move the left foot beside the right foot, extending the entire body into a push-up position (g).

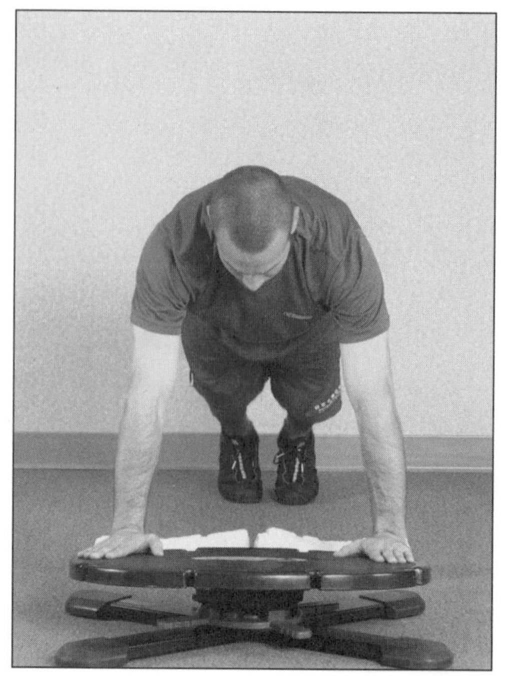

g

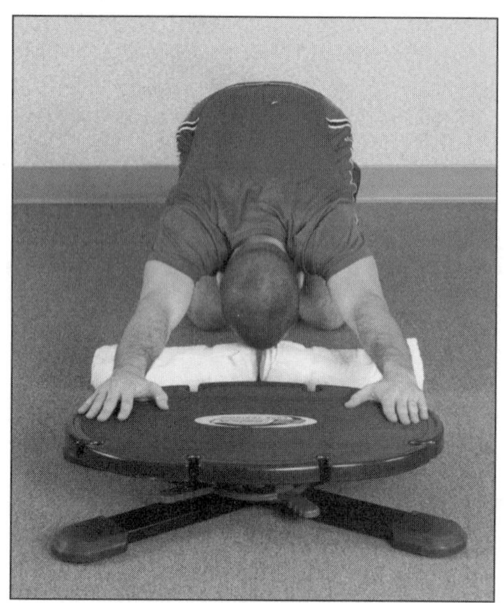

h

Hold the push-up a few seconds and then slowly bend the knees to the floor. Now the weight should be on your hands and knees. Rock back, placing the buttocks on the heels, chest toward thighs, allowing the arms to stretch (h). Remain on the core board. If needed, place a pillow or cushion between the heels and buttocks for comfort.

Twist or rotate the board as far as possible without changing body position by pushing with the right forearm and pulling with the left forearm (i). Maintain a solid and stable core.

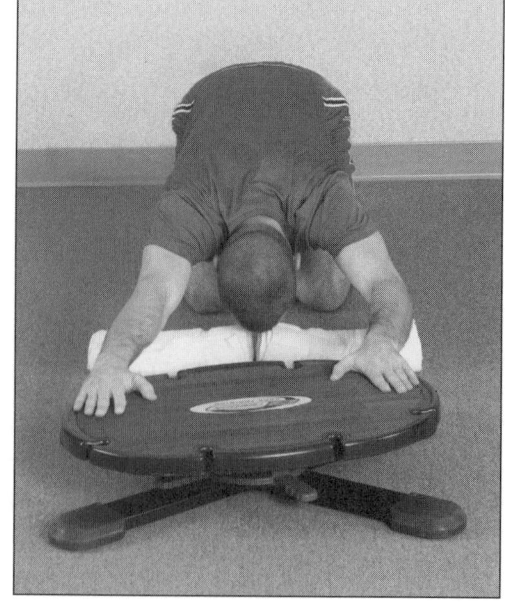

i

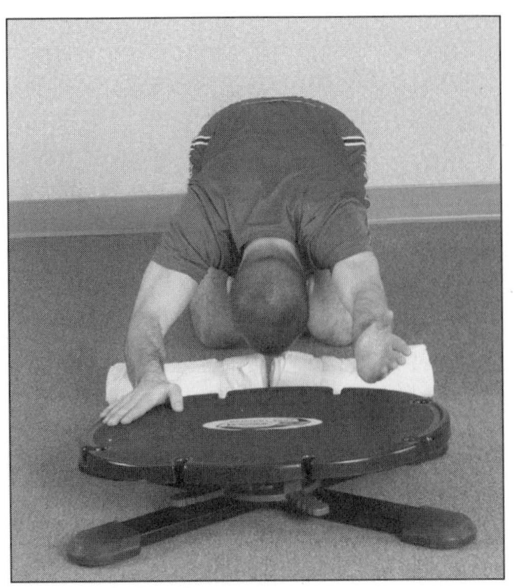
i

Roll the palm of the left arm toward the ceiling while maintaining the twist of the board with the arm (j). Repeat on the other side, then return to the push-up position. Return to the stride position by bringing the right leg forward and then the left leg forward. Now you are in squat position.

Remove the hands from the board and reach overhead as high as possible while keeping the weight on the heels and maintaining a tall spine (k). Return to the standing position (l) and relax the arms.

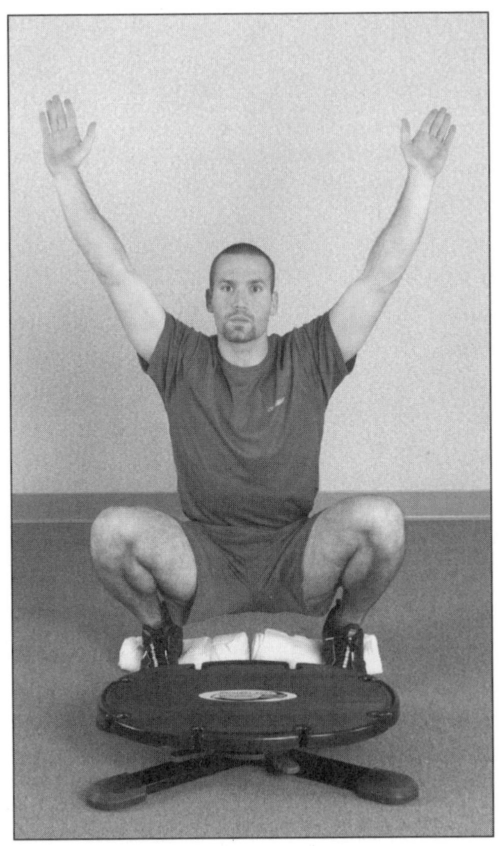
k

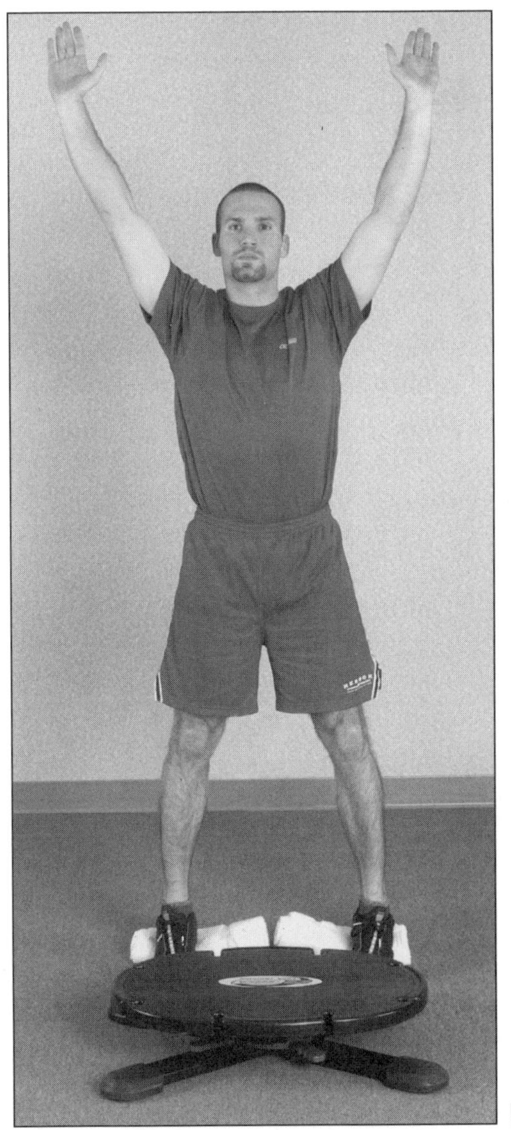
l

HURDLE STEP SEQUENCE

The hurdle step sequence would most benefit running athletes of any distance, cyclists, climbers, martial artists, and jumping athletes. It can be used as a warm-up to running work or plyometrics. This sequence is also beneficial for balance. It will improve weight shifting and weight-transfer ability. If you don't have a core board, stand on the floor.

Stand on a core board, feet side by side and centered, arms at sides (a). Flex the left hip and knee to an angle greater than 90 degrees (b).

With the right arm, pull the left knee and hip across the body (c). Keep the right leg slightly flexed at the knee. Do not rotate the shoulders. Maintain a tall and upright spine. Pull until you feel a stretch through the posterior hip of the left leg. Do not rotate the body. Relax the hip and bring it across the front of the body.

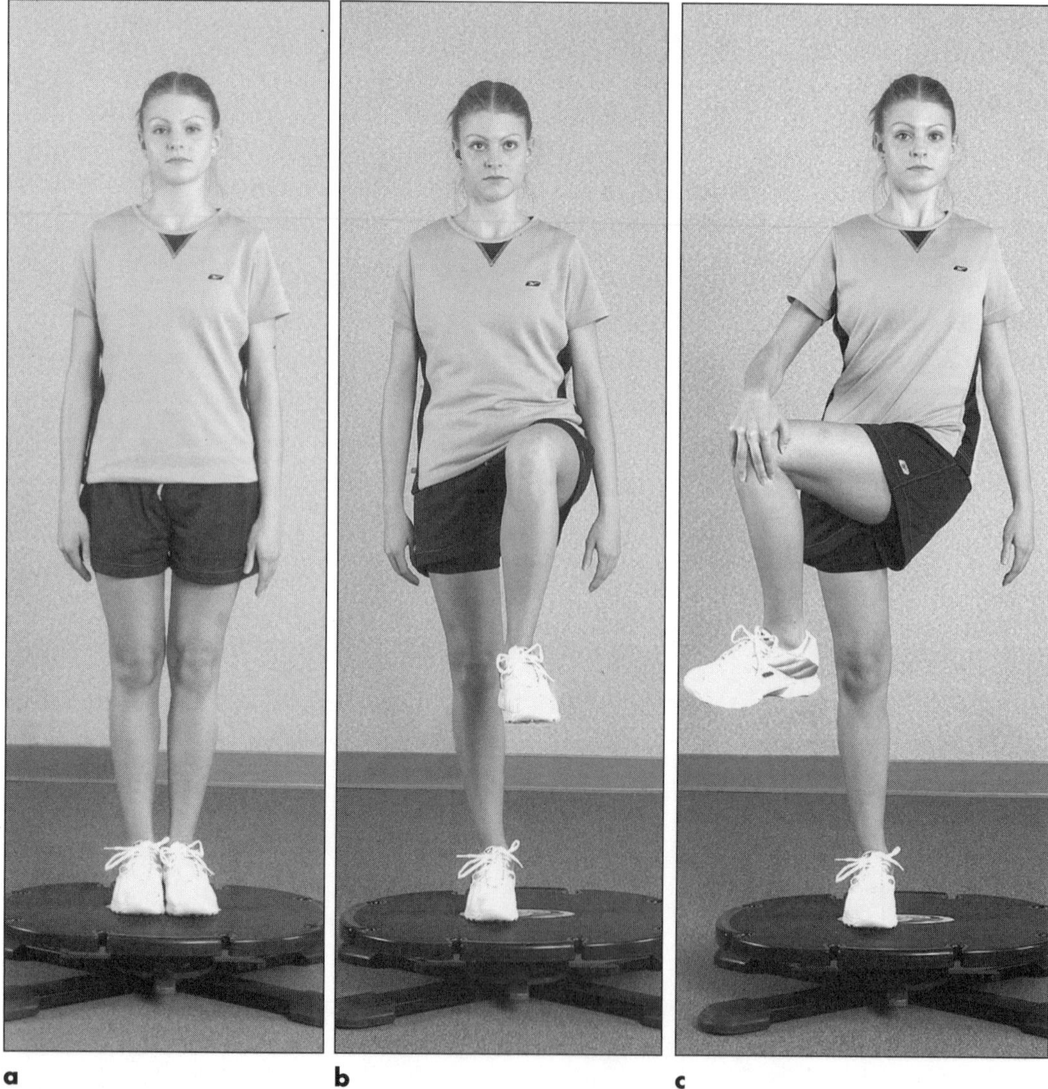

a b c

With the left arm, pull the leg outward (d). Keeping the hip flexed more than 90 degrees, open the hip without rotating the body. Maintain a tall and upright spine. Keep the right leg and knee slightly flexed. Do not rotate the shoulders. Return to the forward hip-flexed position. Perform the same moves on the right hip (e). First cross the hip in front of the body, then open the hip outward.

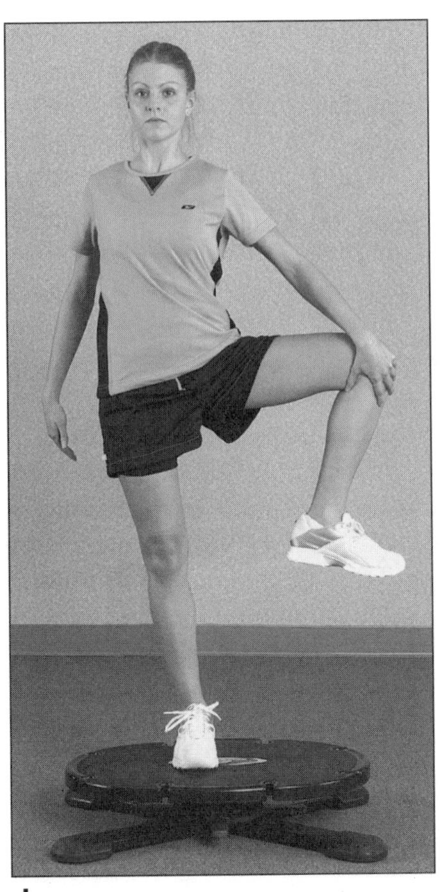
d

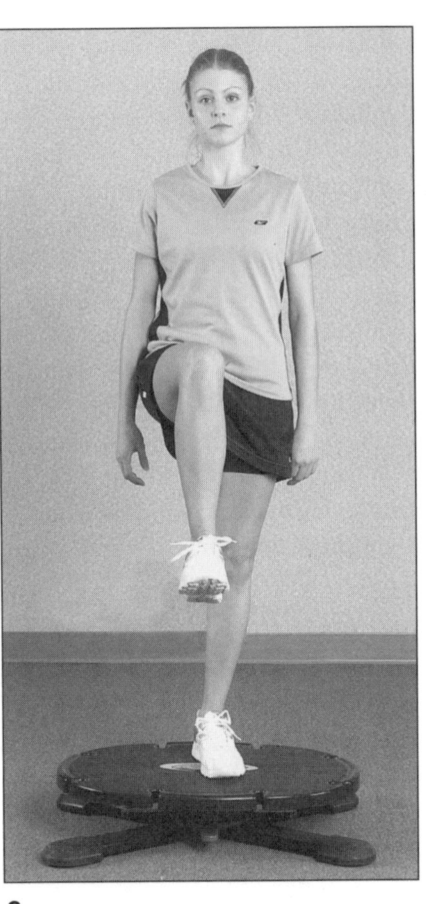
e

If you are on the core board, step back onto the floor one foot behind the core board. Extend the left leg and bend toward the board (f). All your weight should be on the right foot. The heel, knee, hip, spine, and shoulders should be in a straight line.

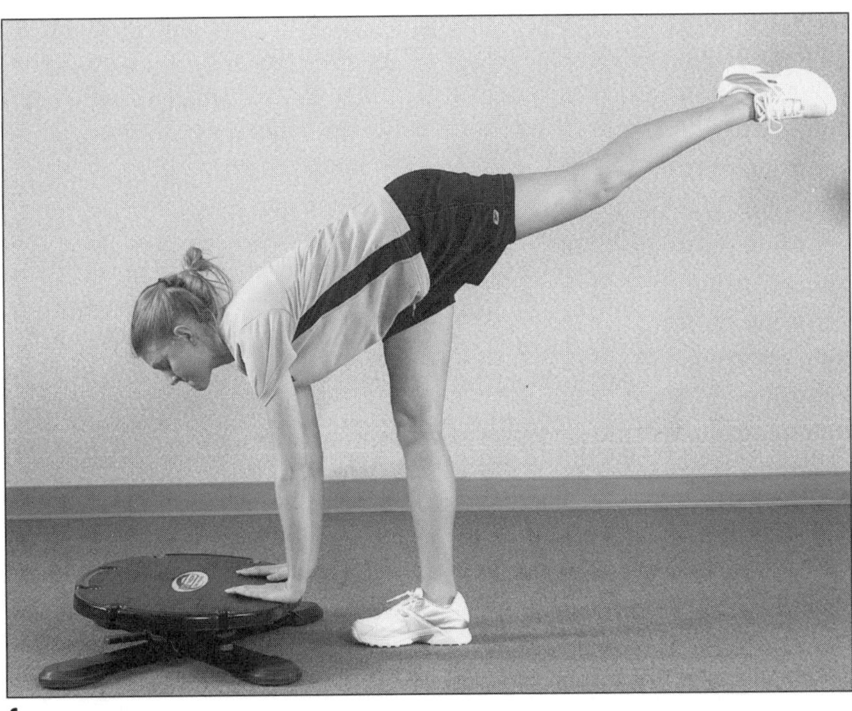
f

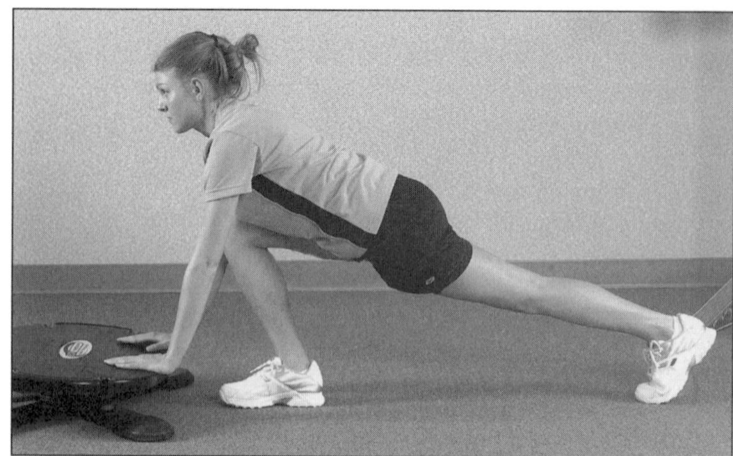

g

Place the hands on the near side of the board or step. Press into the board while elongating the left leg and maintaining a flat spine. Lower into a stride position with the right leg forward and left leg back (g). Move into a push-up position by taking the right leg back (h).

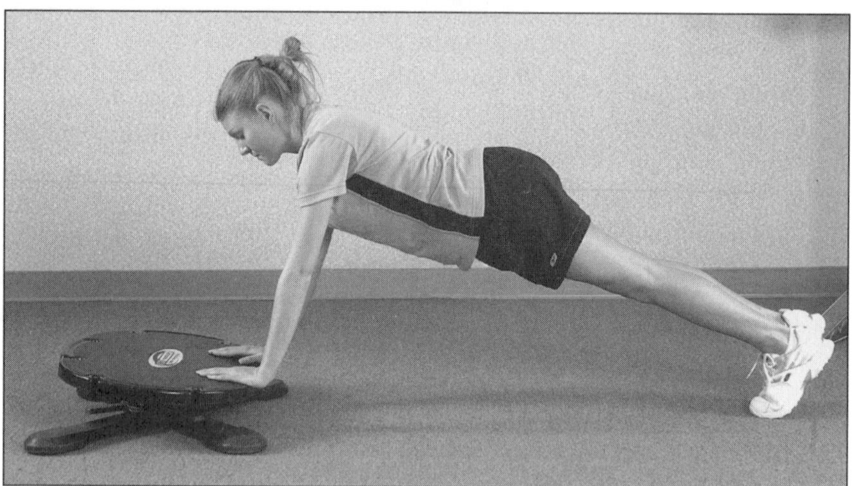

h

From the push-up position extend the spine, allowing the hips to sway toward the floor, but do not allow hips to touch the floor (i). Hold the sway position a few seconds. Return to the push-up position.

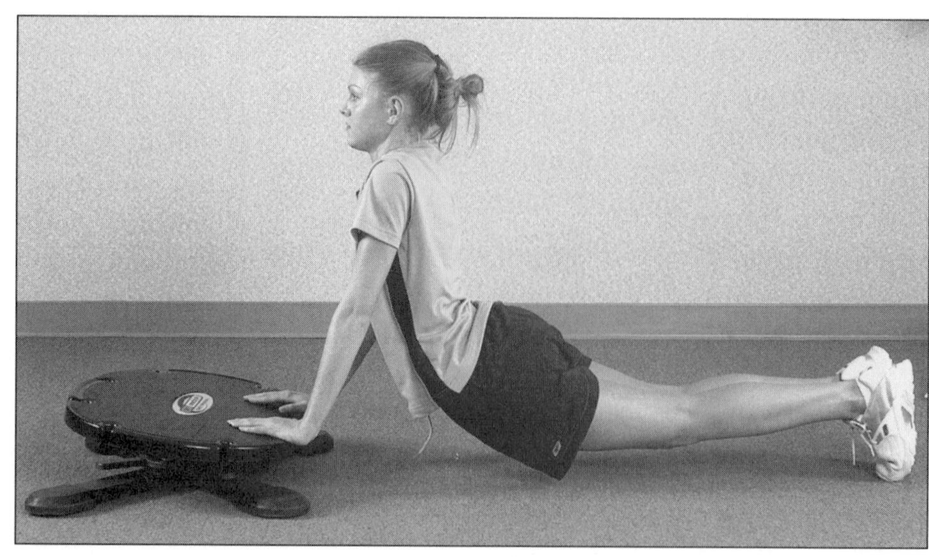

i

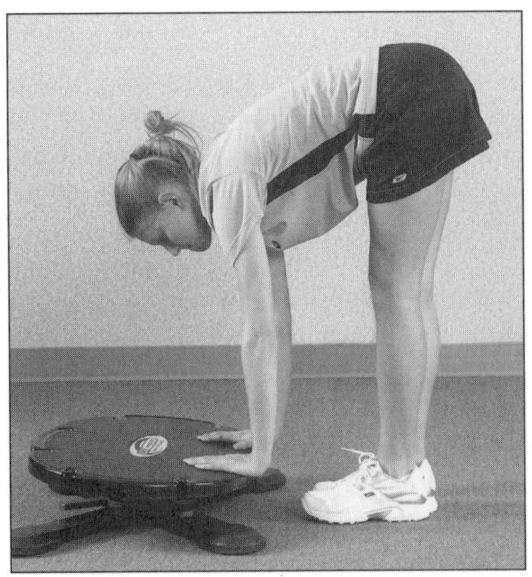

i

Walk the feet forward until you feel a slight stretch in the legs but the heels can maintain contact with the floor, feet slightly wider than shoulder-width apart (j). Maintain pressure on the board to ensure a tilt, which engages the abdominals. Return to the push-up position.

Step forward to a stride position with the left leg forward and the right leg backward (k).

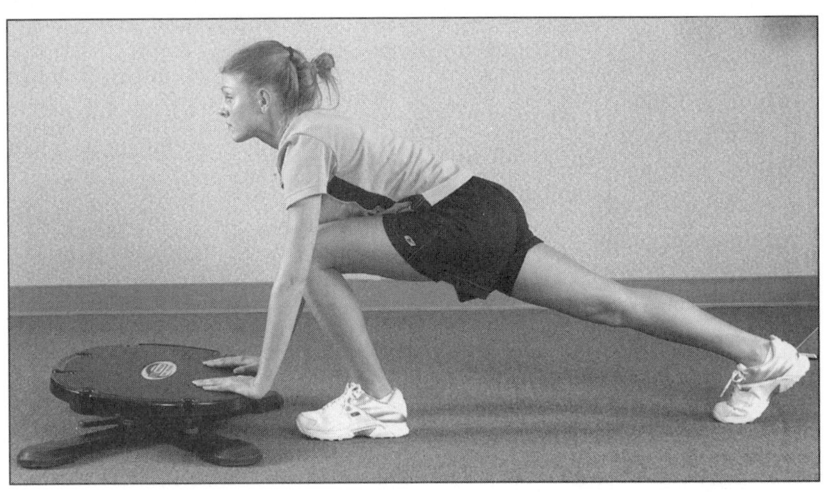

k

Return to the push-up position, but keep the right leg extended at the knee and the hip and point the toes (l). Do not sway or extend the lower back. Flex the knee as much as possible while maintaining maximal hip extension. Maintain a tall spine. Return to the push-up position and repeat on the left side.

Move into a forward bend position, maintaining pressure on the board. Stand up straight. Heel, knee, hip, spine, and shoulders should be in a straight line. Relax the arms.

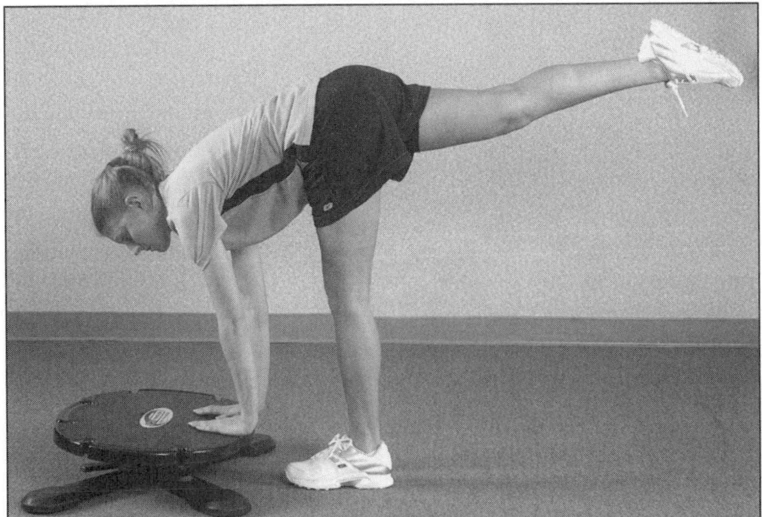

l

LUNGE SEQUENCE

The lunge sequence would most benefit field and court athletes and hockey players who need quick direction changes and acceleration or deceleration. It may also be used to prepare for speed and agility work. If you don't have a core board, you can work from the floor.

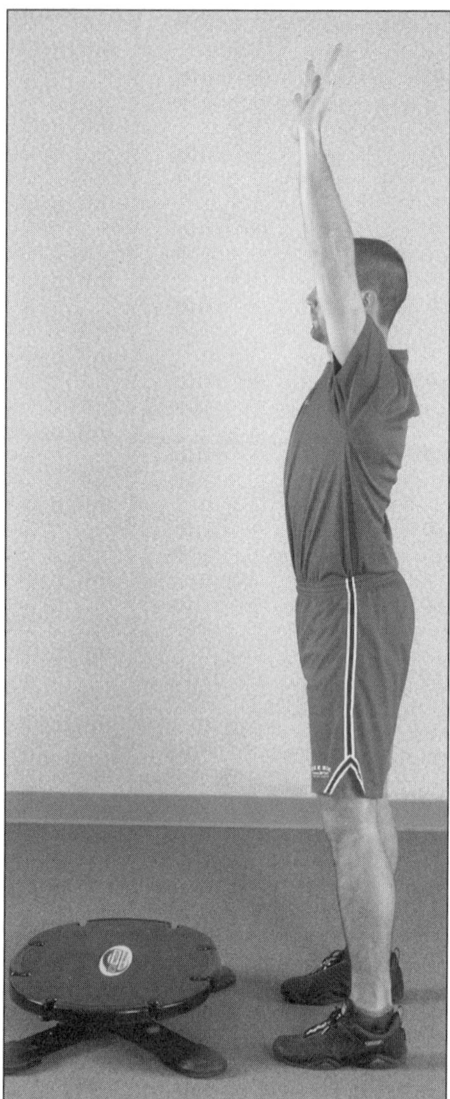

a

Stand in front of a core board, hands reaching up to the ceiling (a). You can place towel rolls under the heels to help with the squat if you need to. Squat with feet slightly wider than shoulder-width apart, approximately six inches away from the core board. Make the body as tall as possible while pulling in the abdominals.

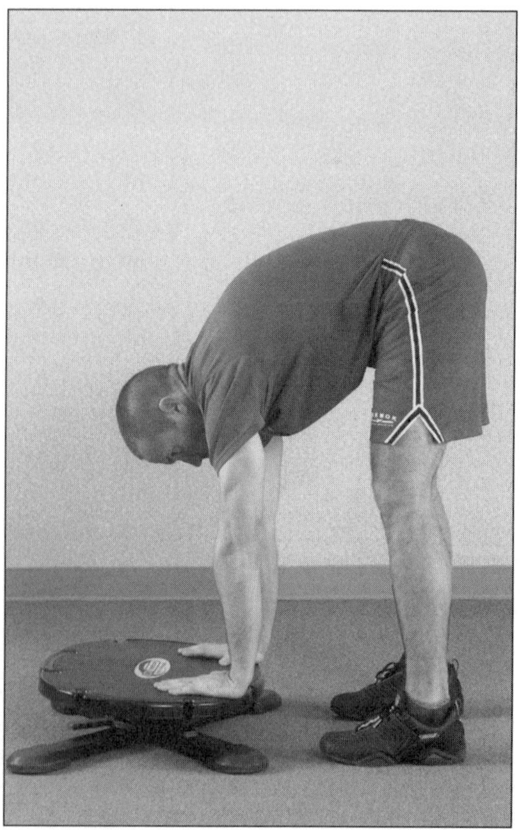

b

Bend forward. Place the hands on the edge of the core board, keeping the knees as straight as possible without hyperextending (b). Let the spine comfortably round and press on the core board hard enough to make it tilt in your direction. Keep abdominals pulled in.

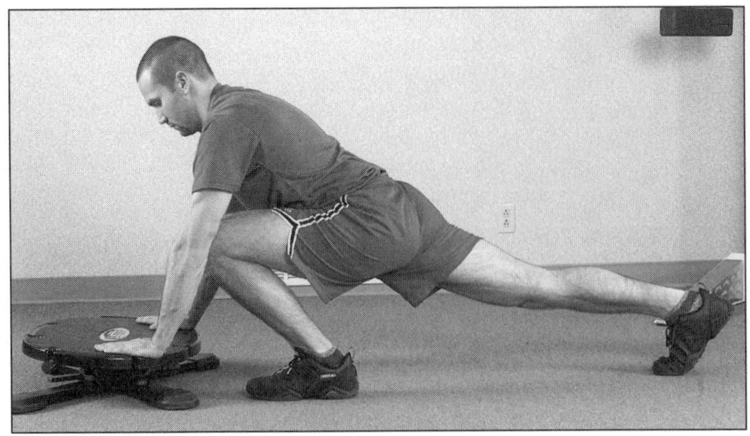

Move into a stride position by extending the right leg, keeping the spine extended, looking forward and bending as deeply as possible through the left knee and ankle (c). The left heel should maintain contact with the floor.

c

Pull with the left arm and push with the right arm to press and turn the board while maintaining the stride position. Maintain pressure with the right arm. Lift the left arm, rotate the spine, and turn the head (d). Hold the hand toward the ceiling with the arm fully extended and palm up. Do not rotate through the hips. Maintain a stable position on the flexed left knee. Return to the stride position.

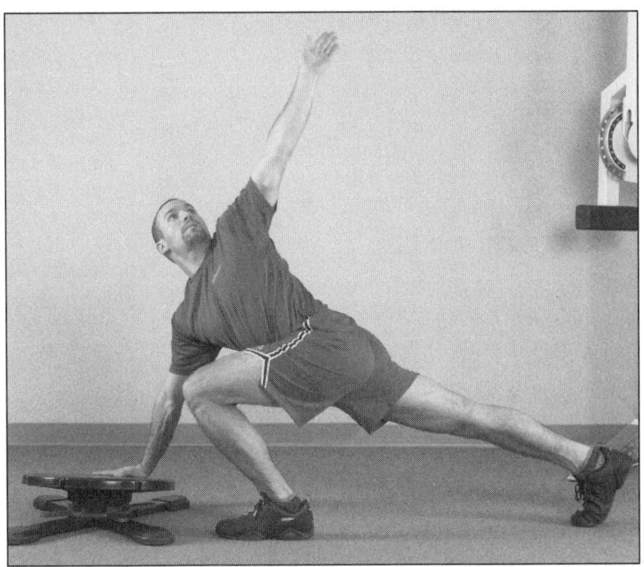

d

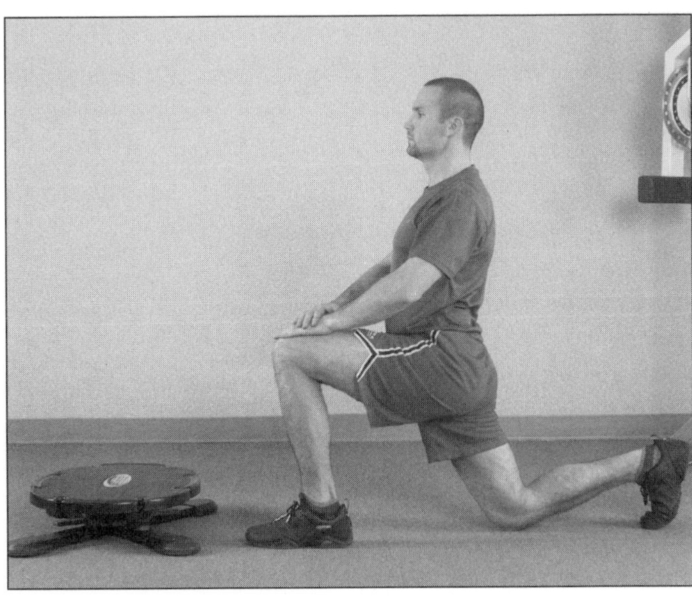

Place the hands on the left knee while bringing the spine upright (e). This is the hip flexor stretch position. Balance with the feet in line, bending the knee and extending the hip. Keep the abdominals pulled in and the trunk erect. Do not hyperextend the spine.

e

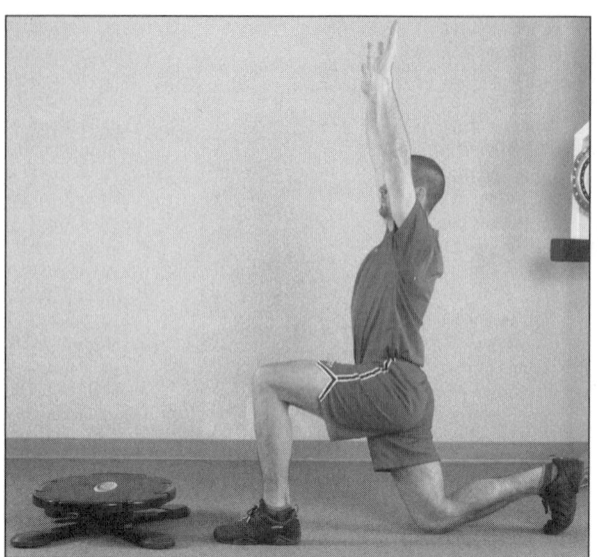
f

Press arms overhead while maintaining an elongated spine (f). Do not hyper-extend the spine.

Rotate the torso toward the flexed knee and hip without any movement in the lower body (g). Keep the knee flexed and the hip stable. Twist the torso as far as possible, turning the head, reaching upward, and maintaining an elongated spine.

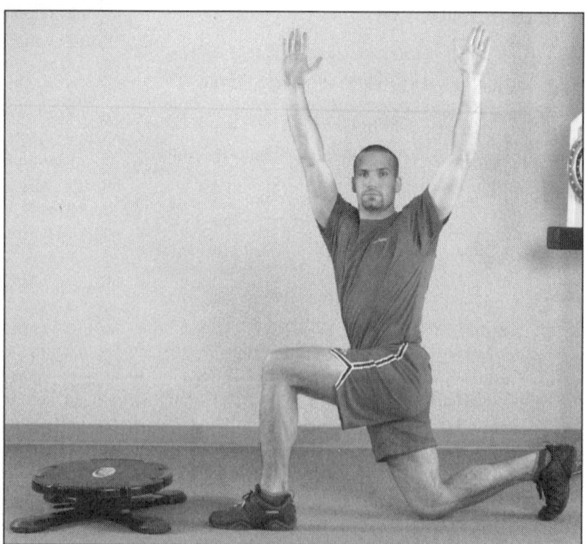
g

Return to the hip flexor stretch position. Balance with the feet in line, bending the knee and extending the hip. Keep the abdominals pulled in and the trunk erect. Do not hyperextend the spine. Return to the stride position.

Step forward into a forward bend. Bring one leg forward and then the other until you are in a forward bend position. Keep the hands on the edge of the core board with knees as straight as possible but without hyperextension. Let the spine comfortably round and press on the core board hard enough to make it tilt in your direction.

While maintaining enough pressure to keep the board tilted forward, go into as deep a squat as possible, splitting the knees wide enough so that they do not touch the elbows. Make the spine as tall as possible while keeping the feet flat and weight on the heels. Keep the board tilted forward.

Remove the hands from the board and reach overhead as high as possible without changing weight on heels. Maintain a tall spine. Return to the standing position with the arms reaching toward the ceiling. Relax the arms.

PART III

STRENGTH AND ENDURANCE

8

Strength and Endurance Testing

In her book *Diagnosis and Treatment of Movement Impairment Syndromes,* Dr. Shirley Sahrmann warns against treating muscle weakness as a lack of strength without first considering movement patterns. She writes, "There are numerous ways in which slight subtleties in movement patterns contribute to specific muscle weaknesses. The relationship between altered movement patterns and specific muscle weaknesses requires that remediation addresses the changes to the movement pattern; the performance of strengthening exercises alone will not likely affect the timing and manner of recruitment during functional performance."

I placed movement pattern testing and corrective exercises before strength and endurance testing and exercises for the same reason. Many strength and endurance problems can be greatly improved by first correcting basic movement patterns. You have likely already initiated corrective exercises for your specific movement pattern problems. It is human nature to want to skip ahead and start the good stuff and train with weight. However, strength and endurance gains will be far greater if you first refine movement patterns. Training for strength and endurance before correcting faulty movement patterns will only reinforce the compensations that have developed. If you have adequately addressed your faulty movement patterns, then you are ready to perform strength and endurance tests. These tests will now more accurately identify strength and endurance problems because altered movement patterns have been removed from the equation.

Mobility and stability lay the foundation for effective training and conditioning, and strength and endurance are the first two cornerstones. Strength and endurance training build a larger reserve of energy. This larger reserve will not automatically create a better athlete, but it will help the athlete practice and perform for longer periods of time, providing more opportunities for the body to learn motor patterns. It is hard for the body to learn skillful movement when fatigued.

Defining Strength and Endurance

Strength and endurance should be thought of as work. Force times distance equals work, and the goal at this level is to produce the greatest amount of work with the least amount of effort. I don't mean "produce the greatest amount of work in the least amount of time." That would be power, which we will get to later. Just as mobility and stability should precede strength and endurance, strength and endurance should precede power, speed, and agility.

Strength is the ability to perform work. It is usually thought of as work intensity and volume over a short period of time. Effective resistance training can produce *hypertrophy*, or muscle growth. Muscle growth is not simply an increase in muscle tissue; the larger muscle is better hydrated and can store more glycogen, which is fuel for muscles. There is also greater circulation throughout the muscle. With strength training, capillaries grow and expand throughout the muscle to maintain adequate blood flow during work and recovery.

Endurance is the ability to perform work for a long period of time. Endurance is usually thought of as work intensity and volume over a long period of time. Endurance training does not usually produce muscle hypertrophy, but it is extremely effective from a cardiovascular standpoint.

Many people think that endurance training simply requires performing an aerobic activity, such as jogging, riding a bike, or swimming, for a long period of time. Actually, interval training—short bouts of exercise followed by short bouts of rest—is the best way to increase endurance. Interval training increases tolerance to fatigue and improves the ability to recover.

Most team sports are anaerobic in nature, not aerobic, meaning they consist of short bursts of activity followed by periods of lesser activity. While weight and endurance training may help with sport-specific performance, the true purpose of strength and endurance training is to provide volume and intensity, or the capacity to train and play at higher intensities for longer periods of time.

Increased muscular strength and cardiovascular endurance allow more opportunities to hone sport-specific skills and tolerate more sport-specific training. They also allow one to recover more quickly because both depend heavily on proper circulation and improved cellular efficiency (or improved metabolism).

Maximum Strength Assessment

Effective testing for strength and endurance will set baselines so progress can be monitored. Even athletes who have scored high on strength and endurance tests but who have taken time off should retest when they decide to return to training. It would be a mistake to return to the same level as before the hiatus was taken without reestablishing baseline scores.

The tests in this chapter have been chosen specifically for their simplicity and effectiveness. It is a good idea for a coach or trainer experienced in testing protocol and safety to guide and monitor the tests. The coach or trainer may also be able to provide feedback regarding weak links and give overall appraisals of strengths and weaknesses.

These tests provide feedback in specific categories of performance. They represent only a small sampling of a large group of tests used to chart performance, but they are enough to provide a basic picture of performance, strengths, and weaknesses. The tests show a general rank against other individuals. Many high schools and colleges keep records on performance for these simple tests and group scores by sex, age, and sport. Researchers have also compiled databases for the same information. The charts included in this chapter will allow you to compare scores to others in similar circumstances. If your sport or group isn't included, use a comparison that is most representative of your group.

Many other factors come into play in assessing total athletic performance, but you need an idea of your basic strength and endurance. The strength and endurance represented by these simple tests does not totally represent the strength and endurance used during competition. Skill, competitive spirit, experience, emotional state, and many other factors come into play during competition. Simply use this information as a guide and remember that whether your scores are favorable, average, or poor, the map is not the territory. A map is just a representation of a particular terrain. Your test scores are only a guide for you to follow and consider.

The tests in the maximum strength assessment need not be done in any particular order. You should use a standard simple warm-up to ready your body for the test and have help from one or more people (depending on the particular test you are performing). The following tests are included in the maximum strength assessment:

1. One-repetition maximum bench press
2. One-repetition maximum squat
3. Local muscle endurance
4. Aerobic capacity

These tests were chosen because they are generally well accepted, are familiar to most athletes and coaches, are easily reproduced with standardized equipment, and include normative data you can use to compare yourself to other people of your age, sex, and sport. If one test stands out as representative of poor performance, consider this area of fitness your weakest link.

The recommendations in the next two chapters will help you build both strength and endurance. As you focus on these exercises and movement patterns, periodically retest, especially those tests where performance was average or poor. Exercises will be extremely functional, focusing on body balance and the fundamentals of strength and endurance. There should be significant carryover between the exercises that you do and improvement in the four basic tests provided in this chapter.

ONE-REPETITION MAXIMUM BENCH PRESS

The one-repetition (1RM) maximum bench press tests for upper-body strength. This test was chosen because the data available will help you rank yourself with others in your same age, sex, and sport category (see table 8.1).

You will need an Olympic-style weightlifting set with enough weight to test your maximum ability. It is best to have plates in a variety of sizes to allow for as little as a five-pound gradation in weight. You will need a standard bench with a bar rack of adjustable height and a spotter.

For the bench press, lie on your back on the bench, eyes directly below the bar. Grip the bar with palms facing away from you, hands shoulder-width apart. The entire spine, including the head, should be supported by the bench. Feet should be flat on the floor with knees bent at 90 degrees. The elbows should be fully extended. Have the spotter help you lift the bar off the rack. Bring the bar down to the chest (figure 8.1a). Wrists should be rigid and in direct line with the elbows. Continue to maintain a flat spine and keep feet flat on the floor. The body should not move, just the arms. The spotter should stay close to the bar but not touch it. Let

Table 8.1 One-Repetition Maximum Data* for Bench Press

Type of athlete	One-repetition maximum (lb)	One-repetition maximum (kg)
NCAA Division I college football players:		
Offensive linemen	385	175
Defensive linemen	377	171
Linebackers	358	163
Offensive backs	335	152
Tight ends	333	151
Defensive backs	307	140
Wide receivers	280	127
Quarterbacks	277	126
College baseball players (men)	233	106
College basketball players (men)	225	102
College basketball players (men)	207	94
College track athletes (women)	103	47
College basketball players (women)	113	51
NCAA Division II college basketball players (women):		
Guards	95	43
Forwards	105	48
Centers	105	48

* Data are either means or 50th percentiles (medians). The two sets of data for men's and women's basketball come from multiple samples.

Adapted from T.R. Baechle and R.W. Earle, *Essentials of Strength Training and Conditioning (2nd ed.)*, 2000, Human Kinetics, page 309.

the bar touch the chest at the bottom of the movement before pushing it up again (figure 8.1b). As the bar is pressed up and the elbows fully extend, there should be no body movement or change in body position. Let the spotter help return the weight to the rack.

To warm up for the 1RM attempt, perform a light set of bench presses, 5 to 10 repetitions, followed by 2 heavier sets of 2 to 3 repetitions. After the warm-up, rest for 2 to 4 minutes. Because the 2 heavy warm-up sets should have been near maximum load, allowing 2 to 3 repetitions, you should have a good idea of what maximum load should be. If you are successful with your first estimate, take another 2- to 4-minute rest break, increase the load by 10 to 20 pounds, and attempt the 1RM again. Repeat until you find your 1RM. Ideally, you will achieve your one-repetition maximum within 5 testing sets.

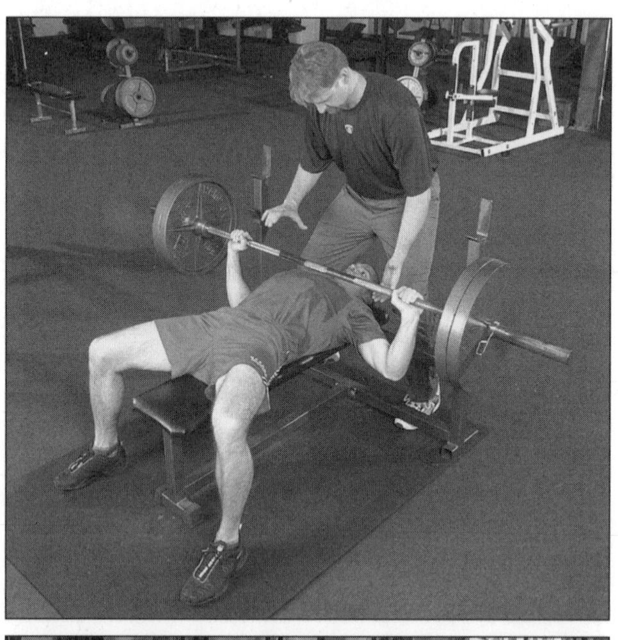

a

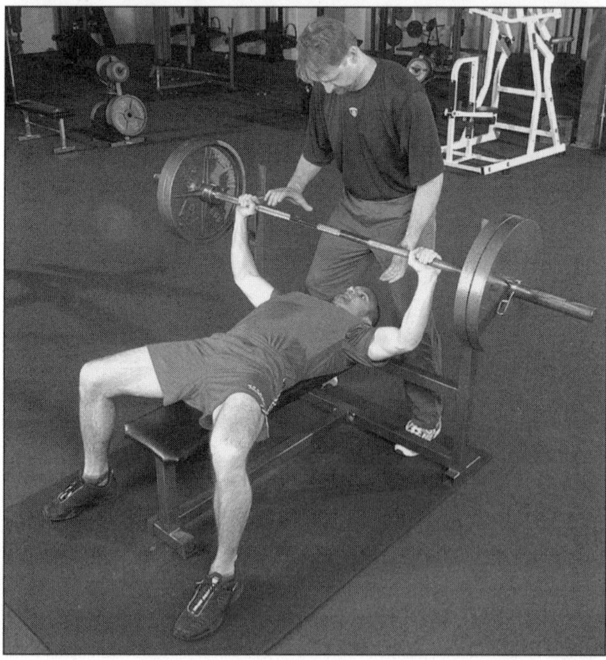

b

Figure 8.1 One-repetition maximum bench press: *(a)* bring the bar to your chest; *(b)* push the bar up.

ONE-REPETITION MAXIMUM SQUAT

The one-repetition maximum squat tests for lower-body and core strength. Use table 8.2 to compare your score to other athletes. You need an Olympic-style weightlifting set and a squat rack. This test should not be performed without spotters, and it is best that you have two. There should be enough weight to accommodate a 1RM lift. Wear appropriate footwear and stand on a flat, solid surface.

With the bar adjusted to your height in the squat rack and spotters on the outside of the rack at the bar ends, grip the bar with palms facing away from you, hands wider than shoulder-width apart. You can use a low or high position. In the low position, the bar rests across the posterior deltoid; in the high position, it rests above the posterior deltoid. If this is uncomfortable, add a towel roll or pad. The bar should not rest on the lower neck. Lift the elbows as high as possible and point them behind you to create an adequate shelf for the back squat. Stand erect and look forward. Tilt the head up slightly. Signal the spotters to lift the bar off the supports. Take two steps back and position the feet shoulder-width apart or wider, slightly

Table 8.2 One-Repetition Maximum Data* for Squat

Type of athlete	One-repetition maximum (lb)	One-repetition maximum (kg)
NCAA Division I college football players:		
Offensive linemen	531	241
Defensive linemen	502	228
Linebackers	476	216
Offensive backs	471	214
Tight ends	464	211
Defensive backs	415	189
Wide receivers	390	177
Quarterbacks	379	172
College baseball players (men)	308	140
College basketball players (men)	302	137
College basketball players (men)	233	106
College track athletes (women)	150	68
College basketball players (women)	182	83
NCAA Division II college basketball players (women):		
Guards	165	75
Forwards	185	84
Centers	220	100

* Data are either means or 50th percentiles (medians). The two sets of data for men's and women's basketball come from multiple samples.

Adapted from T.R. Baechle and R.W. Earle, *Essentials of Strength Training and Conditioning (2nd ed.)*, 2000, Human Kinetics, page 309.

turned out (figure 8.2a). Lower to the down position, maintaining a flat back with the elbows high, chest up and out, looking forward (figure 8.2b). Do not let the heels come up. Do not round the back. Continue flexing the hips and knees in the downward position until thighs are parallel to the floor. Spotters can help if this position causes problems. Once you have achieved the proper depth in the squat, extend hips and knees and maintain the flat back and high elbow position. Once standing, step forward and use assistance from the spotters to reset the weight into the rack.

To warm up for the 1RM attempt, perform a light set of squats, 5 to 10 repetitions, followed by 2 heavier sets of 2 to 3 repetitions. After the warm-up, rest for 2 to 4 minutes. Because the 2 heavy warm-up sets should have been near maximum load, allowing 2 to 3 repetitions, you should have a good idea of what maximum load should be. If you are successful with your first estimate, take another 2- to 4-minute rest break, increase the load by 30 to 40 pounds, and attempt the 1RM again. Repeat until you find your 1RM. Ideally, you will achieve your one-repetition maximum within 5 testing sets.

a

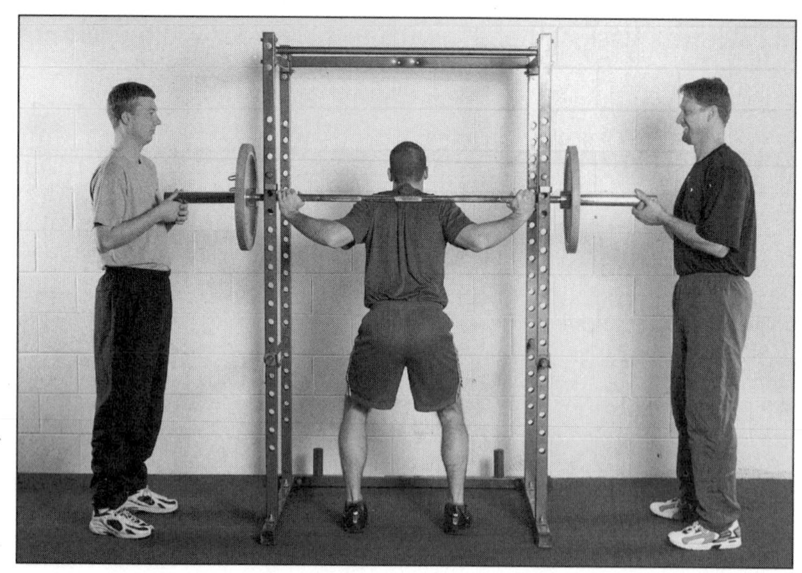

b

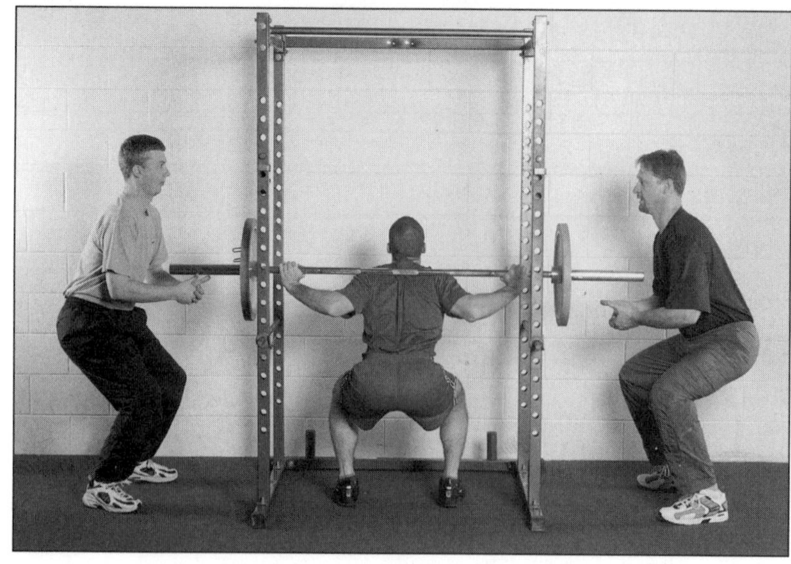

Figure 8.2 One-repetition maximum squat: *(a)* stand with feet shoulder-width apart; *(b)* descend into the squat.

LOCAL MUSCLE ENDURANCE

In this test, you will perform curl-ups for one minute. Use table 8.3 to compare yourself to others in your age group. If you have a testing partner, have your partner keep time with a standard stopwatch. If you are self-testing, use a large clock with a sweep secondhand. Place an exercise, gymnastic, or wrestling mat on the floor.

Lie on your back and flex your hips to 45 degrees and knees just slightly greater than 90 degrees, keeping feet flat on the floor. Arms should be crossed over the chest so that you can feel the outer edges of your collarbone with your hands (figure 8.3a). Flex the neck so that the chin moves toward the chest, and curl the torso toward the thighs until the upper back is off the mat. The feet, buttocks, and lower back should be flat and not move as you perform the curl-up (figure 8.3b). Arms should remain folded across the chest. On the downward movement, allow the torso to flatten back onto the mat.

Perform 4 or 5 practice repetitions of the curl-up before starting the test. When your partner with the stopwatch says "go" or when the secondhand on the clock passes 12, begin performing curl-ups. Continue to curl for exactly one minute, counting repetitions. Lower the back so that the entire upper back and shoulders touch the mat. The chin may remain in a tucked position and the arms should not move.

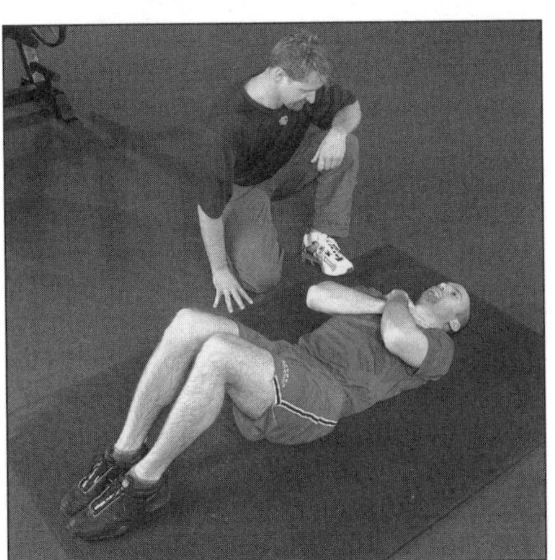

a

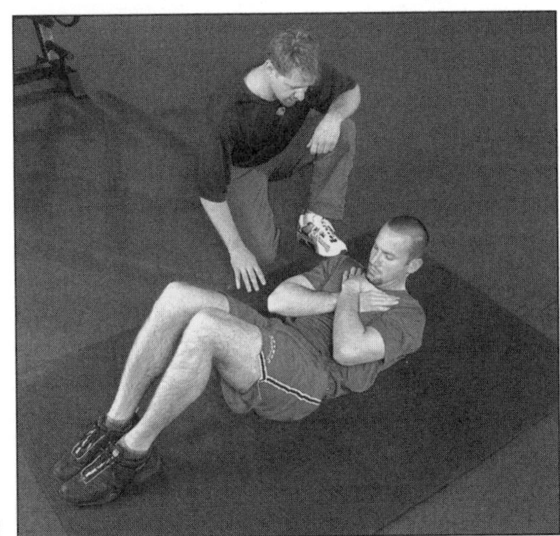

b

Figure 8.3 Local muscle endurance curl-up test: *(a)* lie on the floor with arms crossed over your chest; *(b)* lift the torso toward the thighs.

Table 8.3 Maximum Number of Sit-Ups in 1 Minute

	Ages 20 to 29		Ages 30 to 39	
Percentile	**Men**	**Women**	**Men**	**Women**
99	>55	>51	>51	>42
90	52	49	48	40
80	47	44	43	35
70	45	41	41	32
60	42	38	39	29
50	40	35	36	27
40	38	32	35	25
30	35	30	32	22
20	33	27	30	20
10	30	23	26	15
01	<27	<18	<23	<11

Adapted from E. Harman, J. Garhammer, and C. Pandorf, 2000, in *Essentials of training and conditioning (2nd ed.)*, Human Kinetics.

AEROBIC CAPACITY

The 1.5-mile run is used to test aerobic capacity. Use table 8.4 to compare yourself to others in your age group. You will need a stopwatch or a runner's watch with a digital stopwatch to keep time and a quarter-mile running track or marked, measured 1.5-mile flat course (preferably asphalt or some other good running surface).

Perform a normal warm-up and stretching routine before beginning the test. If you have a partner, start to run when your partner says "go" as he or she starts the stopwatch. Have your partner meet you at the finish area if it is different from the start line so that he or she can accurately record your time. If you are timing yourself with a runner's watch in stopwatch mode, make sure you securely start and stop the watch at the appropriate point. Record your time in both minutes and seconds.

Table 8.4 Times for 1.5-Mile Run

Percentile	Ages 20 to 29		Ages 30 to 39	
	Men	Women	Men	Women
99	<7:29	<8:33	<8:11	<10:05
90	9:09	11:43	9:30	12:51
80	10:16	12:51	10:47	13:43
70	10:47	13:53	11:34	14:24
60	11:41	14:24	12:20	15:08
50	12:18	14:55	12:51	15:26
40	12:51	15:26	13:36	15:57
30	13:22	15:57	14:08	16:35
20	14:13	16:33	14:52	17:14
10	15:10	17:21	15:52	18:00
01	>17:48	>19:25	>18:00	>19:27

All times are given as minutes:seconds.

Adapted from E. Harman, J. Garhammer, and C. Pandorf, 2000, in *Essentials of training and conditioning (2nd ed.)*, Human Kinetics.

9

Movement Imbalance Training

In an article published in *Sports Medicine* in 1992, Knapik and other researchers stated that no clear evidence existed to link tightness or weakness of a particular muscle group with injury, but that a significant amount of injuries were noted in athletes with right-left strength and flexibility imbalances (asymmetries). Through seven lower-body flexibility measurements, the authors showed that an athlete was 2.6 times more likely to suffer injuries if he had a hip extension flexibility imbalance of 15 percent or more.

Few researchers have troubled themselves to look at movement pattern problems and left-right imbalances. Most would rather look at the human body through a microscope, as though through looking at all the parts they can assume the whole. Unfortunately, this is not the way the human body works, moves, or lives. The whole is always greater than the sum of its parts.

You have learned about movement screening, strength testing, and endurance testing. Before going deeper into functional conditioning, take one last opportunity to train any movement imbalance that may remain.

Two proprioceptive neuromuscular facilitation (PNF) patterns are used in this chapter: the *chop* and the *lift*. These patterns combine opposing spiral and diagonal movements of the upper body. These movements are performed in varied lower-body positions to specifically address and identify imbalances in the core. Reducing imbalances in the core with fundamental spiral and diagonal patterns is the best possible foundation for strength and endurance training.

Detecting a muscle imbalance usually requires a thorough musculoskeletal evaluation, and correcting it requires specific exercises designed to rectify or remedy it. The many different ways imbalances can manifest themselves is quite complicated. For our purposes, it is much more appropriate to think of it as *movement imbalance training*.

Thus far, we have covered the many movement patterns of the body and learned how right-left discrepancies can expose performance problems and present a greater risk for injury. In short, we have learned that nothing should be trained that cannot be tested. Because movement can be tested at this level and muscle balance cannot, it makes sense to focus on movement.

Movement training is more functional because if a muscle imbalance is tested and trained and a movement problem is still present, the movement problem must still be trained. On the other hand, usually movement imbalance training also addresses muscle imbalances. Feel confident knowing that taking this approach to training should address 90 percent of underlying problems. Think of it as advanced core training. Until this point all training has been performed without resistance. The following exercises will introduce resistance training. Proficiency with these exercises will lay a functional foundation for the strength and endurance work in chapter 10.

The Chop and Lift

Many different movement patterns could be used here, but for the specific purpose of movement imbalance training I have chosen the chop and lift. The chop and lift is a fundamental movement pattern. Consider it a building block at the ground level of training.

The chop and lift is a dose of reality. Up to this point we have focused on evaluating weak links and problems before exercise or sport-specific training. In this chapter you will see how the exercise *is* the evaluation. Pay attention to what the body is saying and watch for subtle mistakes or greater difficulty when performing the pattern on one side of the body or the other. When these exercises are performed correctly, they are extremely taxing because they use so many different muscles to move through the pattern or to stabilize the body. But because they are so basic, it will be difficult to ignore imbalances. Remember that training is for weak links, not for practicing favorite activities. The chop and lift may feel awkward at first, but use it anyway. You will get used to it.

These movements are based on proprioceptive neuromuscular facilitation (PNF). The central premise of PNF is to allow the body to work in patterns of movement. These patterns are three-dimensional and are often described as diagonal and spiral in nature. The chop and lift is often thought of as an upper-body or trunk-only routine. However, varying foot and leg positions creates balance and weight-shifting reactions that may help identify and remedy movement imbalances in the lower body as well.

Often athletes who do these exercises for the first time say, "I don't feel the burn" or "I don't feel my abs working." This is because these athletes are used to isolation training. When an athlete in training isolates one area or body part for a long time, he starts to think that all training should feel like that, but this is not accurate. When a pitcher throws a baseball, a basketball guard drives in for a layup, a punter kicks a football, a hockey forward executes a slap shot, or a track star runs a 100-meter sprint, does he feel the burn in one body part? Does he feel the abs working? No, because he is executing full-body functional movement patterns. During the chop and lift exercises, one area may feel tired first if many repetitions are performed, but usually this is just fatigue. Often it is generalized fatigue or poor form that limits repetitions.

The movement patterns and positions of the chop and lift exercises have specific rules. Follow each rule to the letter, not to make life difficult but to provide greater objectivity when looking at left-right imbalances. It is my hope that this objectivity will override the need to feel the burn.

Getting Started

Before beginning, follow the recommendations prior to this chapter. Pay attention to the body, watch for subtle mistakes, and note left-right imbalances. Do not begin if you have pain; limitation; or any type of active injury that has not been evaluated, treated, or rehabilitated. It is not mandatory that the movement screen for mobility and stability be perfect; however, it is advisable to correct any significant right-left flexibility imbalances before performing movement imbalance training. In the presence of a flexibility imbalance, the body will do what it has to in order to work around the problem, and in doing so will create strength and endurance imbalances in an attempt to rebalance the system. Do not train for strength symmetry if mobility symmetry is not yet present. However, if the movement screens in chapter 5 reveal no problems with right-left imbalances or basic movement patterns, then move on to the next level of balancing the body: movement imbalance strength and endurance training.

The exercises featured have right-left components to evaluate and train movement imbalances. By training these imbalances you take care of the underlying muscle imbalances that create the movement problem. Remember that muscles do what they are told. If they are doing something you don't like, tell them to do it differently: communicate to the muscle through repetition of posture and movement. The chop and lift requires a basic posture, specific movement, and specific direction of movement. Attention to these details is the key.

Specific equipment is needed to perform these exercises. A high-low cable machine is the most user-friendly piece of equipment with which to perform the chop and lift exercises. On a high-low cable machine, a cable from a low pulley can be pulled up or a cable from a high pulley can be pulled down. A large amount of weight is not needed because a great distance is being covered and so many body parts are being used. Get an appropriate handle attachment, preferably a rigid stick with a secured eyelet in one end. The handle should be attached to the high or low pulley with an appropriate clasp or clip attachment. A long, large-diameter rope attachment can be used if the stick is not available, but the rope requires greater attention to detail and technique and may increase the difficulty of the exercise. A third handle attachment option is a large-diameter rope halved through the clasp and held independently in the right and left hands.

The stick and long rope methods allow slightly greater force and target the core to a greater extent. They give the arms a biomechanical advantage and therefore require more core stability and place greater emphasis on posture. The halved rope uses each hand independently to perform reciprocal patterns. It doesn't allow the same amount of force as the stick or long rope because the halved rope requires a greater range of motion. A wrist spiral movement is needed when a halved rope is used and this creates slightly greater responsibility in the upper body. Try the halved rope once you have gained proficiency with the other two to place greater emphasis on the upper extremities, especially to train for sports that require handling an implement, such as a hockey stick, golf club, baseball bat, or tennis racket. Climbers, rowers, paddlers, mountain bikers, and cross-country skiers may also enjoy a workout that allows slightly greater independent upper-extremity movement.

An elastic tubing system can also be used to create the chop and lift pattern. Use a stick attachment or use the two pieces of tubing independently. It is important, whenever possible, to use the elastic tubing through a pulley system. The pulley system creates more appropriate pull angles. It also allows one to use a much longer piece of elastic. This keeps the resistance from maxing out too quickly and altering the movement pattern.

With a conventional pulley system, the weight does not change throughout the movement, whereas elastic tension builds as elongation occurs. Therefore, starting resistance and ending resistance are not the same. Elastic resistance does not develop inertia. Thus, quicker and brisker movements can be used without the inertia or jerking that would be noted in a pulley system with a one-to-one ratio (one inch of pull through the cable lifts the weight stack one inch). A noninertia pulley system would be considered a four-to-one ratio (four inches of cable pull moves the weight stack one inch). This does not develop inertia and may be more beneficial when performing brisk movements.

Using the Chop and Lift

When building muscle and working on strength, consider force and distance equally. Conventional weight training has made many athletes think that if a large amount of force is applied, regardless of how short the distance, a lot of work will be done. This is not true because they do not go through a full range of motion or do not use perfect technique, which could reduce the amount of distance a weight is pushed or pulled. In fact, this increases force but reduces distance. It is important to get rid of the musclehead mentality. Lift to move better.

The chop and lift covers a lot of distance. Within that distance are areas in which you have a mechanical advantage or disadvantage. You can lift only the amount of weight you can handle in the weakest part of the movement. Because you are covering such a great distance, you may have many weak spots throughout the pattern. Just because you can move the weight initially does not mean that you can complete the full pattern. You may need to reduce the weight to demonstrate good technique through a pattern over the entire distance of the exercise.

The half-kneeling chop and lift is probably the best starting point for movement imbalance training. Take special note of left and right differences with both the chop and the lift. It is best to find a weight that is comfortable for more than eight repetitions and then perform that move for as many repetitions as possible without compensation, loss of form, or excessive fatigue. The left-right differences in those repetitions will indicate the extent of movement imbalance. It is better to have a partner watch you and even hold a dowel or stick against your spine to demonstrate the erect position of the spine throughout the entire movement. When this position is lost or form looks poor, stop performing the movement and record the repetitions.

The assistant should speak up when technique suffers or fatigue starts to show. The participant may or may not be aware of this, so it is important to have external feedback. Once you identify a left-right imbalance in either the chop or the lift, work on that specific movement pattern for approximately one week or at least three sessions. Any changes are probably due not so much to increases in strength but to improvement in coordination and awareness of the imbalance.

You are in the process of breaking a habit developed as a result of activity, a past injury, or even a simple dominance on one side. Look at the left-right differences in the chop and the lift. Both probably will show left-right differences, but choose the movement (either the chop or lift) that had the greatest discrepancy between left and right. By fixing one, you will probably change the other. Target the weakest link. Train only that one movement for one week and then retest the right chop, left chop, right lift, and left lift. Note the differences. If you see improvement but are not completely balanced, continue with the same program. If you do not demonstrate adequate improvement, train both imbalances. Differences of 10 to 15 percent in the ability to perform repetitions are acceptable and considered a result of the fact that most people are more dominant on one side. Anything in excess of 10 to 15 percent is considered an unnecessary movement imbalance and should be targeted.

Most athletes will have a greater difference than 10 to 15 percent. Sport creates imbalances. Even a sport that appears to be balanced, such as running, swimming, or cycling, will often produce or reinforce imbalances. Don't assume a symmetrical sport will create balance; sometimes it strengthens an imbalance.

The tall kneeling chop and lift is the next choice to identify an imbalance. Chances are that if you have done adequate work in the half-kneeling chop and lift, you have fixed any imbalance that would appear in the tall kneeling chop and lift. If you had difficulty with the deep squat in the functional movement screen in chapter 5, it would be worth it to explore movement patterns with respect to the tall kneeling chop and lift. Follow the same format as the half-kneeling chop and lift and remember to compare the right and left side for both movements. If you did not have difficulty with the deep squat, it is appropriate to move on to one of the standing movement patterns.

The scissors stance is probably more functional than the squat stance. However, it is better to look at left-right imbalances in the squat stance first because it is a less complicated pattern and shows left-right differences with greater clarity. Work on the greatest imbalance for one to two weeks, then retest. Move on to the scissors stance chop and lift as part of a maintenance program for movement pattern balance.

Do not think of the chop and lift as a simple cross-pattern exercise. It does not have to look like a functional activity or sport. It is a primitive pattern that exposes the core to three-dimensional stress, incorporating both lower-body weight shifting and upper-body movement. It also works at a speed slow enough to provide feedback about the way you move. This movement pattern is an excellent teacher of stability. It lays a foundation for your other strength training and is by itself a simple reproducible test of left-right movement pattern balance.

Progress through the half-kneeling and tall kneeling chop and lift and spend some time doing the squat stance chop and lift. Progress then to the scissors stance chop and lift and use it one day per week as a warm-up or cool-down activity within a workout. Or make a variation of the chop and lift part of your workout. However you use it, note technique, foot position, and left-right differences in strength and endurance. Strength measures are those that have a resistance that can be performed for 6 to 10 repetitions, whereas endurance measures use a resistance that can be performed for 15 to 30 repetitions. There are many other exercises for muscle imbalance training, but the chop and lift represents a fundamental movement base for all sporting activities.

Chop and Lift Exercises

Two initial positions will be used for chopping and lifting patterns: half-kneeling and tall kneeling. These positions are chosen specifically because they take the leg dominance out of the movement. To be more specific, quad dominance is the problem. For athletes, the legs are often the driving force behind movement. Many times the torso does not get adequately trained, and the legs are used to compensate for the weakness of the torso. So the first order of business is to temporarily take leg dominance out of the movement to reveal a greater left-right difference. Unfortunately, the legs do a great job of hiding the core. If the movement imbalance happens to be within the legs, it will be obvious when the legs are added back into the movement. Start at the core first.

HALF-KNEELING CHOP

Kneel directly perpendicular to the weight stack and pulley system, with the outside knee down and the inside leg flexed 90 degrees at the hip and 90 degrees at the knee. Narrow your base to approximately six inches—the width between the knee of one leg and the heel of the other leg should be within six inches. The cable machine should be fitted with a stick, long rope, or halved rope.

Hold the hips directly under the body. The spine should be erect and the shoulders should be back. A side view shows the ear in line with the shoulder, the shoulder in line with the hip, and the hip in line with the knee. The knee closer to the cable column is up; the knee farther from the cable column is down in the hip-extended position. Arms are elongated. When holding a stick or long rope, the palms should be down (figure 9.1a). When holding a halved rope, palms should be facing each other.

Pull the cable down and across the body into the open space created by the half-kneeling position (figure 9.1b). When using a stick or long rope, pull the stick or rope to the midpoint of the chest with the lower arm. The angle of pull should remain steady from start to finish. Hold the cable close to the body, forcing a bend in the elbows in the middle of the movement when the cable is closest to the body.

Make a conscious transition into a push with the upper arm downward, continuing the same angle of initial pull. Keep the cable close to the body. The angle of the cable should not change during the descent, and its orientation in front of the body should stay the same.

Finish the movement by relaxing the lower hand and pushing through to extension with the upper arm. The shoulders turn minimally or not at all. All of the motion should be in the arms. Just because the trunk and hip are not moving does not mean you are not using them. You are using them in an isometric or stabilized fashion. By pulling down and across the body with the arms, you are imposing a torque both on the core and on the hip of the knee that is down. Your ability to manage this stress and not alter your posture demonstrates stability. This stability is the foundation of your strength and endurance program.

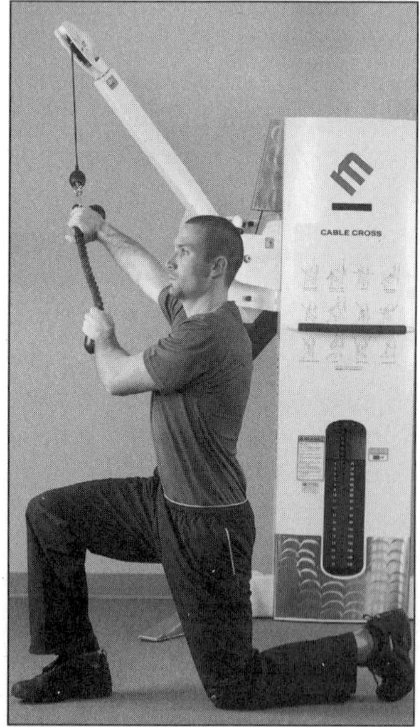

a

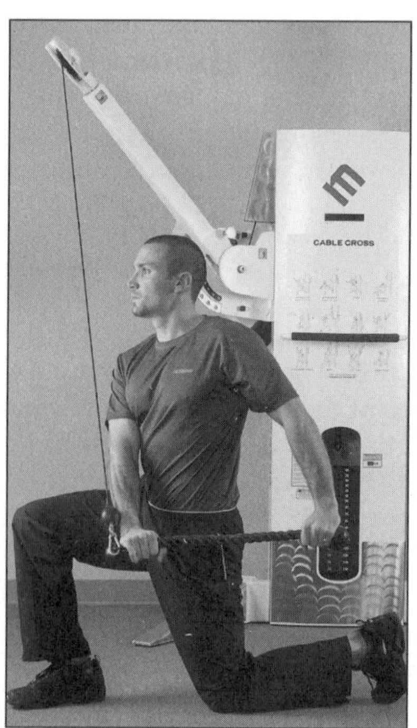

b

Figure 9.1 The half-kneeling chop: *(a)* kneel next to the cable machine and grab the handle, stick, or rope; *(b)* pull the cable down.

A common mistake in the half-kneeling chop is flexion at the hip or in the trunk. Throughout the entire movement, you should feel a gentle stretch over the front thigh in the muscles that flex the hip and extend the knee. These muscles are activated when the trunk is weak. The purpose of this exercise is to maintain a stable trunk while the hip provides a stable base. If the hip is moving, it cannot provide a stable base. If the trunk is moving, the exercise will not develop stability. A gentle stretch across the front thigh demonstrates that these muscles are not being contracted. The minute the stretch disappears, you know you are incorporating the front thigh muscles instead of activating the core muscles. Maintain the front thigh stretch throughout the movement.

This exercise is valuable for making right-left comparisons. Ability to hold the position and the quality of movement are the first things to consider. Then focus on how many quality repetitions can be completed. You may be able to do the same amount of repetitions on each side, but one side may have constant postural movement and poor mechanics.

HALVED ROPE CHOP

The halved rope chop starts in the same basic kneeling position, arms elongated, but with the palms facing each other (figure 9.2a). Pull to the center of the chest as the palms stay together and the elbows split apart. As you push downward rotate your hands away from the body. Palms should face in the direction the cable is being pushed. The arms extend and the wrists roll so that the backs of the hands face each other (figure 9.2b).

The halved rope lift places more stress on the arms, forearms, and wrists and less stress on the trunk. When a stick or long rope is used, the arms generate a larger degree of torque and can handle more load, placing more stress on the core. The core is still worked when the halved rope is used, but the movement incorporates more of a spiral and diagonal pattern in the upper body.

Athletes in sports that use swinging or throwing movements should start with the stick, developing the core first before transitioning to the halved rope to make sure that the forearms and wrists are developed. A good rule of thumb is to start at the core and work out toward your skill. You will always be able to get a better core workout by using the stick; therefore, you may want to use the stick in one workout and the halved rope in another workout. This will allow continual training of the core and develop the upper body for sport specificity as well.

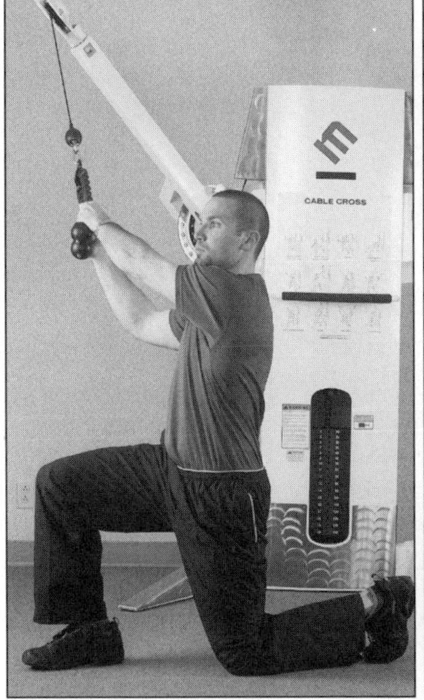

a

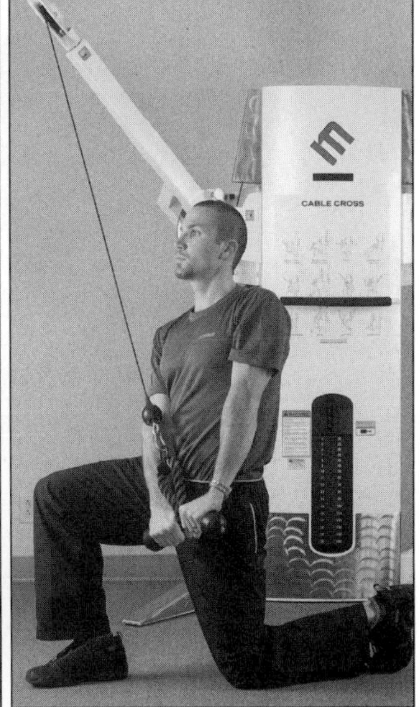

b

Figure 9.2 Halved rope chop: *(a)* begin with palms facing each other; *(b)* rotate hands as you push downward.

HALF-KNEELING LIFT

The half-kneeling lift is basically a reversal of the half-kneeling chop. Kneel directly perpendicular to the weight stack and pulley system with the inside knee down, hip extended, and the outside knee up (figure 9.3a). This puts the open space in the cable's path. Use a narrow base and an erect vertical spine. To get a more vertical line of pull, it may be necessary to elevate the down knee on a 4-, 6- or 8-inch step. This will put you farther from the pulley and allow you to increase the vertical inclination of the cable. Taller people will need more of a vertical path in the chop and lift, and shorter people will need a slightly less vertical path. Once you get the arm movement down, you will feel the natural pattern for you. If you are using a stick or long rope, palms are down; if you are using a halved rope, start with the backs of the hands together.

If using the stick or long rope, pull it up to the center of the chest with the outside arm and then finish with a press of the inside arm (figure 9.3b). The shoulders should have minimal turn. The movement is a total-arm movement. Maintain the front thigh stretch throughout the entire exercise and compare the left and right side for both quality and repetitions.

If using a halved rope, pull up and through to the center of the chest and press through until palms are facing each other. Once again, simply reverse the chop movement.

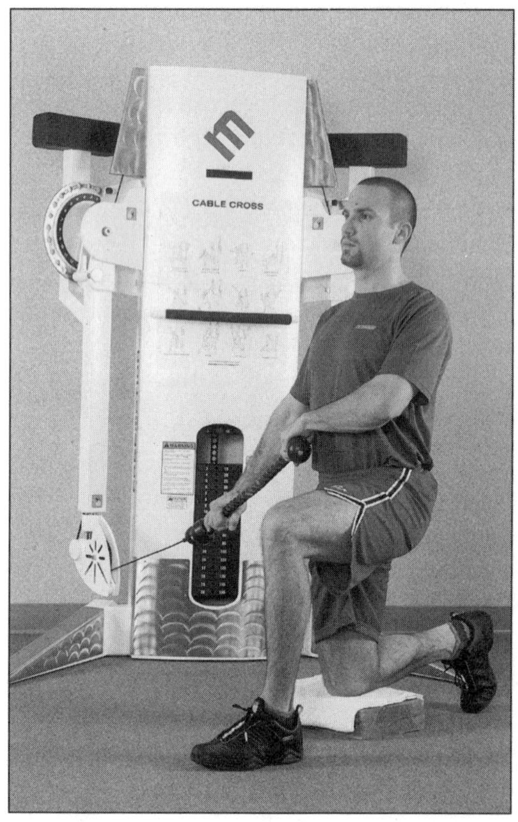

a

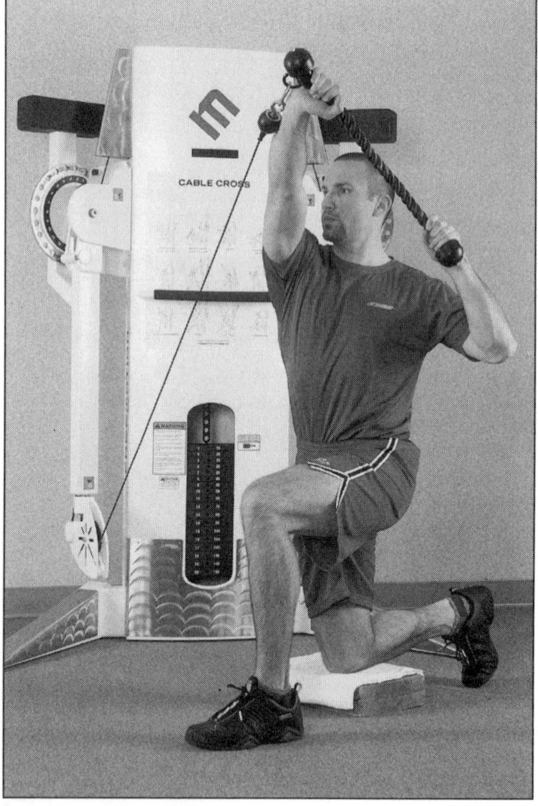

b

Figure 9.3 The half-kneeling lift: *(a)* kneel next to the cable machine; *(b)* pull the cable to the center of the chest and then press with the inside arm.

TALL KNEELING CHOP AND LIFT

To get into the starting position, kneel so that you are sitting on your heels with your torso upright. Extend your knees to so that a vertical line can connect the ear, shoulder, hips and knees from a side view (figure 9.4a). Make sure the hips are fully extended. Follow the instructions for the half-kneeling chop and lift as described on pages 102 and 104, but from the tall kneeling position. Maintain the position throughout the movement (figure 9.4b). Do not flex the hips and do not lose the tall spine position.

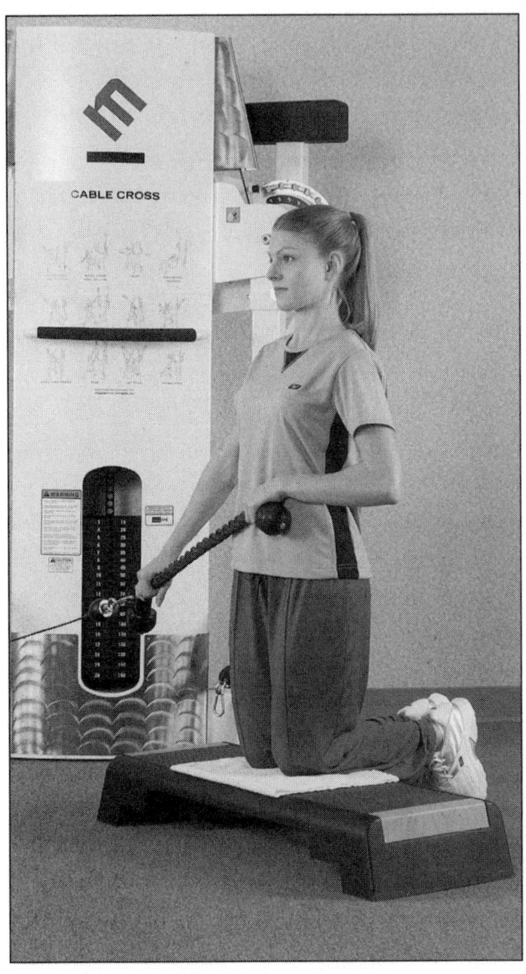

a

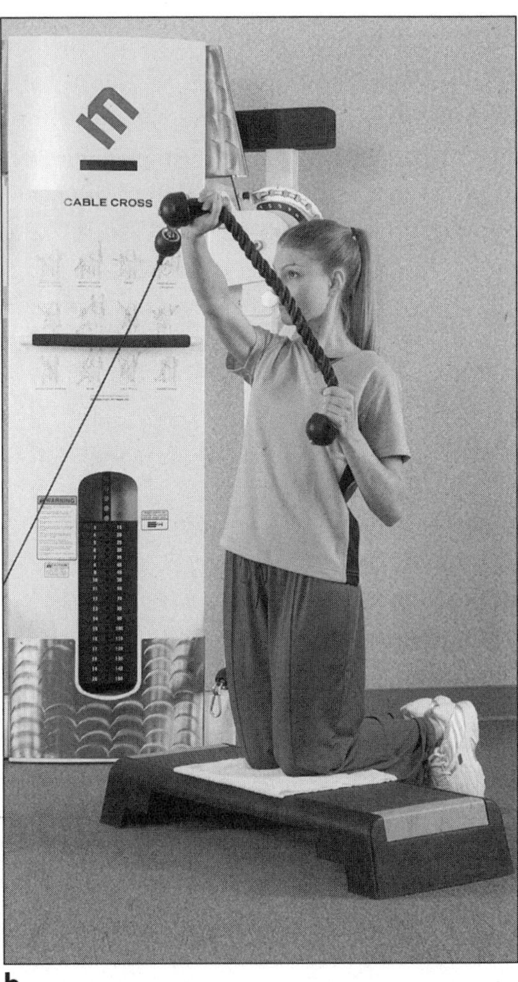

b

Figure 9.4 Tall kneeling chop and lift: *(a)* kneel on both knees; *(b)* complete the chop and lift.

SQUAT STANCE CHOP AND LIFT

The two standing positions for the chop and lift are the squat stance (or modified lunge) and the scissors stance. In the squat position, the feet are slightly wider than shoulder-width apart. Place a foam roll or ball between the feet. Feet point directly forward. Flex the knees and place a roll just below the joint line of the knee (figure 9.5a). The bowlegged position will feel very awkward.

Keep the knees bent and perform the chop and lift using a stick, long rope, or halved rope (figure 9.5b). There should be minimal shoulder turn and no pelvic turn during the spiral and diagonal patterns. Weight will automatically shift as you pull down and across or up and across the body. Therefore, it is not necessary to move the hips or knees. Look for

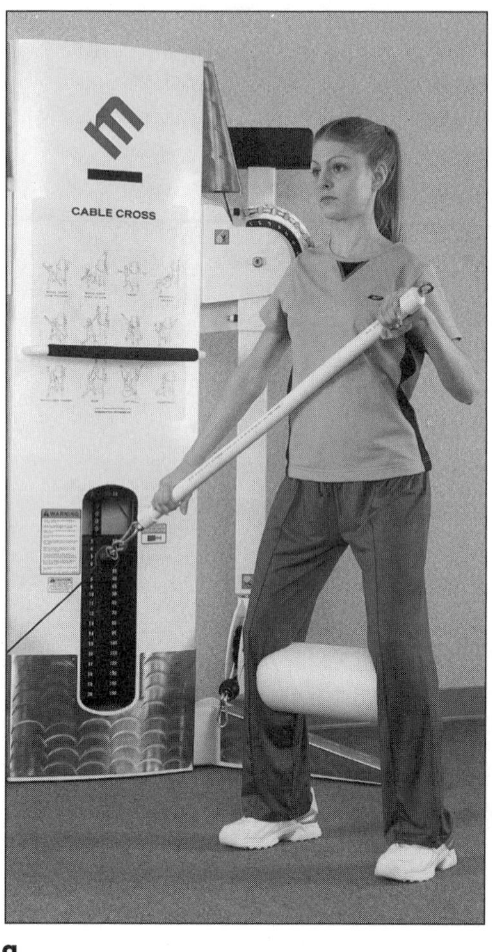

a

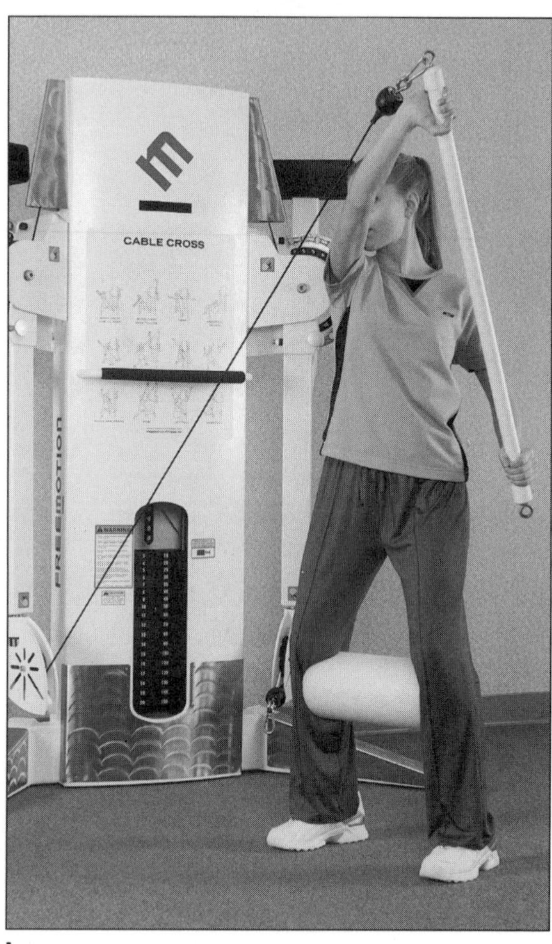

b

Figure 9.5 The squat stance chop and lift: *(a)* stand in squat position; *(b)* complete the chop and lift.

SCISSORS STANCE CHOP AND LIFT

The scissors stance chop and lift requires a ball between the thighs. The ball reduces movement in the lower body and improves weight shifting, balance, and control. The ball will help set a stable base as well as train the legs to transfer energy from the ground to the torso and improve stability. Just because the legs are not moving does not mean the muscles in the legs are not working. They are getting a large amount of work in the form of stability and support for the torso as well as weight shifting. Weight shifting can occur without movement in the lower body.

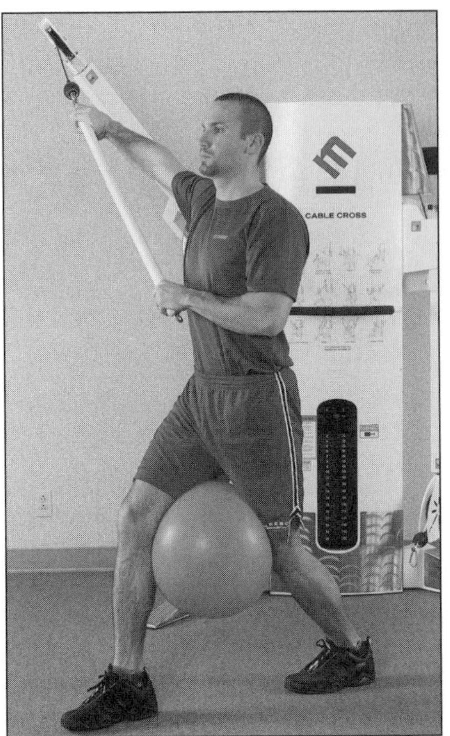

a

Stand in a lunge position with one leg to the front and one to the back. Place a stability ball between the thighs and gently squeeze to hold the ball in place (figure 9.6a). Chop to the open side (figure 9.6b) and lift to the closed side (figure 9.6c). Follow the same instructions for stick, long rope, and halved rope described in the half-kneeling chop and lift. There should be minimal shoulder turn and no pelvis turn. This is predominantly an upper-body activity. Do not change the direction of the cable down and across the body or in front of the body. Compare ability to hold the position and perform the activity on the left and right and count repetitions.

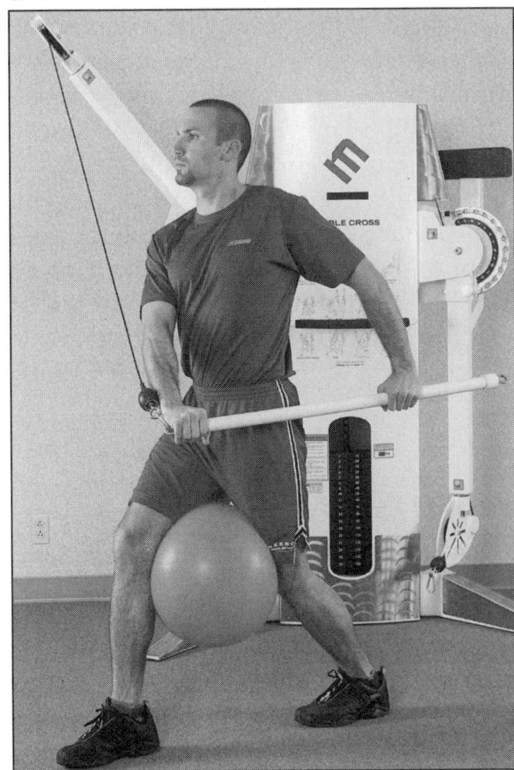

b

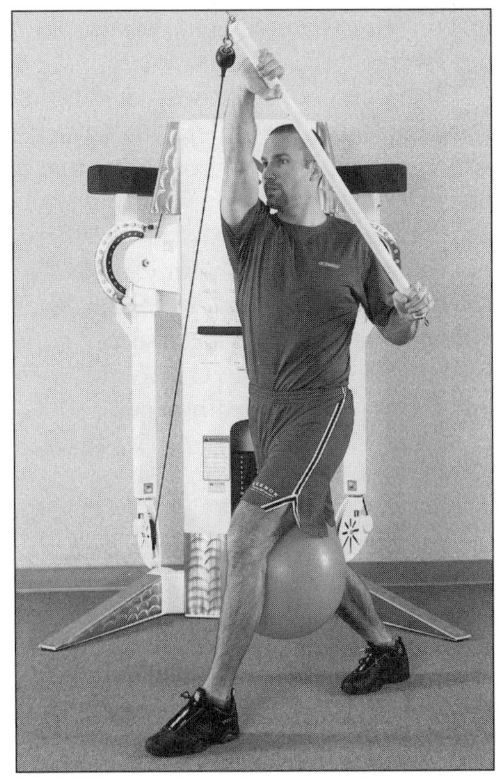

c

Figure 9.6 Scissors stance chop and lift: *(a)* stand in lunge position with a stability ball between your knees; *(b)* pull cable to open side (chop); *(c)* lift cable to closed side.

10

Strength and Endurance Exercises

Support your body and it will support you. When training with weights, you support the body's weight as well as the weight of the dumbbell or barbell you're using. Sitting on a machine and pushing with one body part to isolate one or two muscles does not support the body. Maintaining posture while producing force to perform a lift does support the body.

The key to success in sport is not just producing good movement—it's staying in good position. This could be the universal ready position—ankles, knees, and hips slightly bent—or the position that does not limit the athlete or commit the athlete to just one or two movement patterns. Explosive athletic skill for movement is important, but having a stable, reliable support position to drive from is what makes it possible.

Often fatigue, weakness, and tightness will challenge or affect the support position. This takes the athlete out of the game by throwing off movement. Trying to move effectively with faulty posture is like trying to accelerate a vehicle on snow and ice—no matter how much power is generated, the wheels slip, limiting forward movement. This is the way the body reacts when the muscles that move overpower the muscles that maintain stability. For example, for every muscle that moves the shoulder, there is a muscle that stabilizes the shoulder joint and shoulder blade. For every muscle that allows an athlete to kick a soccer ball or punt a football, there is a strong and stable core that holds the pelvis stable so the hip can anchor and pull through the kick. Don't just train to move—train to support as well.

Simultaneously Improving Strength and Movement

Much of the first part of this book focused on explaining movement. Now let's use this information to understand how strength and movement can be improved together.

Four or five passing tests on the movement screen is a great demonstration of movement patterns that are better than average. However, you don't get off easy. So you have great mobility: but can you control it? You could be at greater risk for injury because your better-than-average mobility will get you into situations that you may be unable to control with your current strength or stability.

Stability is hard to grade. It is a complex system of control, which is much harder to qualify, quantify, and score than mobility. Stability and mobility are interwoven and always linked, especially in athletics. Therefore a good mobility score will indicate adequate stability to a degree, but athletics require great stability. The advanced functional movement screen I referred to in chapter 5 has a more complex grading system and seven screening tests. It is more involved and does require greater stability. Although your stability has not been graded you can become more aware of your stabilizing abilities if you simply redirect your focus when training. Don't just look at your movement—look at your ability to hold a stable position and posture. This chapter will offer many suggestions for training strength and endurance. Each exercise is an opportunity to evaluate and train your own stability.

When you work on the exercises in this chapter, focus on technique. Extra mobility will sometimes allow sloppy, imprecise technique. Use a mirror or training partner to reinforce technique. Always compare the left and right sides of the body. Always work toward balance. Never allow these exercise techniques to serve as stretches. Do not go to the end of your range and try to perform a stretch and a weightlifting maneuver at the same time.

A simple example that often causes problems with people who have good mobility is the lunge. In a dumbbell or straight bar lunge, an athlete with great or even good mobility may try to go too deep, loading the front leg but also trying to get a hip flexor stretch on the rear leg. This is unnecessary and unsafe. Mobility is already good; more strength is needed. This athlete already has range of motion; she needs to control it. She does not need to go up against her end range, because it is adequate. It's OK to train *near* the end range, just not all the way *to* the end range. Joints can be damaged and muscles can be strained. By stopping your movement before end range (if you have normal or excessive range of motion) you will build better body awareness and protection for muscles and joints.

Two or three passing scores on the movement screen is average, but if you're a serious athlete you should try to do better. Consider using lighter weight and better form until your movement screen improves. Chances are that you fall into one of two categories: stiff, or stiff and strong. Either way, it is important to reduce the amount of weight.

If you are stiff, you are going to expend a lot of energy just working against tight muscles. Therefore, the added weight will hurt your ability to perform adequate repetitions using proper technique. If you are stiff and strong, you probably could lift more weight, but because you will be exploring new territory—using free weights and covering a large amount of motion—chances are you will tend to move in shortened ranges and compact positions because this is your comfort zone. You probably have been extremely strong in lifts, such as the bench press, or in seated machine work, such as the overhead press and leg press, but now is the time to open up your body and still maintain your strength. Initially this may be frustrating for someone who has been known as a strong athlete.

Achieving total athleticism means moving away from strengths and confronting weaknesses. In this case, your strength can be your weakness. Strength has been gained, but within a shortened or limited range. This can hurt your power, speed, and agility. It can damage body awareness, make you less efficient, and hurt your endurance and efficiency. It can also prevent you from learning new techniques and advancing in skill because of limited movement patterns.

Take time to execute these lifts, working toward the end range. A gentle stretch is OK, but learn to relax. The stretch is not coming from tight muscles; it is coming from muscles that have been used inappropriately. Strive for perfect technique on every repetition and every set. Keep the spine tall and long. Relax the extremities. Hold the shoulders back and the head upright. Breathe deep and slow, move under control, and feel what is happening.

If a muscle feels tight, it is probably because you are trying to use it at the wrong time, in the wrong sequence, and in the wrong position. Quit using it. In doing so, you may learn which other part of the body you have not been using. Take time and be patient. If you need an ego boost after a couple of weeks, go back to your old routine. Techniques will probably improve, but remember *how* they improved. Then go back to a more functional workout if your goal happens to be more than just bodybuilding.

The exercises in this chapter are taken from classic free-weight moves involving both dumbbells and barbells. The positions can supplement a strength-training program or function as the program itself until the body is balanced and ready to take a more aggressive approach to strength training. Selection of exercises is based on movement screen assessments in chapter 5.

The three classic and fundamental foot positions—the squat, hurdle step, and lunge—will be used as the framework for your strength and endurance program. Each makes a unique, important contribution to your total athletic development. You may feel your sport or your body favors one movement pattern over the other two patterns. You need proficiency in each pattern because each one supports the other two.

Use these exercises to complement the mobility or stability that you have gained. For example, if most of the test results were great but the result on the squat was poor, then use the strength-training routine that targets the squat. The mobility and stability exercises covered in part II should have improved squat performance; now reinforce that improvement by adding strength and endurance to the motion, thereby improving motor learning and motor memory. Also, by developing the movement pattern with strength work you will support the other movement patterns by reducing compensation.

Squat Strength-Training Series

Adding weight to a squat exercise program challenges posture in support positions as well as the movements that come most frequently out of the squat posture. Working on your squat position and movements will increase fundamental strength and provide a much better foundation for advanced strength training.

TALL KNEELING DUMBBELL CURL AND PRESS

The tall kneeling dumbbell curl and press is not as simple as it sounds. Kneel on a well-cushioned exercise mat with adequate thickness for comfort. If you have or have had a knee, shin, or ankle injury that prevents you from staying in this position without pain, move on to the next exercise. Place the dumbbells on benches or stands to your sides so that you can easily grab them.

Lengthen your spine, becoming as tall as possible without hyperextending the back. Pull in the abs but do not hold your breath. This should slightly increase the stretch on the front thighs and hip flexors. Maintain this slight stretch throughout the entire exercise. If you cannot feel these muscles stretching, chances are you are using them instead of the abs to support posture. Leg muscles are for movement; ab muscles are for support and posture. Relax the abs, holding them in. Slightly tighten the buttocks.

Grab the dumbbells, one in each hand (figure 10.1a). Swing the dumbbells down by your sides, curl them, and press overhead (figure 10.1b). Maintain posture and balance the entire time. Find a nice gentle rhythm for the curl and press, a rhythm that keeps you balanced and does not feel awkward. Look straight ahead or follow the weights from eye level upward, but do not look down. Maintain balance with a relaxed but pulled-in abdominal wall and slight tightening of the buttocks. Never lose the stretch on the thighs.

Use a weight you can handle for 8 to 12 repetitions. If you cannot achieve 8 repetitions without losing balance or form or becoming overly fatigued, you have too much weight. If you can exceed 12 repetitions with ease while keeping proper technique and maintaining proper posture, the weight is too light. Perform 1 to 3 sets, depending on weightlifting experience and conditioning level.

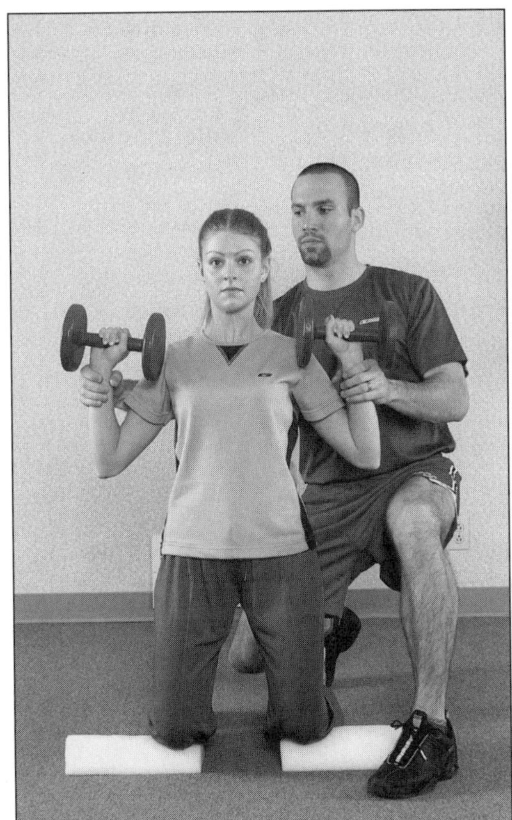

a

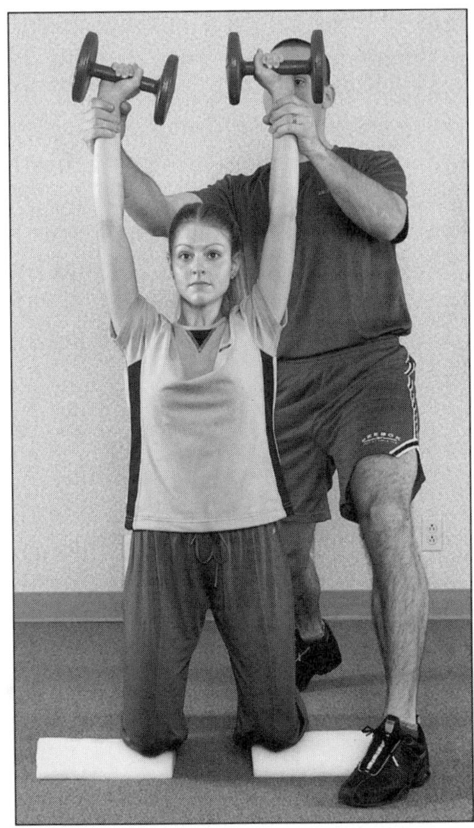

b

Figure 10.1 Tall kneeling dumbbell curl and press: *(a)* while kneeling, grab a dumbbell with each hand; *(b)* press the dumbbells overhead.

DEEP SQUAT DUMBBELL PUSH-PRESS

Stand with feet shoulder-width apart, a dumbbell in each hand. Pull in the abdominals, keeping them relaxed. Breathe. Hold the dumbbells in front of the shoulders so that palms are turned toward each other. If you prefer a more open position, turn palms forward and pull shoulders back.

Descend into a deep squat (figure 10.2a). If this is uncomfortable, you have poor form, or the heels come up, use a slight heel lift. Try a 1-inch heel lift first; if that isn't enough, go to a 1 1/2-inch heel lift. If you feel you need more than a 1 1/2-inch heel lift, return to the mobility and stability routine for the squat and work on improving movement patterns.

Once in a deep squat, check body posture. Make sure the abs are still pulled in. Relax until you feel a stretch in the buttocks or groin. Come out of the squat and return to the start position, then press the dumbbells overhead (figure 10.2b). This is a push-press movement, so use the legs. Bend knees slightly and push through the legs. Lift the dumbbells off the shoulders and overhead. Hold the position, arms slightly wider apart than feet, palms turned toward each other or turned forward. Do not hyperextend the elbows. Lower the dumbbells very slowly while maintaining posture and repeat the entire movement.

The deep squat dumbbell push-press can be very fatiguing because it involves full range of motion of both arms and legs. Remember that work is the result of force times distance. Reducing the force but proportionally increasing the distance results in the same amount of work. If you feel like the weights are too light, consider the distance that weight is being moved. It is not about the weight; it is about strength.

Do not hyperextend the knees, and use the legs as much as needed to propel the dumbbells off the shoulders. As the arms fatigue, you will have to use more leg. This is an important connection for your brain to learn as the body transmits power from the legs, through the torso, and into the shoulders. Performing this exercise will increase efficiency in transmitting power from a double-leg stance.

Use a weight you can handle for 6 to 10 repetitions. If you cannot achieve 6 repetitions without losing balance or form or becoming overly fatigued, you have too much weight. If you can exceed 10 repetitions with ease while keeping proper technique and maintaining proper posture, the weight is too light. Perform 1 to 3 sets, depending on weightlifting experience and conditioning level.

a

b

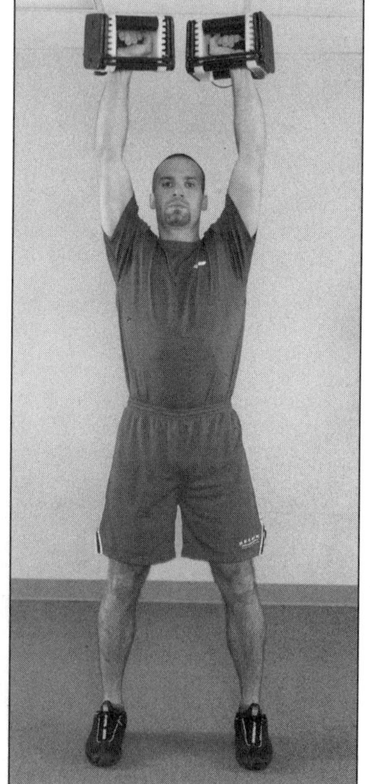

Figure 10.2 Deep squat dumbbell push-press: *(a)* lower into a deep squat position; *(b)* stand out of the squat and press the dumbbells overhead.

SINGLE-LEG SQUAT WITH DUMBBELLS

The single-leg squat with dumbbells is a safe way to overload a single leg without a spotter. You can easily drop the dumbbells at any time during the lift. (Just watch your feet!)

This exercise is often performed with one leg resting on a bench or short table behind the athlete (figure 10.3a). Although this position does isolate one leg, it will hyperextend the back and tilt the pelvis forward in some cases, especially if the bench is too high. The knee should bend more than 90 degrees, and the hip should never hyperextend at the deep point of the squat (figure 10.3b).

Basically, your back should not move. If it does move, here is a way to modify the exercise. You can lift the heel to improve your technique and help with balance if necessary. Use a 1- to 1 1/2-inch heel lift block and reduce the lift by 50 percent until the block is no longer needed.

Keep the knee completely outside the foot at all times, and keep the foot flat on the floor. If you look down at your foot, the knee should be outside the foot and the foot should be in the center of the body, pointing straight ahead. Shoulders and hips should be in line and pointing straight ahead. The back should be erect and tall. Stomach muscles should be drawn in. Relax the shoulders. Let go of the dumbbells if you lose balance, feel pain, or can't complete the repetition.

Use a weight you can handle for 8 to 12 repetitions. If you cannot achieve 8 repetitions without losing balance or form or becoming overly fatigued, you have too much weight. If you can exceed 12 repetitions with ease while keeping proper technique and maintaining proper posture, the weight is too light. Perform 1 to 3 sets, depending on weightlifting experience and conditioning level.

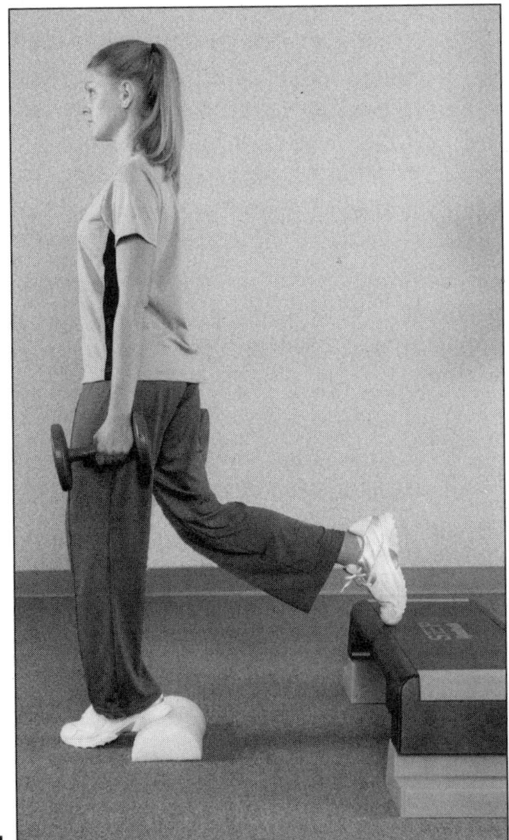

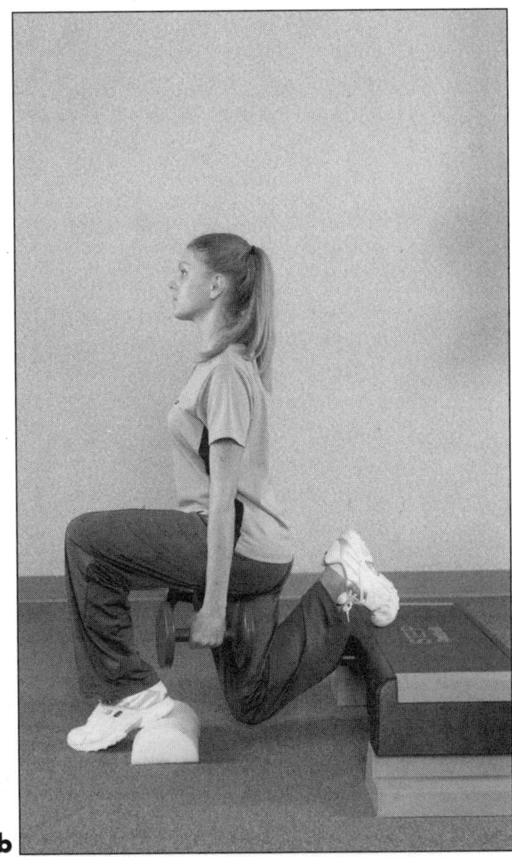

Figure 10.3 Single-leg squat with dumbbells: *(a)* place one leg on a slightly elevated platform; *(b)* lower into the other leg until thigh is parallel with the floor.

DEEP SQUAT PUSH-PRESS WITH BARBELL

The use of the barbell with a straight bar will enable you to increase the speed of the push-press compared to the dumbbell lift. You also will be able to move more weight because the straight bar provides a mechanical advantage.

Standing in a front squat position, hold the barbell at chest height with elbows pointed forward if possible. Descend into a deep squat, using a heel lift if necessary (figure 10.4a). Rise out of the deep squat, keeping a tall spine, pulled-in abdomen, and appropriate foot and knee position. Once you return to the starting position, bend the knees slightly and lift the weight overhead, first with an explosion from the legs and then with the arms (figure 10.4b). Keep the weight overhead and check posture. Slowly lower the weight to the starting position without moving the legs. Do not hyperextend the knees. For some, this is the hardest part of the lift.

This exercise will build strength in the upper body. You can perform a number of negative repetitions without a spotter. The legs help raise the weight, and the arms are overloaded when the weight is lowered.

Use a weight you can handle for 6 to 10 repetitions. If you cannot achieve 6 repetitions without losing balance or form or becoming overly fatigued, you have too much weight. If you can exceed 10 repetitions with ease while keeping proper technique and maintaining proper posture, the weight is too light. Perform 1 to 3 sets, depending on weightlifting experience and conditioning level.

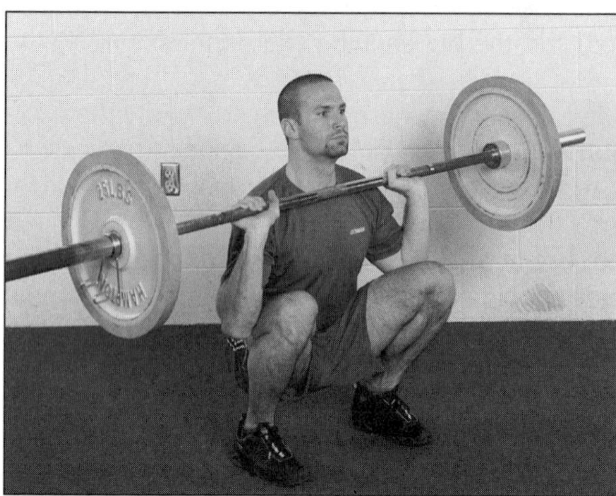

a

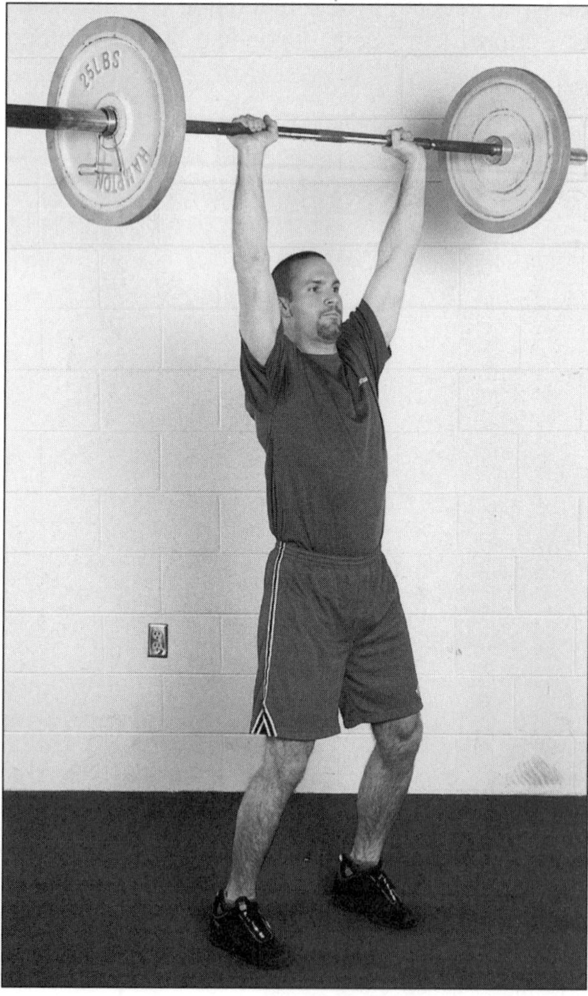

b

Figure 10.4 Deep squat push-press with barbell: *(a)* lower into a deep squat; *(b)* rise out of the squat and lift the barbell overhead.

FRONT SQUAT

There is absolutely nothing wrong with back squatting, one of the three major lifts from powerlifting. The back squat is an excellent way to overload the legs. However, it is not a natural form of lifting. In real life, no one ever sets weight on your shoulders and then asks you to stand up.

Keeping the weight in front of you will limit the amount of weight you can lift. This may explain why the front squat is less popular than the back squat. If lifting a lot of weight is important to you, consider powerlifting. If you are concerned about leg strength for fundamental athletic development, add the front squat to your routine.

Foot position is very important. A narrow squat focuses more on the front thigh and knee because it causes the knee to flex more. A wider squat with the feet turned out focuses more on the hip because it reduces the amount of knee flexion and increases the amount of hip flexion and abduction. It is best to explore both positions, even if it requires you to change weight.

Arm position is also important. Find a comfortable arm position to support the weight. A towel roll or pad around the bar is helpful. The arms can be crossed holding the bar with palms facing you (figure 10.5a) or uncrossed with palms facing upward and elbows facing away (figure 10.5b).

Use a weight you can handle for 8 to 12 repetitions. If you cannot achieve 8 repetitions without losing balance or form or becoming overly fatigued, you have too much weight. If you can exceed 12 repetitions with ease while keeping proper technique and maintaining proper posture, the weight is too light. Perform 1 to 3 sets, depending on weightlifting experience and conditioning level.

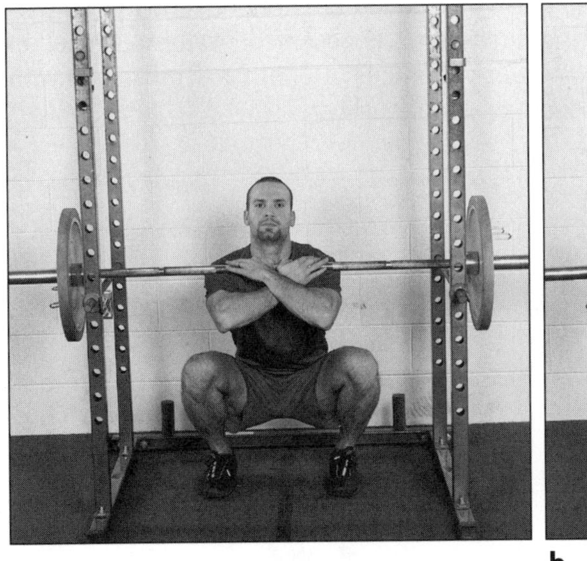

a

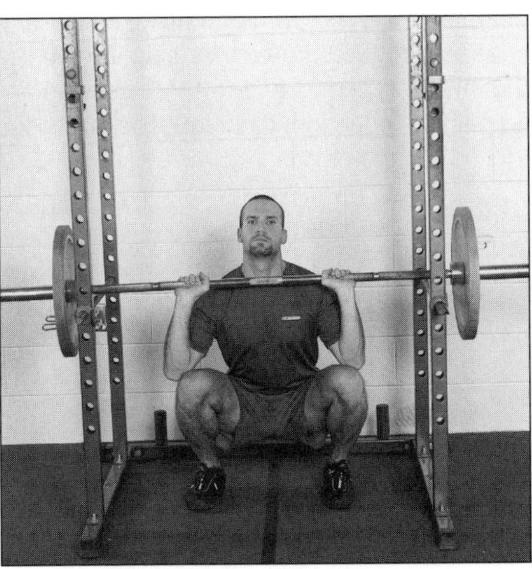

b

Figure 10.5 Front squat: *(a)* hold the bar with arms crossed and palms facing you or *(b)* with arms uncrossed, palms turned up, and elbows turned out.

Hurdle Step Training Series

If the hurdle step presented some difficulty, perform the mobility and stability movement exercises first to correct this movement pattern. Once it has been corrected, the exercises in this section are excellent for improving strength, coordination, and muscle memory.

TALL KNEELING FLEXION AND EXTENSION WITH STEP

Do not use a large amount of weight with this exercise. With one shoulder, you will do a stiff-arm lift for shoulder flexion; with the other, you will do a stiff-arm extension.

Kneel on a well-cushioned exercise mat with adequate thickness for comfort (figure 10.6a). If you have or have had a knee, shin, or ankle injury that prevents you from staying in this position without pain, move on to the next exercise.

Lengthen your spine, becoming as tall as possible without hyperextending the back. Pull in the abs but do not hold your breath. This should slightly increase the stretch on the front thighs and hip flexors. Maintain this slight stretch throughout the entire exercise. If you cannot feel these muscles stretching, chances are you are using them instead of the abs to support posture. Leg muscles are for movement; ab muscles are for support and posture. Relax the abs, holding them in. Slightly tighten the buttocks.

Hold a dumbbell in each hand. Slowly swing the left arm forward like a pendulum until it is directly overhead. At the same time, pull the right arm back but allow the elbow to bend, taking the right shoulder into maximum extension. The right arm can remain straight, if you prefer. The dumbbell will point down. The arms should arrive in the end position at the same time.

As the arms are moving, shift weight to the left knee and step forward with the right leg, moving into a half-kneeling position (figure 10.6b). The narrower the stance, the greater the difficulty and challenge. For the narrow stance, the foot and knee are aligned as closely as possible. Hold the position. Return the arms and legs to the starting position.

Using a manageable weight is very important. Keep the weight low because all of your weight will be shifted to one knee. Use a heavy-duty exercise mat. If kneeling causes any discomfort, move on to the next exercise.

Note any left-right differences, ability to perform repetitions, and tendency to lose balance. Strengthen the weaker side if a left-right difference is observed. Perform one set on the strong side and two to three sets on the weak side until strength is symmetrical with respect to repetition, technique, balance, and movement quality.

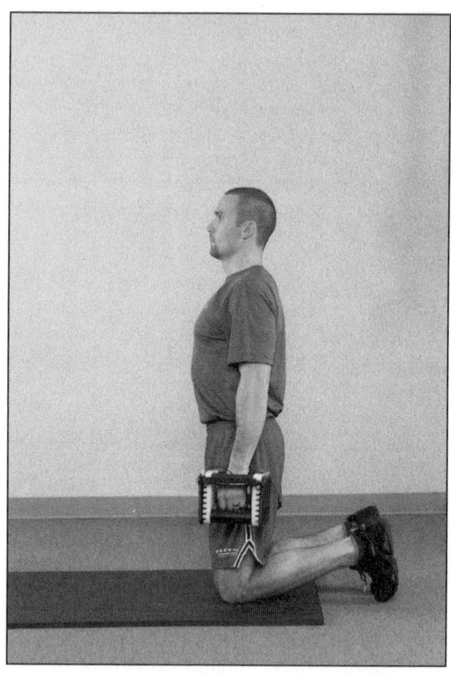

a

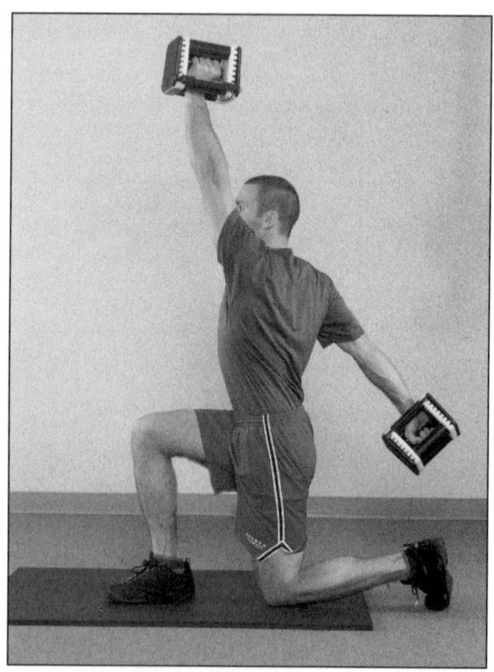

b

Figure 10.6 Tall kneeling flexion and extension with step: *(a)* kneel on a mat with a dumbbell in each hand; *(b)* as the left arm swings forward, step forward with the right leg.

Use a weight you can handle for 8 to 12 repetitions. If you cannot achieve 8 repetitions without losing balance or form or becoming overly fatigued, you have too much weight. If you can exceed 12 repetitions with ease while keeping proper technique and maintaining proper posture, the weight is too light. Perform 1 to 3 sets, depending on weightlifting experience and conditioning level.

DUMBBELL STEP-UPS

Use a bench or step-up box that is at the level of your knee or slightly lower, depending on ability. The higher the step, the harder the exercise. Make sure you can perform this move on each side before adding dumbbells.

If using dumbbells, hold them to your sides. Step up onto the box, right leg first (figure 10.7a), then step down. The right foot should never leave the box and the left foot should never touch it. Once the left foot touches the floor, descend slightly by bending the left knee as far as possible while keeping the left heel on the ground (figure 10.7b). A slight descent before each step-up teaches you to relax and gives a subtle stretch before the movement. You will feel a slight stretch in the left calf, left thigh, or maybe the right buttocks.

Straighten the left knee and lift the left heel. Complete the motion by pulling yourself onto the box with the right leg as you lift the left leg off the ground. Balance on the right leg until it is straight but not hyperextended. Return to the start position.

Keep abs pulled in and keep the spine as tall as possible. Perform 6 to 10 repetitions on each side and take note of poor balance, poor technique, or the inability to perform an equal number of repetitions. If one side is weaker, perform 2 or 3 sets of 6 to 10 repetitions on the weaker side and 1 set of 6 to 10 repetitions on the stronger side.

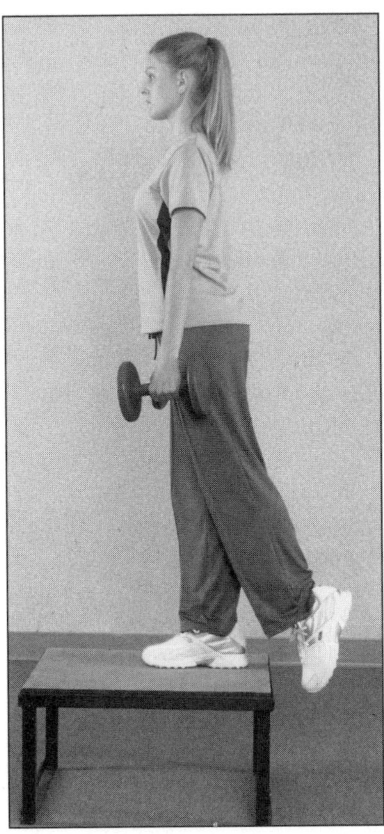
a

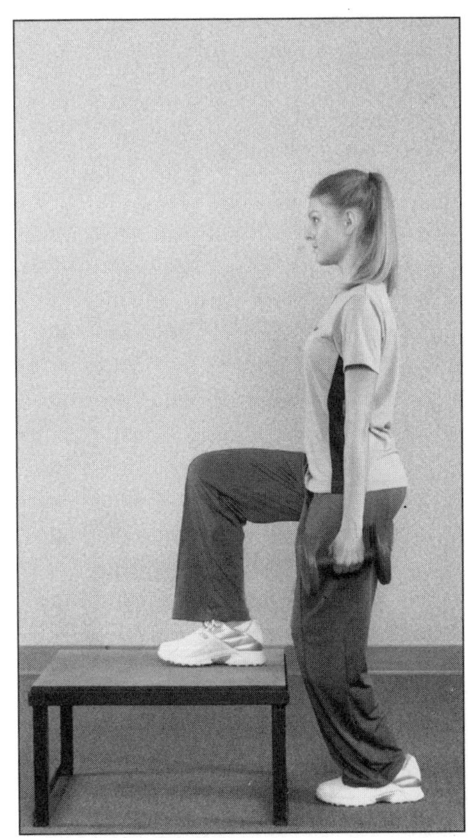
b

Figure 10.7 Dumbbell step-ups: *(a)* step up onto box; *(b)* step down and bend knee as far as you can while keeping heel on the ground.

SQUAT RACK SINGLE-LEG HEEL RAISES

This exercise uses a straight bar held across the shoulders in the back squat position. Stand with feet about shoulder-width apart. Slowly bring them together until they are touching (figure 10.8a). Lift the left knee into the air until the hip and knee are flexed 90 degrees (the hurdle step position; figure 10.8b). Remember your posture—tall spine, abdominal wall pulled in. Do not tighten the thigh; tighten the glutes. Do not hyperextend the knee. Slightly bend the knee only. Keep the spine tall; it may help to focus on a point in front of you. Do not look down.

If this is awkward or too difficult and you feel you will lose balance, then place the left heel on a box. Pull the foot up so only the heel is in contact. Do not rest the whole foot on the box. If you do you will have a tendency to push off with the left foot. Lower your body 2 to 3 inches by bending your right leg. Then straighten the right knee, but do not lock it. Continue to make yourself taller by lifting the right heel as high as possible. As you go onto the toes, do not lose balance. Hold position and lower slowly.

This exercise will not only develop calf muscles but will create comfort in balancing on one leg with weight. Focus on keeping the spine tall and abdominal wall drawn in, keeping shoulders and head relaxed. Do not focus on legs.

If you notice a right-left difference, work the weak side for 2 to 3 sets and perform only 1 set on the stronger side. Use a weight you can handle for 15 to 25 repetitions. If you cannot achieve 15 repetitions without losing balance or form or becoming overly fatigued, you have too much weight. If you can exceed 25 repetitions with ease while keeping proper technique and maintaining proper posture, the weight is too light. Perform 1 to 3 sets, depending on weightlifting experience and conditioning level.

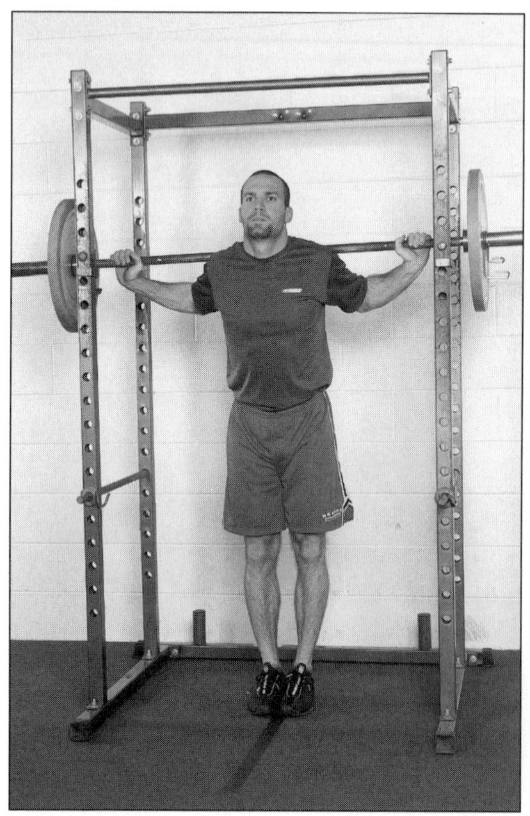

a

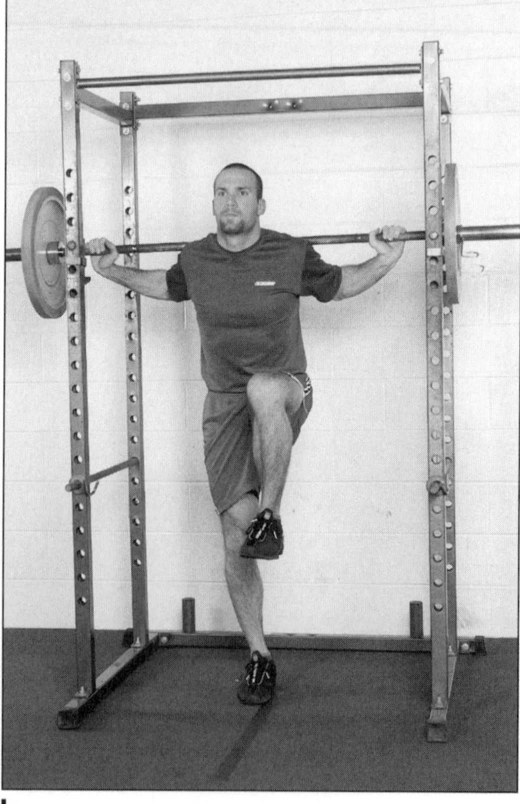

b

Figure 10.8 Squat rack single-leg heel raises: *(a)* bring feet together; *(a)* lift the knee.

SQUAT RACK SINGLE-LEG QUARTER-SQUATS

Place a 3-foot piece of tape, pointing forward, in the center of the squat rack. Stand in a back squat position with feet shoulder-width apart and lift the weight. Place the right foot on the tape and move the left foot behind with the toe pointing toward the ground (figure 10.9a).

Your goal is to get the left toe on the tape. However, you can use a wider base at first if you need to. Work toward a narrow base before increasing the weight.

Keeping the spine tall, lower into a quarter-squat position with all of the weight on the front leg, equally distributed between heel and toe (figure 10.9b). Feel the weight just in front of the heel. Remember to keep the knee to the outside of the foot at all times. Do not hold the knee directly over the foot. Keep the foot pointed straight and forward with the tape; do not let it turn outward. Keep the spine tall, look forward, and do not focus on the leg. Relax the shoulders and neck and use the abs to help balance the weight. Note weaknesses, poor balance, or poor technique.

Perform 2 to 3 sets. If you notice a problem on one side, perform 1 set on the stronger side and 2 to 3 sets on the weaker side. Use a weight you can handle for 6 to 10 repetitions. If you cannot achieve 6 repetitions without losing balance or form or becoming overly fatigued, you have too much weight. If you can exceed 10 repetitions with ease while keeping proper technique and maintaining proper posture, the weight is too light. This exercise will clearly show right-left differences. Always perform a set on the stronger side because it serves as a proper example for the weaker side. Take note of what you are doing correctly and try to replicate it on the weaker side. The strong side also serves as a warm-up to the weaker side and provides a continual comparison so you can mark improvement.

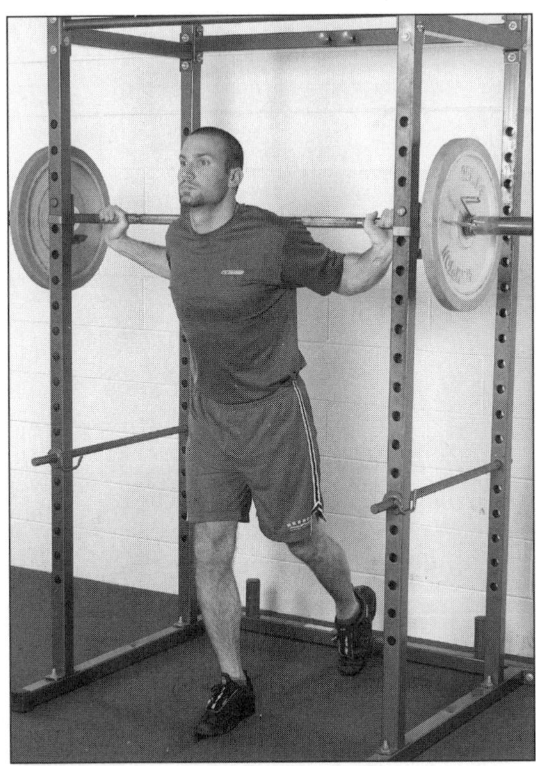

a

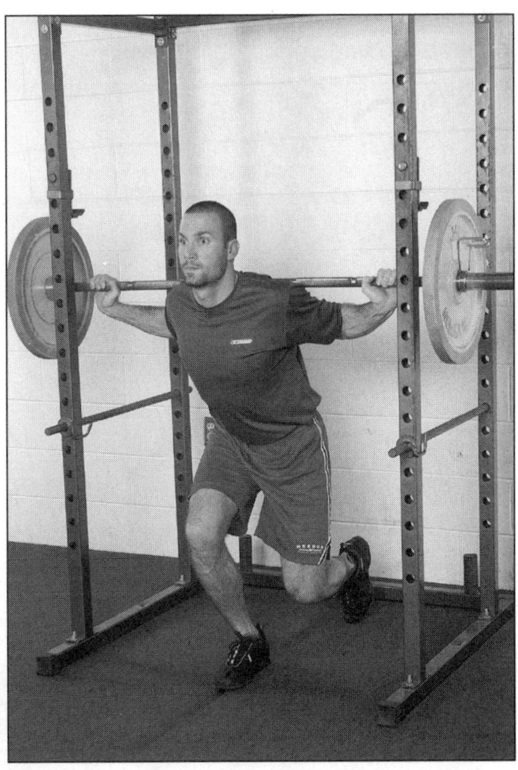

b

Figure 10.9 Squat rack single-leg quarter-squats: *(a)* move feet into lunge position; *(b)* descend into a quarter squat.

Lunge Training Series

If the lunge presented some difficulty, perform the mobility and stability movement exercises first to correct this movement pattern. Once it has been corrected, the exercises in this section are excellent for improving strength, coordination, and muscle memory.

HALF-KNEELING DUMBBELL CURL AND PRESS

Get into a half-kneeling position with foot and knee nearly on the same line (figure 10.10a). Pull in the abs and hold the spine tall until you feel a slight stretch on the thigh of the down hip. Maintain this stretch for the entire exercise. The stretch means that you are using the abs appropriately and are not contracting the quadriceps or hip flexor, which would hurt form. Slightly contract the buttocks and make sure the spine stays erect through the entire exercise.

With a dumbbell in each hand, swing the arms down to your sides, curl your arms, and press the dumbbells overhead (figure 10.10b). Press the weights overhead and return to the starting position while maintaining balance, posture, and technique.

If the half-kneeling position is more difficult on one side, perform 2 to 3 sets on the weaker side and 1 set on the stronger side. You may feel more tightness in the quadriceps on one side or the other. Relax. Part of the reason the leg feels tight is because you are trying to use it. Learn to relax it. Use the spine and core, not the legs, to balance.

Use a weight you can handle for 8 to 12 repetitions. If you cannot achieve 8 repetitions without losing balance or form or becoming overly fatigued, you have too much weight. If you can exceed 12 repetitions with ease while keeping proper technique and maintaining proper posture, the weight is too light. Perform 1 to 3 sets, depending on weightlifting experience and conditioning level.

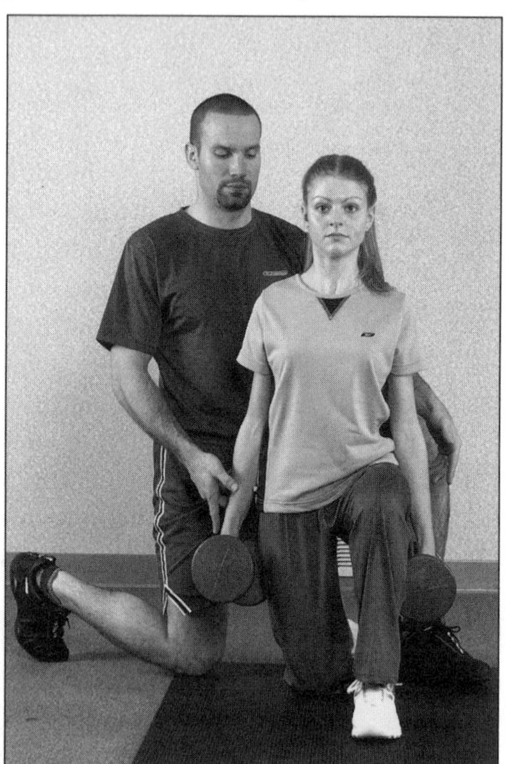

a

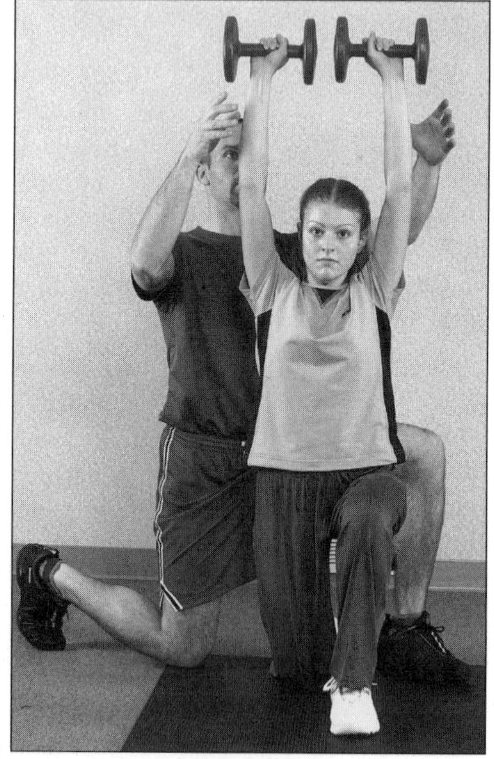

b

Figure 10.10 Half-kneeling dumbbell curl and press: *(a)* get into half-kneeling position; *(b)* press the dumbbells overhead.

DUMBBELL LUNGES

The dumbbell lunge is simple. Begin with feet side by side. You can choose to step forward or backward before sinking into a lunge. Both movements are advantageous, and a set of each movement for each leg is adequate (2 total sets on each side). Extra sets can be added if needed. Try to use a narrow base, which can be marked with a piece of wide tape. Note weaknesses, poor technique, or loss of balance. Hold dumbbells at your sides with a tall spine posture and abs pulled in (figure 10.11a).

If you step forward, do not look down, but allow your foot to find the line (figure 10.11b). Initially you can use a mirror to help find the tape, but after a little practice you will know where your foot is. Do not push out of the lunge with just the legs. Use a tall spine to pull yourself out of the lunge and back to the starting position. Do not hinge at the waist or use momentum to pull out of the lunge. Keep the spine still and tall.

If you step backward, find the line with your foot, keep the legs relaxed, and maintain a tall spine. If you observe a left-right difference, perform 2 sets on the stronger side and 4 sets on the weaker side.

Use a weight you can handle for 8 to 12 repetitions. If you cannot achieve 8 repetitions without losing balance or form or becoming overly fatigued, you have too much weight. If you can exceed 12 repetitions with ease while keeping proper technique and maintaining proper posture, the weight is too light. Perform 1 to 3 sets, depending on weightlifting experience and conditioning level.

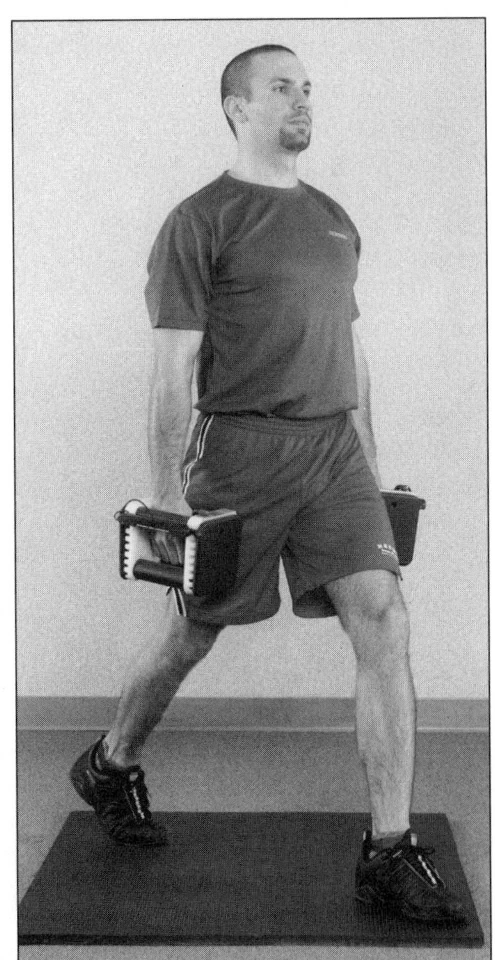

a

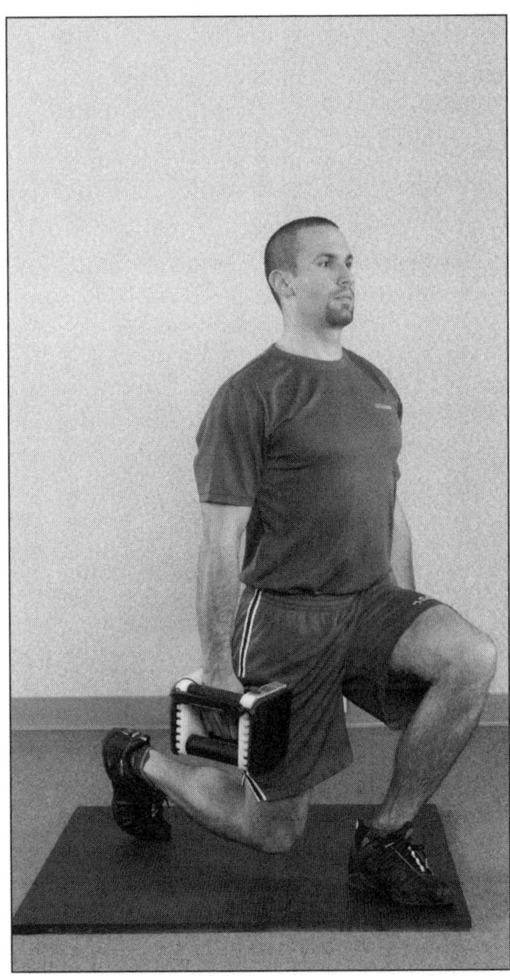

b

Figure 10.11 Dumbbell lunges: *(a)* hold dumbbells to your sides; *(a)* step forward into a lunge.

STRAIGHT BAR LUNGE STEP

Stand in a back squat position with a straight bar resting comfortably across the shoulders, gripping the bar comfortably. Execute either a forward or backward lunge. A slightly wider base than in the dumbbell lunge may be needed because the center of gravity is higher with the weight across the shoulders.

Step forward or backward (figure 10.12a), or perform one of each, as in the dumbbell lunge. Lower the body as far as possible into the lunge position without the rear knee touching the ground (figure 10.12b). Look for the 90-degree position at the front knee and you will be in good form. Use a wider stance to start and you will feel strong and stable. As you gain strength, balance, and stability, narrow your base. Make sure you can narrow the base on either side.

Maintain an erect spine and pull the abs in. Do not struggle through the movement by twisting, jerking, or moving the spine unnecessarily. If you have to twist, it probably means you need to reduce the weight.

Look for left-right differences. If there is a left-right difference, work the weaker side for 4 sets and the stronger side for 2 sets. Use the front and back step equally and do not play favorites. Usually the least favorite exercises will produce the most benefits if performed correctly. Remember, an unfamiliar movement pattern will feel better with practice.

Use a weight you can handle for 8 to 12 repetitions. If you cannot achieve 8 repetitions without losing balance or form or becoming overly fatigued, you have too much weight. If you can exceed 12 repetitions with ease while keeping proper technique and maintaining proper posture, the weight is too light. Perform 1 to 3 sets, depending on weightlifting experience and conditioning level.

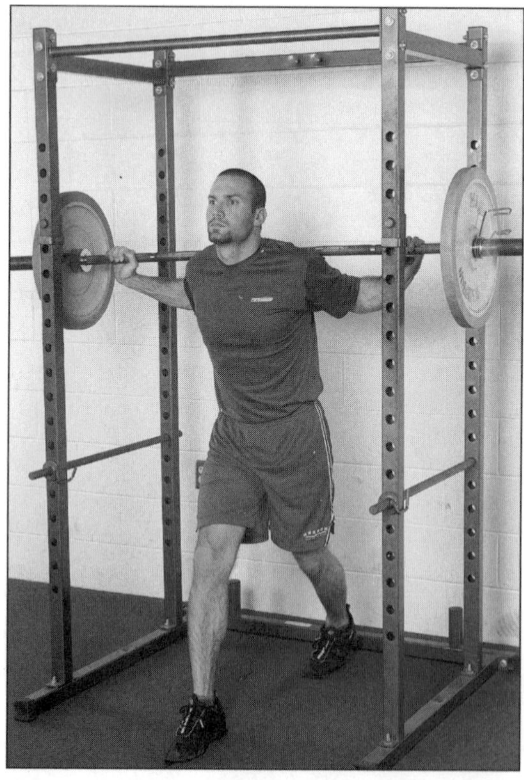

a

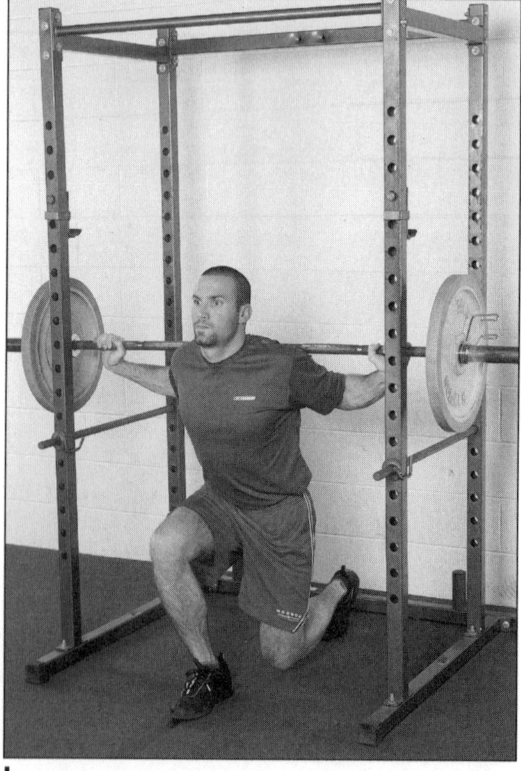

b

Figure 10.12 Straight bar lunge step: *(a)* step backward from a back squat position; *(b)* lower the body into a lunge position.

SCISSORS STANCE SQUATTING

This exercise uses the same back squat straight bar position as the straight bar lunge step and should be performed in a squat rack.

Get into a lunge stance, but reduce the distance between the feet by a quarter to a third to increase stability (figure 10.13a). Drop into a half-squat, keeping the hip of the trailing leg in extension and the spine tall and erect (figure 10.13b). The rear heel can come up.

Narrow the base and note right-left differences in balance, technique, and strength. Perform 2 to 3 sets on the weaker side and 1 set on the stronger side.

Use a weight you can handle for 8 to 12 repetitions. If you cannot achieve 8 repetitions without losing balance or form or becoming overly fatigued, you have too much weight. If you can exceed 12 repetitions with ease while keeping proper technique and maintaining proper posture, the weight is too light. Perform 1 to 3 sets, depending on weightlifting experience and conditioning level.

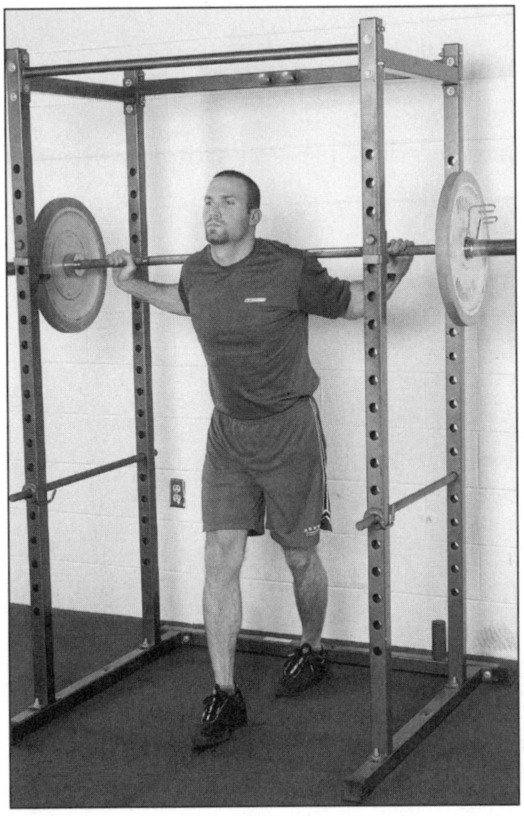
a

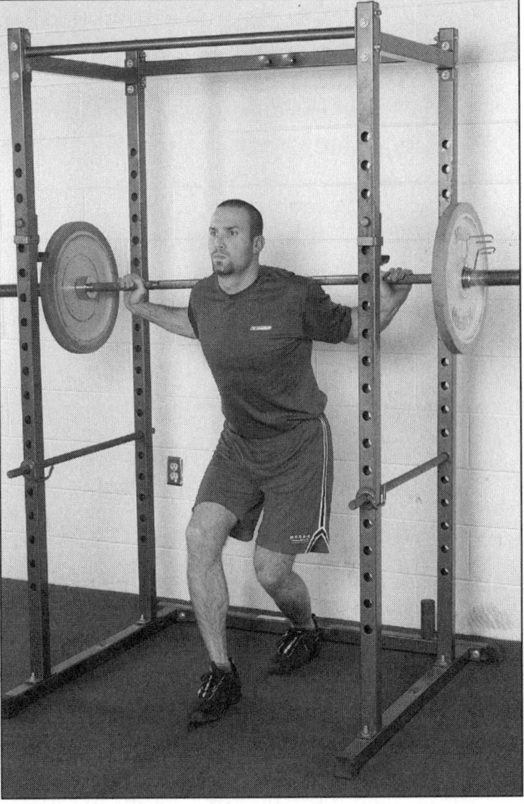
b

Figure 10.13 Scissors stance squatting: *(a)* get into a modified lunge stance; *(b)* descend into a half-squat.

You may have noticed the predominance of lower body work, and it is intentional. Most athletes will benefit from more lower body work, particularly single-leg work. If you do not have a spotter, I recommend a safety squat device such as a Smith Machine, which will help you balance and will assist with proper alignment.

Lower-body strength training will have positive effects on the core and upper body. Exclusive upper body training does not have the same carryover. The upper body strength exercises discussed are basic and generally follow a vertical orientation, which promotes better posture and better core development.

Most conventional upper-body training revolves around push and pull exercises, but it is better to get a postural base first, following the vertical training proposed in this chapter. Once you have developed a postural base and developed your core, you can progress to more upper body work. Equal amounts of push- and pull-up sets will be a great addition if you're just getting started. If you want to progress into more advanced strength training, I suggest equal amounts of push and pull movements. Push and pull movements give you great muscular development, and you should not need to isolate particular muscle groups. Here are my suggestions:

Push movements

- Seated dumbbell overhead press
- Incline dumbbell flys
- Incline dumbbell press
- Flat-bench or decline dumbbell press
- Flat-bench or decline dumbbell flys
- Close grip straight bar flat or decline bench press
- Standing press downs with cable
- Functional supersets: incline, decline, and standard push-ups; dips (with spotter if needed)

Pull movements

- Wide grip lat pull down with palms facing away
- Close grip lat pull down with palms facing you
- Bent-over dumbbell row
- Seated low row with cable
- Standing lateral front raises with dumbbells
- Laying dumbbell pullovers
- Upward rows with cable
- Functional supersets: wide-grip pull-ups with spotter; close grip pull-ups with spotter

Supersets are used to increase muscular development by overloading activity on already fatigued muscles. This technique is often used in bodybuilding to pump up muscles, but it is also great for creating better circulation in the muscle. By using what I call *functional supersets,* you will gain body control in the presence of fatigue. No weight is used because the weight is you. Perform a push or pull movement for 8 to 12 reps, and follow it quickly with the suggested superset. It is not necessary to superset every exercise. I recommend using supersets the last two or three exercises of your push or pull workout.

Endurance Work

Endurance work is often called *aerobic work,* which means that the body functions using oxygen at a steady metabolic state without exaggerated changes in heart rate or respiration. Endurance work is exactly what it sounds like—work. It provides exercise volume to improve stamina and combat fatigue, maintain alertness, and teach relaxation while moving and recovering quickly during rest breaks.

Interval training sounds almost paradoxical—working in short bursts of fairly intense activity with a set recovery time, and then doing it again. Exercising in intervals, challenging the body to recover and repeat over a series of exercises, is the best way to improve endurance for field and court sports. Other terms to describe endurance include *stamina* and *staying power.* Endurance is needed to keep the athlete on top of her game. Even if the game is marathon running or another sustained aerobic activity, it has been proved that training in intervals of higher intensity for shorter duration is the best way to improve performance.

Jumping Rope

My goal is to make the tests and exercises in this book practical and efficient. Therefore, I want to incorporate as many *collateral benefits* as possible into the interval program. Collateral benefits complement the musculoskeletal system, improve posture, and simulate the reactions and speed of any chosen sport. Jumping rope fits the bill perfectly. Many have dismissed jumping rope as too simple to be considered a viable exercise option, probably due to today's flashy fitness and conditioning equipment market.

I know that even if I make an extremely strong case for jumping rope, many of you will skip over (pardon the pun) this section and go to a more glamorous plyometrics routine or, even worse, move directly into speed and agility work, thinking that jumping rope is a waste of time. People who never learned to jump rope or have a tough time with the technique are embarrassed because of their poor form and constant mistakes while jumping. This is precisely what makes jumping rope great.

Jumping rope is barely possible with poor form or poor technique. Everyone will make consistent mistakes and be interrupted by a rope that catches on a foot. The rope is the coach. Jumping rope is what I call a *self-limiting exercise.* Participants are limited in their ability to perform the exercise by lack of technique. In other words, truly poor technique will prevent the participant from performing the exercise, so bad movement patterns cannot be reinforced. This is the most important reason for jumping rope. It is possible to perform sprints, shuttles, and agility work with poor form as long as times are adequate. Other forms of popular endurance work such as jogging, cycling, and rowing can also allow poor form without supervision and coaching. Poor form can be reinforced without the athlete ever realizing it.

Jumping rope allows many athletes to self-train effectively, whereas self-training or training with a partner using running or sprints sometimes has too many uncontrollable variables. The jump rope is extremely portable and allows for position variations. Running, wind sprints, cycling, and rowing can provide a workout, burn calories, and improve stamina, but possibly by sacrificing technique, hurting reaction times, and altering ready position. Jumping rope, on the other hand, reinforces three basic movement patterns from the movement screen in chapter 5—the squat, hurdle step, and lunge—while providing a workout, burning calories, and improving stamina.

Variations can be performed to work on left-right differences. This is not possible in running or sprinting because both sides must work equally to propel the body forward. It is easy to focus on a weak side while skipping rope.

The three basic movement patterns used in a weight-training program will be used in a jump rope program:

1. **Squat stance:** Both feet placed side by side or slightly apart
2. **Hurdle step stance:** Single-leg stance in a stride position with one leg held at 90 degrees at both the hip and knee

3. **Lunge stance:** Also called the *scissors stance;* one foot in front and one foot behind, narrowing the base of support

These three key foot positions are used in most field and court sports. Regardless of skill level in any field or court sport, I recommend jumping rope as an excellent training tool that is both efficient and effective for reinforcing good movement patterns. Jumping rope will also help to develop great speed and agility and a power foundation for sports performance.

For swimmers and cyclists and other athletes who may feel jumping rope is not sport specific or functional, I still recommend rope work because it is an excellent way to cross-train. Athletes in sports such as ice hockey, cross-country running, Olympic-style weight lifting, and alpine skiing also benefit from the quick footwork involved in jumping rope. The stamina displayed by elite boxers and wrestlers has long stood as a testament to the effectiveness of jumping rope.

Distance runners, dancers, martial artists, and athletes in paddle sports may feel that jumping rope is not the best choice for improving stamina, but I disagree. Although jumping rope may not seem sport specific, it is extremely posture specific. It improves the ability to maintain a long spine and actually has far less impact than sprinting or jogging. I encourage endurance athletes who are not involved in field or court sports to study the literature and continue to explore the added benefits of interval training to complement sport-specific training.

Much of the impact of jumping rope is taken through the leg muscles. The erect posture and long spine forces the abdominal muscles to hold the midsection tight and work in perfect coordination with the back muscles to form the same kind of internal pressure as a weight belt.

Many athletes heel strike when running; heel striking jars the joints, and only a select few runners can do it correctly. At low mileage, jogging with heavy heel striking will not adversely affect the body. But working on endurance, performing intense intervals, and improving stamina requires a lot of work. Only a prototypical runner with a lean frame and exceptional technique would be able to run enough to benefit the legs and cardiovascular system without exposing the body to greater risk from musculoskeletal breakdown. Jumping rope combats this by forcing the athlete to land on the toes and use the untapped power in the calves and the combined power of the quads, hamstrings, glutes, and core.

The agility and quick direction changes needed in many sports require quick reactions and excellent footwork. This is not possible if the heel is planted on the ground. Major knee injuries are often noncontact injuries, caused by a twisting of the knee without any outside force. This is a result of sloppy training, poor body awareness, or unnecessary fatigue during competition, which reduces body awareness and forces greater stress on the knees. Although the knee is often the victim of injury, it rarely is the culprit. If the foot is planted and the ankle and hip are stiff, there is only one place for rotation to occur—the knee. Unfortunately, the knee was not designed to rotate as primary motion. Jumping rope teaches the athlete to stay on the toes and keep the calf ready for action, increasing his chance of pivoting on a good strong foot with most of his weight on the toe.

Consider one last fact about jumping rope. It takes less training time to jump rope than to run for the same benefits. Because jumping rope requires greater technique, it incorporates more muscles, both the muscles that move and those that hold the body stable. Jumping rope requires a greater expenditure of energy. Turning the rope increases the level of intensity. Periodic rest breaks are incorporated into the routine. Total time jumping rope is far less than total time in a continuous running or jogging workout. This results in greater workout intensity and reduced mechanical stress from impact at the same time.

Jumping rope is a natural choice for interval work. It provides an opportunity to practice breathing techniques that allow quicker recovery, which will help during a time-out situation or other rest break during competition. Experiment with your breathing and see which type (slow and deep, smooth and relaxed, and so on) will get you ready to jump again in the shortest amount of time.

Jumping rope toughens the body. It proves that quickness comes from staying relaxed in the extremities while keeping the spine erect and the abdominals drawn in and reinforces this pattern in your body. Pulling in the abs does not require holding the breath or tightening the stomach as if anticipating a blow to the gut. However, the more the trunk is held in the appropriate position and the more the extremities are relaxed, the quicker and more powerful movements will become.

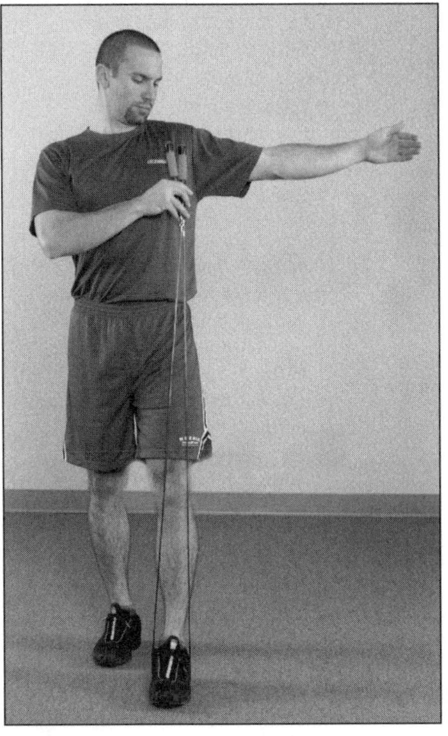

Figure 10.14 Measuring the jump rope.

First, measure the jump rope (figure 10.14). Stand on the rope with the left foot in the center of the body directly under the body and pull the handles of the rope up to your armpits. The handles should just graze the inside of the top of the armpits and go no higher than the top of your shoulders. Adjust the rope accordingly.

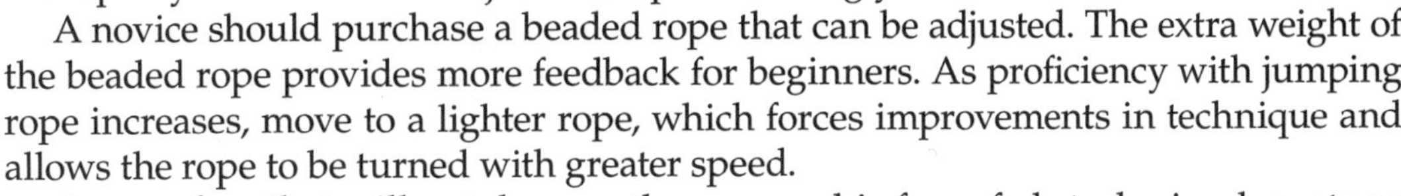

A novice should purchase a beaded rope that can be adjusted. The extra weight of the beaded rope provides more feedback for beginners. As proficiency with jumping rope increases, move to a lighter rope, which forces improvements in technique and allows the rope to be turned with greater speed.

Any surface that will not damage the rope and is free of obstacles is adequate as long as it is flat and fairly hard. Wooden floors, tile floors, asphalt surfaces, and concrete surfaces have all been used. Asphalt and concrete are rough on the texture of the rope and will break down the rope at a quicker rate. Another solution is to cut a small piece of plywood, 3 or 4 feet square, and lay it over grass that has been closely mowed. The grass will hold the board slightly above the ground, providing a forgiving surface while still allowing the rope to turn without catching on grass or other obstacles. This is a great alternative for the athlete on turf who wants to cross-train at practice.

Jumping rope can be used in conjunction with other activities. If running road work is deemed necessary, take the rope along. Create a personal interval routine, using a light jogging rest break as one interval and a vigorous bout of rope jumping as another. Use jumping rope as a complementary cross-training tool with cycling, swimming, exercise machines, and the slide board.

For all three foot positions, train in intervals. Experiment by going for 15, 20, or 30 seconds as fast as you can turn the rope. Rest for twice the amount of time you jumped, then try to jump the same amount in the same time to keep the intensity of each set near maximum. Find an exercise-to-rest ratio that you can use for 4 sets or more. Interval training is not just about timed exercise and timed rest. If you do not perform at a maximum level of intensity you will not push the anaerobic system to a higher level, which you must do to increase endurance. The aerobic system performance depends on the condition of the anaerobic system. Train this system and endurance will take care of itself.

SQUAT STANCE

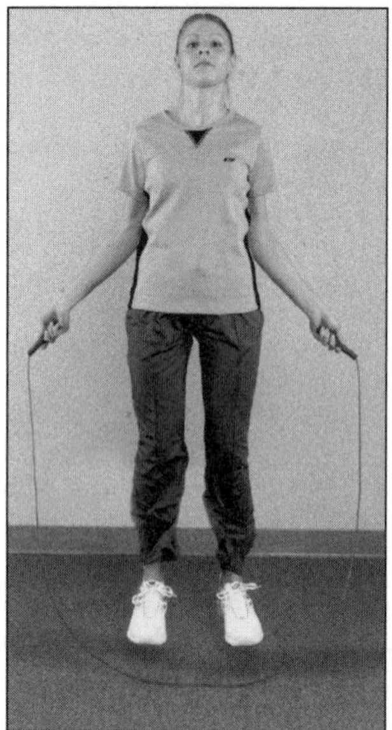

Figure 10.15 Jumping rope with the squat stance.

With feet slightly less than shoulder-width apart and the rope hanging behind the heels, swing the rope overhead and skip rope with equal weight on each foot (figure 10.15). Do not tighten the stomach muscles, but hold them in. Hold the spine tall, keep the shoulders back, and look forward with the head up straight and eyes forward. Keep your knees slightly bent and land on the toes, but not in an exaggerated way. Jump only high enough to clear the rope. If you find yourself double jumping (two skips to every rope turn), turn the rope faster.

If you cannot clear the rope for more than 10 repetitions, hold both handles in your dominant hand. Turn the rope with one hand and jump when you hear the rope strike the floor. This way you do not have to clear the rope but you learn to match the rhythm of the rope. Once you can complete at least 30 to 40 repetitions, switch the rope to your nondominant hand.

The motion of the arm or wrist is not what turns the rope. Once the rope starts turning (it's OK to use your wrist to get started), the up-and-down movement of the body keeps it in motion. Therefore, once the rope is spinning the wrist can relax by the side with very little circular motion. The momentum of the body going up and down should turn the rope. Keep it going fast enough with a little boost from your wrist action as needed.

The squat stance is the fundamental position for rope jumping. All other movements and foot positions will spring from your ability to perform this move. Even if mobility and stability testing did not reveal a problem with the squat, this is a good movement to start with if you have never jumped rope before. Learn to jump rope from the easiest position before working on a difficult position.

HURDLE STEP STANCE

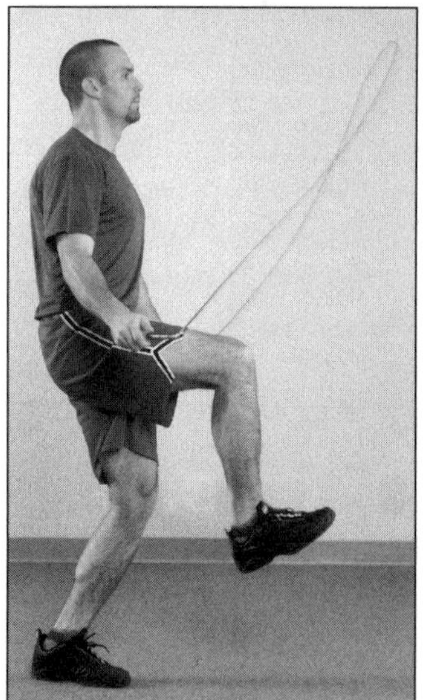

Figure 10.16 Jumping rope in the hurdle step stance.

Put all of your weight on one leg, slightly bending the knee. Shift most of the weight to the toes. Keep the spine tall and erect. Lift the other leg, bending it 90 degrees at the hip and knee. Swing the rope and skip over it, keeping the lifted leg as still as possible (figure 10.16). If this is difficult, start with a double-leg jump and then lift your leg.

If you still have difficulty clearing the rope as you jump, try both handles in one hand until you gain your rhythm. Take particular note of the lifted leg. Pretend you are balancing a flat rock on top of your lifted thigh. Keep the body rigid enough so that you can jump on one leg while holding the other leg in a position that would not cause the rock to fall. This improves core stability and helps improve stride by teaching you to relax one leg and stabilize the core while pushing off the other leg.

Work both legs equally unless you have greater difficulty on one side. Perform more sets on the weaker or slower side until both sides are equal.

LUNGE STANCE

The last position involves a modified lunge stance. Because a wide stance would not allow you to clear the rope, bring your feet closer together in a lunge position (one foot in front and one behind). The stance looks like someone water skiing on a slalom ski. Hold the spine erect and tall. The weight should be evenly distributed on both toes. Swing the rope and skip over it, lifting the front foot first, then the back foot (figure 10.17).

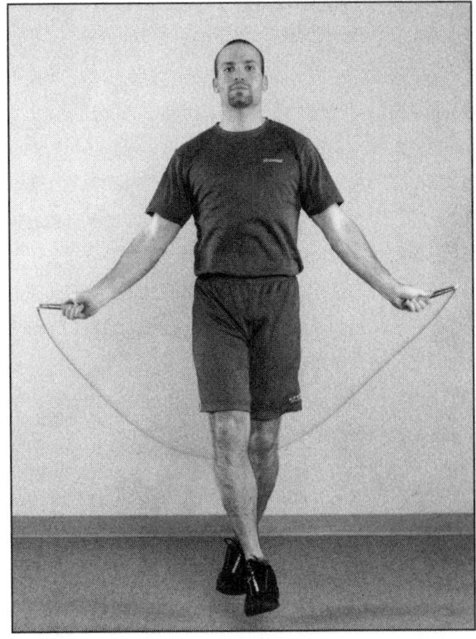

Figure 10.17 Jumping rope in the lunge stance.

Work both stances equally unless you have greater difficulty on one side. Perform more sets on the weaker or slower side until both sides are equal.

The hurdle step and lunge stances provide a good chance to compare left-right abilities. Count repetitions for each set of exercises and note whether the move is more difficult to perform on one side. Lack of coordination and stamina within a particular movement pattern may cause inefficient movement by increasing fatigue and hurting technique. During the rest interval, try stretching or mobility and stability exercises to reinforce the difficult movement pattern. For example, if you have difficulty jumping rope while standing on the left leg in a hurdle step position, perform the stride stretch on the left side between jumping sets.

Hill Running

Although many consider hill running to be as boring as jumping rope or running laps in the gym, it is an excellent foundation exercise. Hill running automatically induces the forward lean needed for proper sprint mechanics, explosive movements, and lateral agility work. Without realizing it, the athlete gets closer to the ground because he has to lean forward on an incline. The hill automatically teaches the athlete to bend the ankles, knees, and hips to a far greater extent to allow forward movement while keeping a tall spine and pulled-in abs.

The hill exaggerates the runner's stride. The runner has to pick up the front foot and stride high so that he does not catch the toe on the ground while simultaneously extending the rear hip as far as possible to get an adequate pushoff to accelerate up the hill. Basically the runner performs a scissors move or an exaggerated hurdle step; the changeover from the left to right leg also incorporates the lunge.

Many athletes have used bodybuilding and nonfunctional weight training to develop a lower body that is stronger than the core, and this breaks a law of nature. It is not possible or advantageous for the limbs of a tree to be stronger than the trunk, nor is it possible or advantageous for an athlete to perform efficiently if the strength and power in the legs exceeds the strength in the core. The exaggerated stride necessary in hill running will fatigue those who have poor mobility patterns identified by a poor movement screen score. Relax and move the legs.

The arm movement in hill running is a great way to learn to stabilize the core and move the legs. The abs balance the power between the upper and lower body. The arms counterbalance what the legs are doing. The spine must stabilize these two forces to maintain balance. Do not tighten the abs when running. This only limits the natural rotation needed to maximize stride length. Use the counterbalance of the arms. Exaggerating upper-body movement automatically elicits improved abdominal reactions as a counterbalance to the legs.

If the legs are already overdeveloped, tight, or excessively strong compared to the upper body and core, the body makes up for the lack of strength by increasing speed. Try pumping the arms faster or holding a small weight in each palm (for example, a roll of quarters or up to a two-pound dumbbell). Reduce the weight and increase arm speed as you improve.

Increasing arm speed will increase leg speed and improve spine stability. Imagine parallel bars as you run up the hill. Throw the arm out and grab the bar, pulling through as you step with the opposite leg. By using weights, increasing arm speed, and visualizing parallel bars, you will slowly improve running technique by naturally using the arms and not just arbitrarily swinging.

Hill running is low impact compared to flat running. The runner has to overcome gravity to accelerate up the hill. The incline causes the ground to come up to meet the feet, so the landing is lower impact than in flat running. Therefore, the hips can be trained extremely hard. It's possible to challenge the stride with every sprint without beating or pounding the body. It's easier on the joints, which is vital when working on technique. Hill running promotes toe running. It promotes forward leaning and arm pumping. It is hard to cheat the hill.

Hill running is a natural interval. After sprinting up the hill, you need to get back down so that you can do another sprint up the hill. Many techniques can be used to get down the hill, but running should not be one of them—not yet. Try a side step to stretch the groin; step backward, elongating the stride; or simply walk down the hill using an effective form of breathing to facilitate recovery before the next hill sprint. The interval is built in.

The best hill will have closely mowed grass that is well packed and free of obstacles. A good substitute is any (safe) paved incline, ramp, or grade free of traffic. An incline treadmill is not an option for many biomechanical reasons. It does not adequately simulate what the hill and gravity naturally do. A treadmill does not allow a free arm swing or a natural stride. Also, because the treadmill is driven by a motor, runners have the tendency to run faster than natural in an incline position. This reinforces poor biomechanics and creates a risk of injury.

Many athletes use stadium stairs or staircases to substitute for hill running. If this is all that is available, work with what you have. With stairs, you have to worry about foot placement, and there is a slightly greater chance of injury because the stair length may not be matched to your natural stride. If a hill or an incline is not accessible, pulling a sled is probably the next best thing. I recommend pulling the sled rather than running stadium stairs or steps. Many conditioning catalogs offer sleds that can be weighted or unloaded. They also offer excellent harnesses. Start with the sled attached to a waist belt. Use the forward lean and arm speed to move the weight. It is best to slightly overload the sled so that you do not overrun. You have to constantly pump the legs and arms. As you develop strength, look into a shoulder harness, but do only half as much shoulder harness training as waist training. Part of acceleration is allowing the natural arm swing to occur. When you resist through the shoulders, you reduce this. However, it may be advantageous for football linemen, wrestlers, rugby players, and other athletes who have to push with the upper body and drive with the lower body.

PART IV

POWER, SPEED, AND AGILITY

11

Power, Speed, and Agility Testing

In the book *What Makes Winners Win* by Charlie Jones, baseball great Tony Gwynn recounts, "There were always coaches who said that I couldn't do something. I couldn't throw, I couldn't hit with power, I couldn't run, I couldn't field my position. I think that's one of the reasons I've been successful, because they can measure everything you do on the field, but they cannot measure what's inside of you and what drives you. It's easy to cheat yourself and do just enough to get by, but that's what everybody can do, just enough to get by. But those who want to be successful and maintain that level of success have got to push a little bit harder and do a little bit more."

I think Tony is trying to say that you should not simply define yourself by the things you measure but by how you plan to deal with the measurable goals you have set for yourself. The testing and ranking that you will do in this chapter with respect to your power, speed, and agility will show you where you are now. Where you decide to go and how you decide to get there is what will define you.

Defining Power, Speed, and Agility

Power equals work divided by time. This concept can be confusing. Two people who max out on the bench press at 375 pounds demonstrate the same strength because they move the same weight over the same distance. However, a closer analysis may show that one athlete has excellent technique and brisk movement and takes 2 to 3 seconds to perform the lift from start to finish while the other athlete may struggle with poor form, taking 10 to 15 seconds to perform the same lift. From a work standpoint, these athletes display the same strength, but the athlete who takes less time demonstrates greater power.

Consider another example. Two athletes display the same strength in the squat rack but differ greatly in jumping ability. Even though the athletes demonstrate the same amount of strength, the better jumper demonstrates better power. Therefore, a person can show power not simply by gaining strength but by taking the strength he has and learning to become more efficient, coordinated, and smooth with his movements.

Think of power as adding quickness to strength and speed to endurance. You should have a good strength base before adding quickness, and you need to develop endurance before adding speed. The word *agility* is often coupled with the words *power, speed,* and *quickness;* but the best definition for agility is "quickness under control." An example of good agility is extreme accuracy and power when throwing, swinging, or punching or quick acceleration, deceleration, or direction change when running, jumping, or cutting. By moving quickly and efficiently, you emphasize timing and coordination in a workout. Usually relaxation, timing, and coordination allow a person to move with more power, not just harder or more forcefully. Testing for power, speed, and agility allows you to track your baseline and continuously monitor efficiency.

Power, Speed, and Agility Assessment

The tests in this chapter have been chosen specifically for their effectiveness. It is a good idea for a coach or trainer experienced in testing protocol and safety to guide and monitor the tests. The coach or trainer may also be able to provide feedback regarding weak links and give overall appraisals of strengths and weaknesses.

These tests provide feedback in specific categories of performance. These tests represent only a small sampling of a large group of tests used to chart performance; but they are enough to get you started and provide a basic picture of performance, strengths, and weaknesses. Data tables are included so that you can compare your scores to those of others in your sport. Many other factors—such as skill, competitive spirit, experience, and emotional state—come into play in assessing total athletic performance.

The power, agility, and speed assessment includes the following tests:

1. **Power tests:** One-repetition maximum power clean, vertical jump
2. **Agility tests:** T-test, hexagon test
3. **Speed tests:** 120-yard dash, 300-yard shuttle

POWER TEST 1: ONE-REPETITION MAXIMUM POWER CLEAN

This test assesses anaerobic maximum muscular power and high-speed strength. This test was chosen because the data available will help you rank yourself with others in your same age, sex, and sport category (see table 11.1).

You will need an Olympic-style weightlifting set to accommodate your maximum or perceived maximum lift with weight in 5-pound gradations and a lifting platform clear of obstructions and other weight-training equipment. You should wear normal weight-training footwear and the platform should have a nonskid surface.

Place your feet approximately shoulder-width apart with toes turned out slightly. The bar should be approximately 1 to 2 inches from your shins and over the balls of your feet. Squat down while maintaining a flat back so that you can comfortably grab the bar wider than shoulder width with your arms comfortably outside your knees (figure 11.1a). Your elbows should be fully extended and you can readjust the bar to maintain the 1-inch distance from your shin. The shoulders should be relaxed. The chest should be up and out and you should be looking forward or slightly downward.

Lift the bar off the floor as you extend the hips and knees. The torso should remain in the same flat-back position. The hips and shoulders should move upward at the same rate. Keep the elbows fully extended and raise the bar in a vertical plane very close to the shins

Table 11.1 Power Clean Data for Athletes in Different Sports

Sport	1RM power clean (lb)	1RM power clean (kg)
College baseball (men)*	207	94
College basketball (men)*	192	87
College track (women)*	106	48
NCAA Division IA college football (starting players)**		
Quarterbacks, running backs, fullbacks	264	120
Tight ends, wide receivers	259	118
Offensive linemen	294	134
Defensive tackles, defensive ends	298	135
Linebackers	305	139
Defensive backs	269	122
NCAA Division IA college football (non-starting players)**		
Quarterbacks, running backs, fullbacks	241	110
Tight ends, wide receivers	237	108
Offensive linemen	280	127
Defensive tackles, defensive ends	274	125
Linebackers	297	135
Defensive backs	247	112

* Values are either means or 50th percentiles.
** Values are means.

Adapted from Harman, Garhammer, and Pandorf 2000.

but not touching them. Raise the bar above the knees as you continue to extend the hips and maintain a flat spine. Keep elbows extended. Slightly flex the knees and set the body for the second pull phase.

In a brisk movement, extend the hips and knees and plantar flex the ankles as if you were jumping. The movement should quickly and crisply accelerate the bar upward. The bar can remain near or in contact with the front of the thighs and should remain as close to the body as possible while the back remains flat and the elbows remain extended. As the shoulders reach their highest elevation in a shrug position, the elbows should flex and the body should be pulled under the bar. The continual pull of the arms should last as long as possible until the body is under the bar and ready for the catch phase of the movement.

In the catch phase, simultaneously flex the hips and knees into a quarter-squat or slightly deeper position. The elbows should be pointed forward with the upper arm as close to parallel to the floor as possible. The bar should rest on the clavicles and anterior deltoids and the palms should be pointing toward the ceiling (figure 11.1b). The torso should remain in a flat-back and erect position. The feet should remain flat and the head should be in a neutral position looking forward or slightly up.

In the lowering phase, you can either take a step forward and rack the weight on a squat rack that has already been adjusted to your shoulder height or you can gradually lower the weight through your arms and allow a controlled descent to your thigh. Flex the hips and knees to cushion the impact of the bar on the thighs. With the elbows fully extended, squat down until the bar is replaced on the floor.

It is generally recommended that you perform a light set with 5 to 10 repetitions followed by 2 heavier sets of 2 to 5 repetitions (if needed) before the 1RM attempt. Following the warm-up, rest for 2 to 4 minutes and estimate your maximum lift. Since the heavy warm-up sets should have been near your maximum load, you should have a good idea of what your maximum load will be. If you are successful with your first estimate, take another 2- to 4-minute rest break and make a 10- to 20-pound load increase and attempt the one-repetition maximum again. Repeat until you find your 1RM. Ideally, you should achieve your 1RM within 5 testing sets.

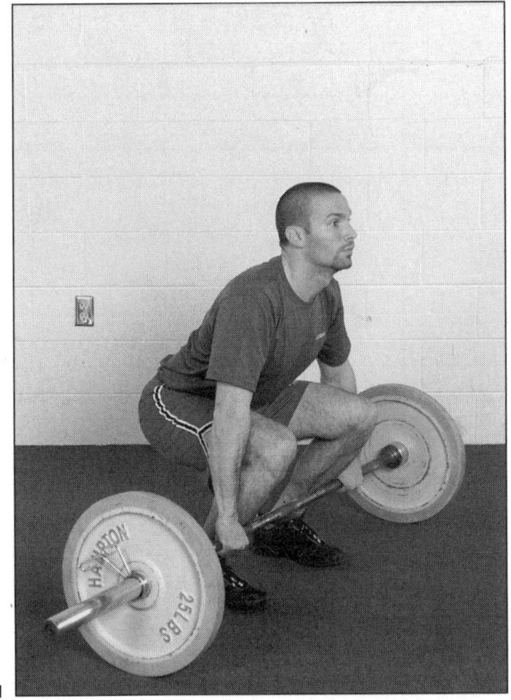

a

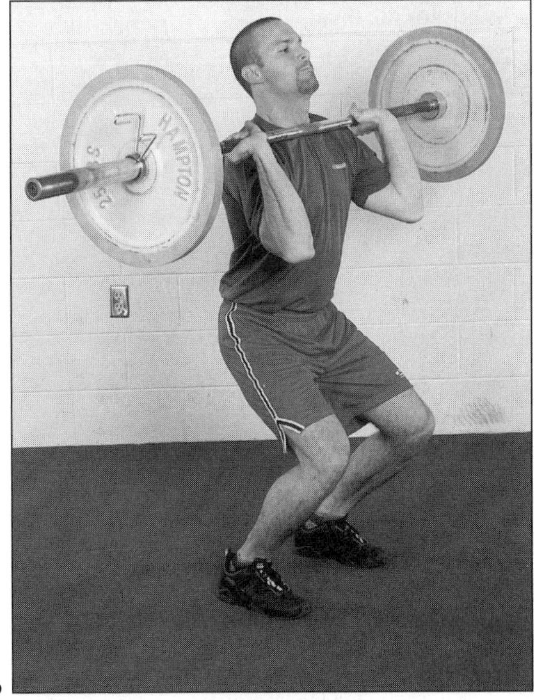

b

Figure 11.1 One-repetition maximum power clean: *(a)* squat down to grab the bar; *(b)* catch the bar.

POWER TEST 2: VERTICAL JUMP

The data shown in table 11.2 will help you rank yourself with others in your same age, sex, and sport category.

Find a flat surface to jump from that provides good traction, is free of obstructions, and is near a smooth wall that is higher than your maximum jump. Get chalk or powder that is a different color than the wall and a measuring tape or yardstick.

Rub chalk on the fingers of your dominant hand and stand away from the wall with about 6 inches between your shoulder and the wall. Stand with your heels flat and feet together.

Table 11.2 Vertical Jump Data for Athletes in Different Sports

Sport	Vertical jump (in.)	Vertical jump (cm)
NCAA Division I college football		
Split ends, strong safetys, offensive and defensive backs	31.5	80
Wide receivers and outside linebackers	31	79
Linebackers, tight ends, safetys	29.5	75
Quarterbacks	28.5	72
Defensive tackles	28	71
Offensive tackles	25 to 26	64 to 66
Offensive guards	27	69
College football	21	53
College basketball (men)	27 to 29	69 to 74
NCAA Division I college basketball (men)	28	71
College basketball (women)	21	53
NCAA Division II college basketball (women)		
Guards	19	48
Forwards	18	46
Centers	17.5	44
Competitive college athletes (men)	25 to 25.5	64 to 65
Competitive college athletes (women)	16 to 18.5	41 to 47
Recreational college athletes (men)	24	61
Recreational college athletes (women)	15 to 15.5	38 to 39
College baseball (men)	23	58
College tennis (men)	23	58
College tennis (women)	15	38

Values are either means or 50th percentiles.

Adapted from Harman, Garhammer, and Pandorf 2000.

Reach as high as you can onto the wall and make an initial mark (figure 11.2a). Make sure the mark is visible before you perform the vertical leap. If the mark is visible, prepare for the vertical leap by squatting without stepping or moving the feet. Explode as high as you can, arm fully extended overhead, and place a second mark on the wall at the height of your jump (figure 11.2b). Perform three vertical jumps and take the best of the three trials to the nearest half-inch.

You can also do a ratio test with the vertical jump by comparing a single-leg vertical leap on the left to a single-leg vertical leap on the right. Look for differences greater than 10 to 15 percent. Follow the instructions for the vertical leap, except jump off one leg only. For safety, land on both feet. If you have a difference between the right- and left-leg performance of greater than 15 percent, you should focus on single-leg performance until the difference is below 15 percent. Otherwise your double-leg jumping assessment is limited by the side that is performing poorly.

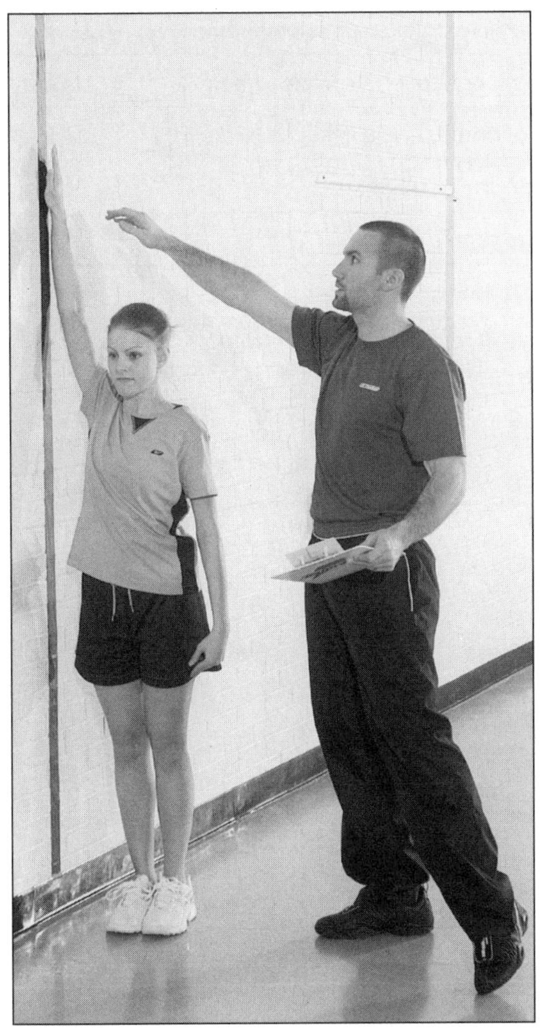

a

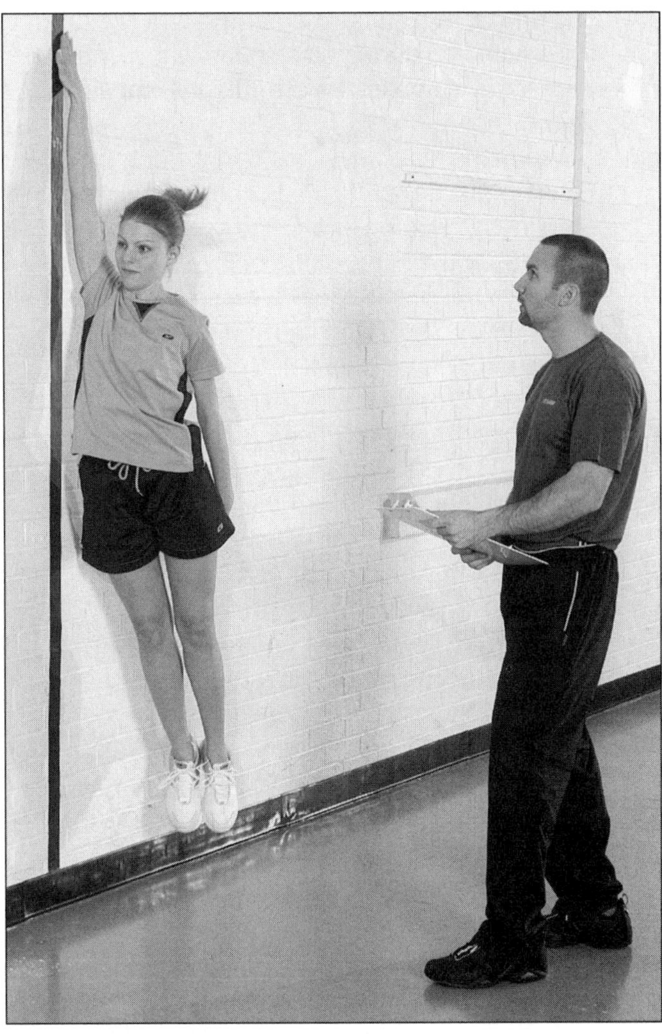

b

Figure 11.2 Vertical jump test: *(a)* make the initial mark on the wall; *(b)* jump up and mark the wall at the height of your jump.

AGILITY TEST 1: T-TEST

The data shown in table 11.3 will help you rank yourself with others in your same age, sex, and sport category.

You will need four cones, a stopwatch, a flat floor that provides good traction and is free of obstructions, and a person who can serve as a timer and spotter. Place two cones 10 yards apart to indicate the first line of the T-test (figure 11.3). Place the other two cones exactly 5 yards to the left and right of one of the cones. This should create a perfect T with cones at the end of each line and at the intersection of the two lines. You should go through a standard warm-up and set of stretches before this full-speed, vigorous drill.

When the timer says "go," sprint along the first line, starting at the first cone you placed (cone A). Sprint forward to the second cone (cone B) at the intersection of the two lines. When you arrive at cone B, touch the base and quickly shuffle to the left to cone C. As you shuffle, remember to face forward and never cross the feet. Touch the base of cone C with your left hand, change directions, and shuffle back past cone B to the last cone (cone D). Touch the base of cone D with your right hand. Change directions again. Shuffle to the left for 5 yards and touch the base of cone B with the left hand. Then run backward past cone A as quickly as possible. The timer stops the watch the moment you pass cone A. Be careful as you run backward. It is a good idea for the timer to be in position to catch you or slow you down, or to have a mat to soften the blow if you trip and fall.

Perform two trials of the T-test and take the best time. Times will be recorded to the nearest tenth of a second. Do not count the time on the test if you cross your feet, fail to face forward the entire time, or miss touching the base of any of the cones.

Table 11.3 T-Test Data for Athletes in Different Sports

Sport	Time (s)
College basketball (men)	8.9
College basketball (women)	9.9
Competitive college athletes (men)	10.0
Competitive college athletes (women)	10.8
Recreational college athletes (men)	10.5
Recreational college athletes (women)	12.5
College baseball (men)	9.2
College tennis (men)	9.4
College tennis (women)	11.1

Values are either means or 50th percentiles.

Adapted from Harman, Garhammer, and Pandorf 2000.

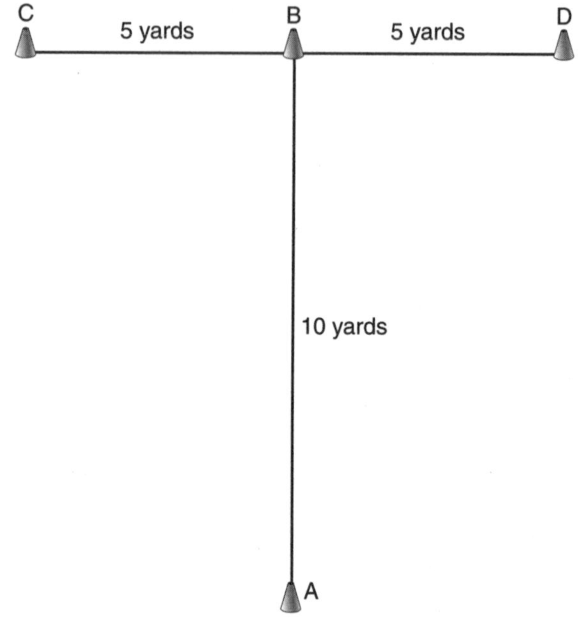

Figure 11.3 Setup for the T-test.

Adapted, by permission, from D. Semenick, 1990, "Tests and measurement: The t-test," *NCSA Journal* 12(1):36-37.

AGILITY TEST 2: HEXAGON TEST

The data shown in table 11.4 will help you rank yourself with others in your same age, sex, and sport category.

You will need adhesive tape that contrasts with the color of the floor or surface, a standard stopwatch, and a flat floor clear of obstructions with a nonslip surface.

Create a hexagon on the floor using the adhesive tape in 24-inch lengths (figure 11.4). Each of the six sides will intersect at 120-degree angles. Start in the center of the hexagon and remain facing in the same direction throughout the entire test. On the "go" command, the stopwatch starts. Hop to the side in front of you and perform a double-leg hop over the line. Hop back to the center then hop to the next side, working in a clockwise sequence until you have hopped over each of the six sides three times. The stopwatch will be stopped when you return to the center of the hexagon after your third time around the hexagon. If you land on a line, lose your balance, or have to take a step, stop the test and restart after resting for 1 to 2 minutes. The score will be the best time of three trials. Remember, there must be 18 total jumps free from mistakes to constitute a valid test.

Table 11.4 Hexagon Test Data for Athletes in Different Sports

Sport	Time (s)
Competitive college athletes (men)	12.3
Competitive college athletes (women)	12.9
Recreational college athletes (men)	12.3
Recreational college athletes (women)	13.2

Values are either means or 50th percentiles.

Adapted from Harman, Garhammer, and Pandorf 2000.

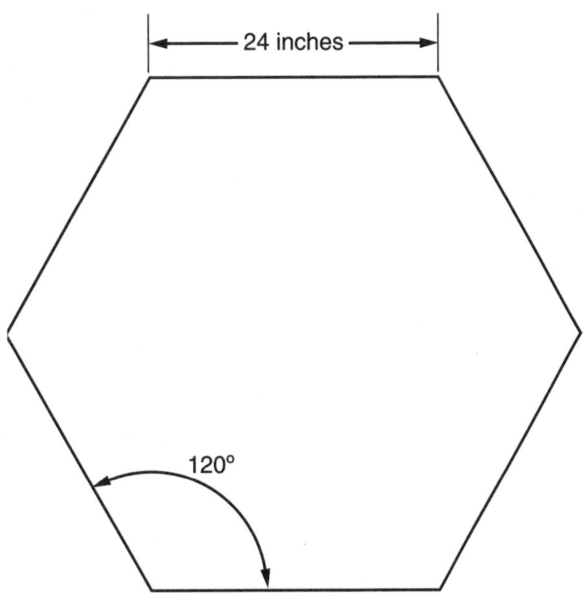

Figure 11.4 Setup for the hexagon test.

Adapted, by permission, from K. Pauole, K. Madole, J. Garhammer, M. Lacourse, and R. Rozenek, 2000, "Reliability and validity of the t-test as a measure of agility, leg power, and leg speed in college age males and females," *Journal of Strength and Conditioning Research* 14.

SPEED TEST 1: 120-YARD DASH

I personally think that this is one of the most ingenious and practical tests because, to quote the authors of *Sports Speed,* it "provides information on practically all phases of sprinting, speed and quickness including the start, acceleration, maximum speed and speed endurance with just one sprint." This test will take a little extra setup time and requires some minor calculations, but I feel that it has applications in nearly all sports. Running movement is fundamental and if it is not a part of your sport it can still be an effective means of cross-training and balancing the body. It is important to understand where your sprinting strengths and weaknesses are. Arbitrarily running wind sprints will not expose or isolate your weakest link with respect to sprinting.

You will need approximately 130 to 140 yards free of obstructions, preferably on a safe running surface, such as a track or a well-groomed turf. You will need three timers with stopwatches at the 40-, 80-, and 120-yard marks. To help the timers, you can also stretch a piece of tape across your running path at these positions. As you break the tape, the timer will know to mark the time.

Start in a sprinter stance or a three-point football stance. On the "go" command from the first timer at the 40-yard mark, begin to sprint. Sprint as fast as you can throughout the entire 120 yards and through the 120-yard mark; do not decelerate until you have passed the last timer. The first timer stops the watch as you pass him at the 40-yard mark. At this exact instant, the timer at the 80-yard mark starts his watch and stops it when you cross the 80-yard mark. At the 80-yard mark, the timer at the 120-yard mark starts his watch and stops it as you pass the 120-yard mark. Record the three times—the stationary 40 (0 to 40 yards), the flying 40 (40 to 80 yards), and the 80 to 120 time.

To assess acceleration, subtract flying 40-yard time from stationary 40-yard time and record the difference. This difference is your time delay required to accelerate. If there is more than a 0.7-second difference, it is recommended that you improve acceleration. This can be accomplished by balancing the body, by building a strength base, and by building a power base specifically with plyometrics, power movements, heel running, jumping rope, and sprint-starts.

To quickly ascertain how fast you should already be sprinting in a 40-yard dash from a stationary start, add 0.7 seconds to your flying 40-yard dash time. With appropriate acceleration training, this is what your 40-yard dash should be.

Next calculate speed endurance. Compare your flying 40 time to your 80 to 120 time. If these scores happen to be the same or almost the same, you are in excellent physical condition, according to the authors of *Sports Speed,* to "sprint a short distance such as 40 yards repeatedly during soccer, football, basketball, rugby, lacrosse or field hockey without slowing down due to fatigue." If these two scores differ by more than two-tenths of a second, target speed endurance in your training. The authors of *Sports Speed* say, "Speed endurance is easy to improve. You only need to sprint short distances 2 or 3 times per week and keep a record of how many repetitions you sprinted, how far you sprinted, and how much recovery time you took between each repetition. The rest is easy. On each workout, you simply increase the sprint distance and decrease the recovery time between each repetition. In a period of 6 to 8 weeks, your speed endurance scores will be better."

SPEED TEST 2: 300-YARD SHUTTLE

You will need two stopwatches, a measured course of 25 yards free of obstructions with a nonslip surface, and tape or cones to mark the lines at each end of the 25-yard course (figure 11.5).

Perform a standard warm-up and stretch routine before testing. On the timer's "go" command, sprint the length of the 25-yard course, touch the line with your foot, and return to the starting line. Touch the starting line with your foot and sprint back and forth until you complete six round trips. Immediately after you cross the finish line after the sixth trip, the second stopwatch is started. Record the time of your 300-yard shuttle. Rest for 5 minutes. After exactly 5 minutes, report to the starting line to repeat the 300-yard shuttle test. Take the average of the two 300-yard shuttle sprints and record times to the nearest tenth of a second.

The two times (fresh shuttle compared to the shuttle after the 5-minute rest) should be close. This will demonstrate good recovery and speed endurance. Of course this will not be accurate if you do not try as hard as you possibly can on each test.

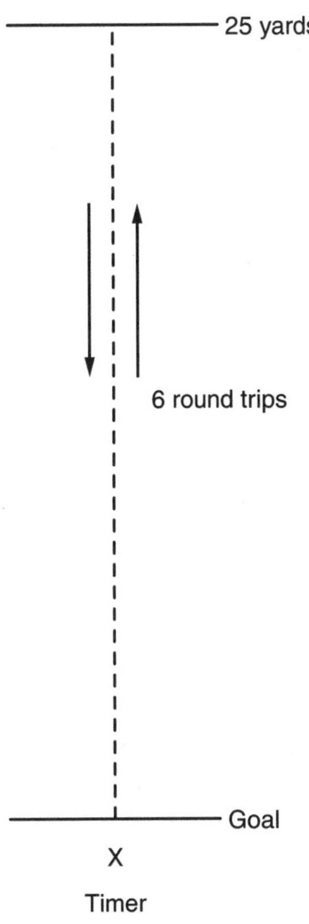

Figure 11.5 Setup for the 300-yard shuttle test.

Adapted, by permission, from G.M. Gilliam, 1983, "300-yard shuttle run," *NSCA Journal* 5(5):46.

12

Speed and Quickness Training

Developing endurance is not just about aerobic conditioning. Anaerobic conditioning is fundamental to most sports. It's important for athletes to develop the ability to recover from quick bursts of explosive activity. Endurance for sports is not about how long you can maintain a steady state of activity; it is the capacity to explode, react, recover, and maintain skill no matter what you're up against.

Buddy Lee provides a good example of this point. He trained as a wrestler and cross-trained at such a high intensity level that no one could keep up with him—he could wear down most opponents in the first period. This was part of his strategy: to wrestle his opponent at an intensity level that took him away from his comfort zone, forcing him to wrestle Buddy's way. Buddy's conditioning was purely anaerobic, and it allowed him to compete at a high level during regulation time and overtime.

As you read this chapter and consider what you will be doing with your speed and quickness training, use the words of George Allen to keep your perspective: "Do the ordinary things in an extraordinary way."

Learning to move with speed and quickness is difficult. To be successful, start with activities that are simple and save yourself the frustration of trying to move quickly through a difficult activity. Pick a basic activity, one that may even be considered boring, and then move faster and faster until the body begins to feel the quickness. Learn to breathe, relax, and recover between sets.

In this chapter you will work with a basic power move for the upper body (power push-ups) and lower body (rope jumping for speed). The challenge is to significantly improve your ability with both. Resist the desire to move to the next chapter and do the more specific drills. Your ability to move with speed, power, and quickness has as much to do with your mental state as your physical state. There are many things you can do to improve your speed and quickness immediately. You can balance your body with a more individualized and specific warm-up. You can reduce your tension and anxiety by breathing slower and deeper before the activity and during recovery. Don't tell your body to move fast; *let* you body move fast. Learn to do these things with simple activities and you will gain the ability to do them with more advanced movements and skills.

Instead of remembering many things about technique in a given activity, you can change just one thing that seems to have an overall correcting effect. I have watched many great sprint coaches at work, and the best are able to reduce instructions to one or two simple comments. I have gotten many athletes to produce better sprint times by simply telling them to pump their arms faster and farther or exaggerate the arm movement. I could have told them to hold the spine taller, stabilize the pelvis better, pick up the knees higher, explode through hip extension with more force, and reduce wasted movement caused by head bobbing. But because exaggerating the arm swing fixes all of those problems in most cases, why bog the athlete down with all of those other instructions?

When an average athlete (not an elite sprinter) exaggerates the arm movement, the core becomes more stable. The arms automatically counterbalance the legs. The swing of one arm creates a counterrotation between the hip and shoulders that complements the work of the core stabilizers. Swinging the arms faster and farther produces greater stability throughout the core, which usually results in greater mobility of the hips, which improves stride, cadence, symmetry, and rhythm.

My point is that in many cases you can do one thing to fix many biomechanical problems. In the strength and endurance training section, I talk about a tall spine for that very reason. A tall spine helps you do many other things correctly.

Start with these two drills. Learn what you can do to quickly improve performance. Write down the things you did to move faster and recover quicker and take those things to the advanced drills in the next chapter. If you go to the next chapter without that knowledge, you will still do well, but the best of the best have and use that knowledge every day. If you can't learn to do the simple things fast, do you really have a foundation for the advanced skills?

I meet many young pitchers who are pretty good for their age. Many complain of shoulder, elbow, and low back pain. Some have poor mobility, but few can do one push-up with a clap. These young athletes can control a baseball with a fast, explosive movement but cannot control their own bodies with the same quality. I use the push-up with the clap to show them that they have a lot of work to do with respect to total conditioning. Most pitchers who specialize early will never make it to any level of pitching significance simply because they focus on the skill of pitching before they consider the mobility, stability, balance, and power that will keep them efficient and effective for the long haul.

Jumping Rope for Speed

In chapter 10 I introduced jumping rope as a method of interval training to improve endurance and stamina. It's basic, fundamental, safe, and self-limiting (meaning it's impossible to do incorrectly). It is extremely difficult to turn the rope fast and have poor posture and poor mechanics at the same time. So take time to learn the rope. Review and reread the jump rope program basics in chapter 10 (pages 125 to 127). Perform the basic moves as fast as possible and use multiple sets to increase work volume.

Use jump rope work to create speed intervals in the same way endurance intervals were performed. Endurance work is about volume, and speed work is about performance. So lengthen your rest breaks and go for greater speed in your rope turns. The purpose for the longer rest is to gain enough recovery to nearly equal your fresh (first set) speed performance.

Plyometrics Training

Plyometrics is another good way to increase speed and quickness. One of the oldest upper-body plyometrics moves is a push-up with a clap. Again, some athletes may consider this move basic or boring, but learning it can be very enlightening when trying to learn to move with speed and quickness.

PUSH-UP WITH A CLAP

Begin down on the floor in a traditional push-up position (figure 12.1a). Accelerate as you push up off the floor, lifting both hands at the top of the move and clapping them together (figure 12.1b). Quickly return both hands to the floor to catch yourself, then repeat the move. Three to 4 sets of 5 to 15 repetitions will give you a good upper-body power base.

If this is difficult, start with the hands on a stable, elevated surface, such as a step or bench. This will shift more of the weight to the feet and allow quick movement with less stress on the arms. Progress to lower elevations as you exceed 15 repetitions with good form.

For example, start on the third step on a standard set of indoor or outdoor stairs. As strength and power develop, move to the second step, then the first step. Eventually you will not need the elevated surface.

a

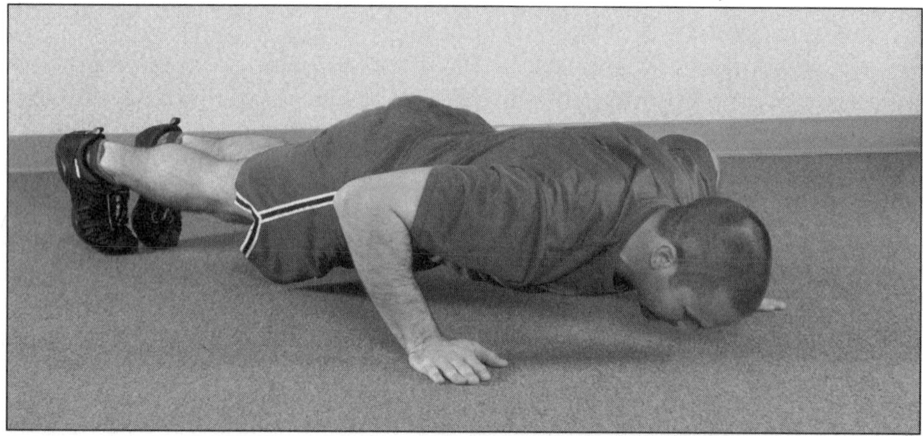

b

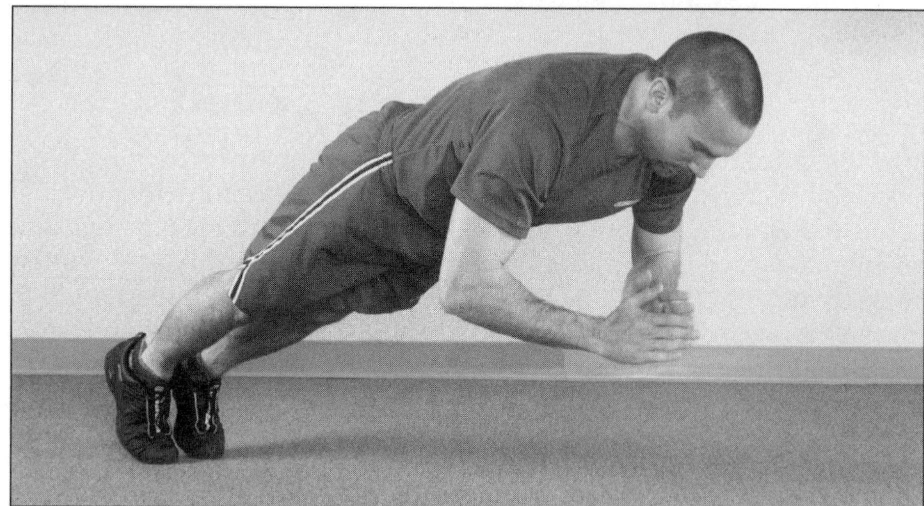

Figure 12.1 Push-up with a clap: *(a)* begin in push-up position; *(b)* when you push up off the floor, lift both hands and clap.

SHOULDER-TAP PUSH-UP

If the push-up with a clap is difficult, try a shoulder-tap push-up. The move looks the same, but instead of lifting both hands off the ground and clapping them together, leave one hand on the floor and lift the other hand across the body, tapping the chest or shoulder on the opposite side (figure 12.2). Quickly return the hand to the original position and repeat the push-up, lifting the other hand and tapping the chest or shoulder. This move challenges the trunk and teaches the muscles of the core to kick in appropriately when weight is shifted to one arm. After a week or two of doing the shoulder-tap push-up, try the push-up with a clap.

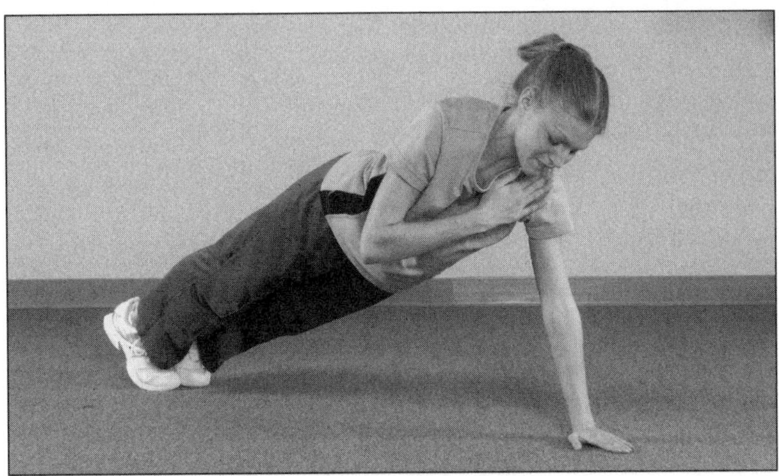

Figure 12.2 Shoulder-tap push-up.

SHORT-ARM PUSH-UP

If you have never done push-ups before and find both of these exercises extremely difficult, it isn't necessary to do a full-depth push-up. Bend the elbows halfway and go through the motion only in the upper half of the range (figure 12.3). This is a short-arm push-up. Some consider it cheating, but it's only cheating if an athlete continues to train this way after getting strong enough to move on to regular push-ups. Use the short-arm push-up to develop proficiency and stability in the shoulder and trunk, then move on to a full range of motion and add the clap.

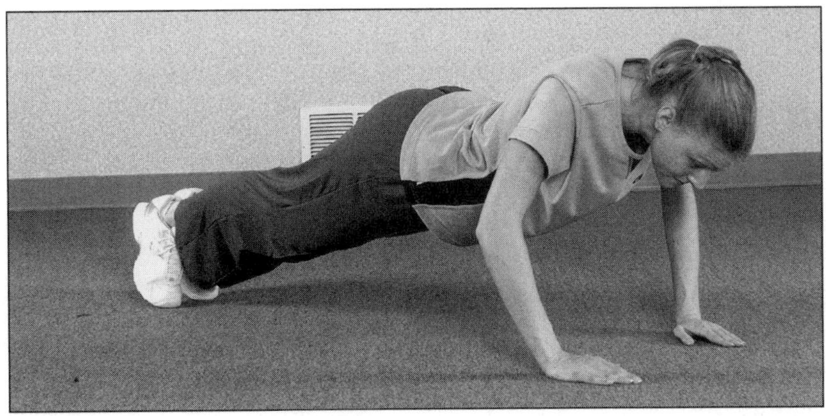

Figure 12.3 Short-arm push-up.

PLYOMETRICS PUSH-UPS

You will need a 5- to 8-pound medicine ball. Start in a normal push-up position, only place the hands closer together on top of the medicine ball (figure 12.4a). Elbows are extended. Knees are straight. The entire spine is straight with no sag in the lower back. Eyes are focused on the medicine ball.

Quickly move the hands from the medicine ball to the floor at a slightly greater distance than shoulder width (figure 12.4b). Flex the elbows as you descend, allowing the chest to nearly touch the medicine ball. When your chest nearly touches the medicine ball, explode by extending the elbows with enough force to propel back to the starting position. Quickly move your hands back onto the medicine ball. At the height of the explosive movement, the hands should be slightly higher than the medicine ball, allowing you to come back onto the medicine ball and resume the starting position.

To make the exercise easier, reduce the size (diameter) of the ball. Increase the size of the ball to make the exercise more difficult. If you can comfortably perform 8 to 12 repetitions, you have chosen the right ball. If you cannot complete 8 to 12 repetitions with good form, try a smaller ball. If you can perform more than 15 repetitions with good form, try a larger ball. Perform 3 to 4 sets with rest breaks between sets, not to exceed 2 minutes.

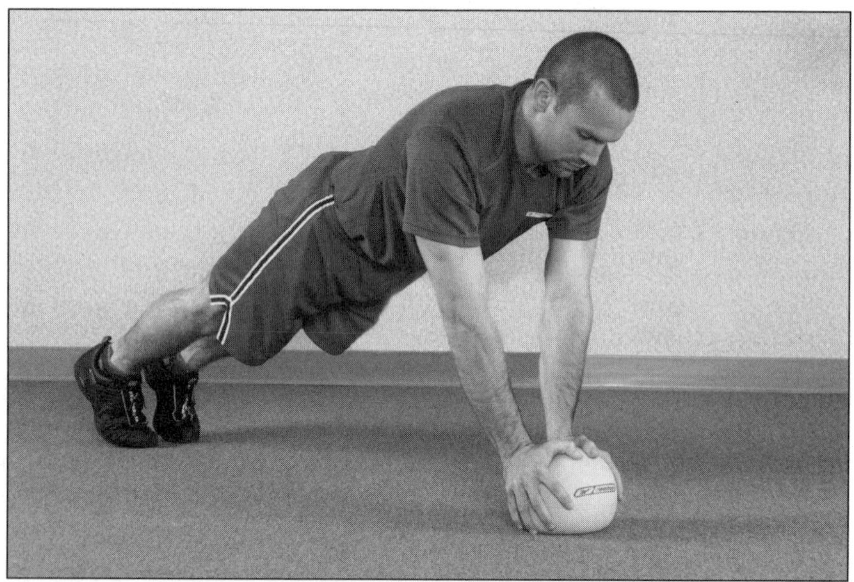

a

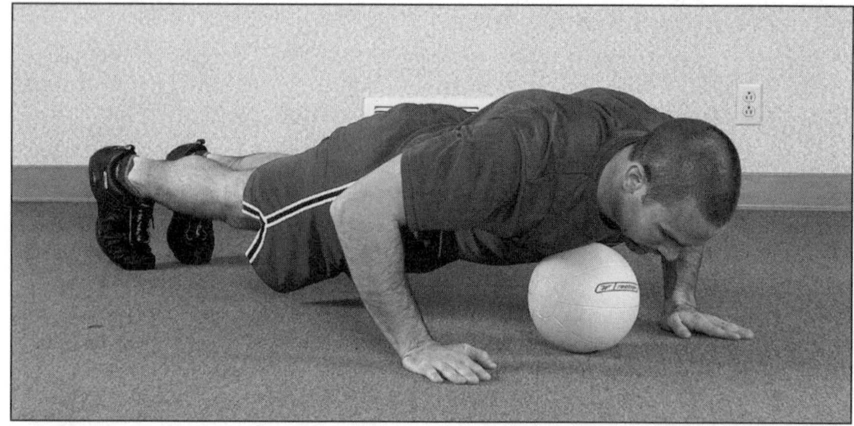

b

Figure 12.4 Plyometrics push-up: *(a)* begin in push-up position with hands on a medicine ball; *(b)* move hands from ball to floor.

Learning to Relax

The push-up with a clap and the shoulder-tap push-up are two basic activities that are safe and require little time, space, and equipment. While doing these exercises, consider the fundamental essence of becoming quicker and developing speed—learning to relax in a situation that normally does not encourage relaxation. Body stress and tension only deplete energy and misdirect focus.

Most great athletes have a ritual that helps them focus. An infielder may fiddle with a spot on his glove. An elite tennis player may adjust the racket strings after a hard shot even though the strings do not need adjusting. A football kicker or punter may take a deep breath and shake his head right to left before the snap. A batter might swing a heavy bat. A golfer may do trunk twists while holding a club across her shoulders.

Between each set of jumping rope or push-ups, develop a relaxation ritual. It may be as simple as leaning left and right and stretching the back or leaning forward and backward and performing toe touches and backbends. It may mean pacing back and forth with eyes closed and focusing on the movements just performed. It doesn't matter what the ritual is; it matters what the ritual *does.* It should redirect focus and help the athlete relax. When developing a ritual to use between bouts of speed, quickness, and power, consider these four words: *relax, recover, recall,* and *repeat.*

- **Relax.** Any ritual should promote relaxation. Control breathing. Increase the amount of air inhaled and exhaled, and reduce breathing speed. Clear the lungs completely instead of just huffing and puffing between sets. Close the eyes and imagine the movement just performed. Or pick an object or spot in space and focus on it. Initially, music may help promote relaxation. Many athletes train with music, but music cannot be reproduced in competition. This is one reason any ritual should come from inside the athlete, not from an outside source. Many athletes talk to themselves or chant. Some athletes hum or sing. It doesn't really matter as long as it creates relaxation.
- **Recover.** Recovering from a bout of explosive activity is partly about relaxation and partly about focusing on a weak link. If that weak link is flexibility, for example, then it's best to pick a few stretches to do between sets, such as calf or quad stretches, upper-back stretches, or entire movement patterns, such as squatting or lunging. If the exercise itself causes anxiety or nervousness, it will develop tension in the muscles. A good way to gauge tension is to stretch or explore movement patterns before the exercise and then repeat the stretch or movement after the exercise to see whether certain muscle groups became tense or tight. This may be part of the athlete's natural response, so recovery requires more than just breathing and lowering heart rate. It means making sure the musculoskeletal system feels loose, relaxed, and ready for another bout of exercise. Figure out what you need to do to lose the tension.

Someone with left-right differences may want to stretch only the stiff side. Those who are just generally stiff should pick the stiffest movement pattern and work on improving that movement pattern as part of recovery. Relax and continue breathing.

If flexibility is not a problem, stability may be. Those with stability problems tend to get sloppy in technique as fatigue sets in. The problem is not moving too little—it's moving too much. A great stabilizing activity is to stand on one foot and pull the opposite knee all the way to the chest. Most people will think that this stretches the hip and knee in the leg being pulled up, but actually it works the stabilizers in the standing leg. Standing on one leg brings in the trunk muscles. It reinforces proper posture as long as a tall, elongated spine and correct body alignment are maintained. To achieve additional stability in the upper body, reach as high as possible with the arm on the same side as the standing leg. Don't reach back; raise it straight up. You should almost feel a stretch in the armpit. Note the stability on one leg compared to the other side. Work to make both sides equally stable. Remember to breathe and relax. This does not require many muscles. It should feel natural. Stay tall, breathe deeply, don't round your back, and don't wobble.

- **Recall.** So far, we have not asked much of the mind. Try to recall the activity just performed, not so much from a technical standpoint but rather from a perspective of feel. What were different body parts doing? Where was the main focus? What minor adjustments should be made now that you know what it felt like? Should you relax more? Should you keep the spine taller or more elongated? Should you move the rope faster or widen the hands in the push-up? Recall the activity. Consider small changes to be made and run through them in your mind while going through your ritual.
- **Repeat.** The final step is to repeat the activity in your mind and visualize how you would do it differently. If you would not do it differently, repeat the previous activity in your mind. If you plan on making a subtle change or adjustment, repeat the activity a few times in your mind before doing it.

That's your ritual. Although rituals may look different on the outside, most champions do the same four things automatically. Some focus more on relaxation or recovery. Some focus completely on the mental imagery of the activity just performed and the one they are going to do next. Most do all four steps; the ratio and the order don't matter much. By incorporating these concepts into your ritual, you will create a home base, a place you can go to recover, a place that you have been many times before in training, a place you can go to during competition.

The key is to eliminate overanalysis and force yourself to feel things you do not naturally feel. The body wants to relax and recover. The mind has no problem recalling a simple activity that it just did, which is why it is important to pick simple activities. If you cannot teach yourself to relax, recover, and repeat a jump rope or push-up activity, how can you find success in a more complex movement? Use what you learn here with power, speed, and agility drills in chapter 13.

Recognize that speed and quickness training occurs just as powerfully when recovering and relaxing between bouts of exercise as it does when actually executing the moves. It can be helpful to pick other activities not related to your sport. Many athletes use table tennis and racquetball to maintain quickness and alertness. One-on-one basketball is also an excellent way to learn to manage quickness and speed. These activities can be used to learn to relax under pressure, to be quick without being tense, and to remember to breathe and maintain good posture while performing an activity. A simple cross-training game like table tennis or racquetball can have positive effects when it comes to the way the brain and emotions deal with other situations that require speed and quickness. But don't just play. Use what you have learned and make it work.

Heart Rate

Those who have never trained with a heart rate monitor will be amazed at how the heart rate fluctuates depending on activity. Usually there is a lag at first, meaning that an increase in activity only slightly increases heart rate. After activity stops, even when the athlete is completely at rest, the heart rate remains elevated. The heart is paying back an oxygen debt and replacing nutrients that were depleted from the muscles. Better conditioned athletes recover more quickly from exercise.

Using a heart rate monitor during jogging or while jumping rope is an excellent way to condition the body for athletics and for dealing with stress. Pick a high and low range for heart rate—for example 80 percent to 60 percent of maximum heart rate. Jump rope or jog a brisk, almost sprinting pace until you hit 80 percent of maximum heart rate. Ease up or do nothing at all until you hit 60 percent of maximum heart rate. Then sprint or jump rope briskly again.

Work back and forth within the range and use breathing, relaxation, and posture to recover quickly. When you can cover more distance or complete more jumps within the range, you will know you are becoming more efficient. In other words, you are accomplishing more within the same heart rate range. Only efficient use of muscle and coordination between the limbs and trunk cause this improvement. Pay attention to mechanics, posture, and breathing while exercising and recovering. You will maximize benefits in a very short bout of exercise.

Staying Relaxed

Competitive games such as beach volleyball, racquetball, one-on-one basketball, and tennis or table tennis teach athletes to move quickly and relax. Don't just go out there to crush your opponent. Go out there focused on staying as relaxed as possible regardless of the score. Use fundamental techniques and execute. Use this as an opportunity to stay relaxed no matter what the outcome. Staying relaxed does not mean moving slowly or not going for the kill shot. It means using posture, breathing, and movement to be as efficient as possible and recover as quickly as possible.

A telltale sign of athletic fatigue is breathing through the mouth. Coaches and seasoned athletes always look for fatigue in their opponents in posture, breathing, or movement. Make sure your posture, breathing, and movements always show your opponent a fresh and invigorated body ready for action. This is probably the most intimidating thing an opponent can notice in the later stages of a match or game.

If you are playing one of the games I have suggested and are already a superior competitor compared to your opponent, disadvantage yourself. In racquetball and tennis, use only your forehand or only your backhand. In basketball, make all your shots with your nondominant hand. In volleyball, use an easy serve or don't spike the ball. These simple changes will make the game more competitive and create more stress for you to overcome. Use this opportunity to maintain composure and learn to relax more efficiently.

13

Power, Speed, and Agility Drills

Michael Jordan, one of the greatest American athletes, had to work hard to keep his body in shape. "I've taken the physical strengthening of my body seriously," Jordan said. "Before this stage, I had my youth to live off and rely upon. Now it's not quite the same. As you grow older, the body starts giving you signals that you've got to listen to and do things that are correct. I just feel that physically I've got to be in the best shape possible to be able to do my job." It takes a lot of work to make things look as easy as the great ones do.

The power, speed, and agility drills in this chapter are basic drills, not sport-specific drills, but they will develop a foundation that will support the needs of any sport. It is important for all athletes to learn to move quickly in basic patterns. Once basic quickness is established, the athlete can move to more complex patterns.

Power Moves: Squat, Hurdle Step, and Lunge

These drills are based on the same movement patterns developed in earlier chapters. Continue to work on the movement patterns that present the greatest difficulty, but feel free to perform all the drills.

Go into these drills with balanced movement patterns. Do not move into power, speed, and agility work with significant limitations or asymmetries between left and right sides. With faster movement, the body needs to be as efficient as possible. If limitations and asymmetries exist, the body is forced to compensate. This compensation will allow completion of the drill, but it will not develop a sound base on which to develop full potential.

Warm-Up

Begin with a personal warm-up, dealing with flexibility movements as well as movements to wake up the neurological system, such as skipping rope or doing push-ups with claps (page 144). After an individualized stretching program and core warm-up exercises, try performing old-fashioned jumping jacks or completing the four-step warm-up that follows.

DOWN AND OFF

Start in a high knee or hurdle step position. Extend the hip and knee downward and bounce the ball of the foot against the ground or floor and quickly bring the hip and knee back into a hurdle step or high knee position (figure 13.1). Use a brisk, explosive contraction of the calf muscle to drive the knee and hip back into the high knee or hurdle step position. As the ball of the foot bounces off the ground and the knee is pulled up, throw the opposite arm up as well to simulate a running motion. Perform a set of 12 repetitions with each leg.

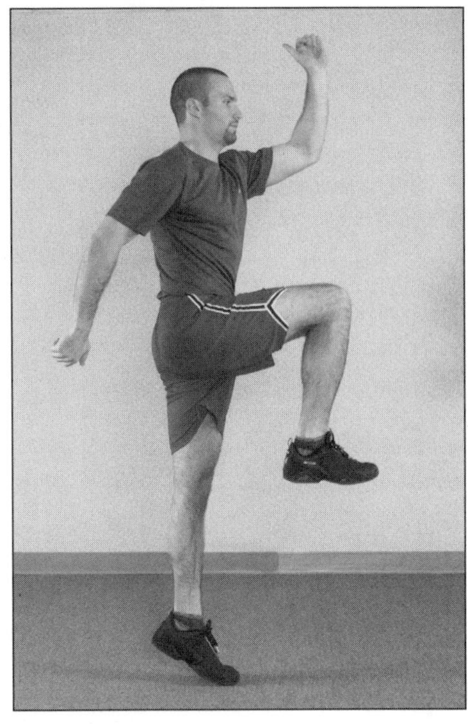

Figure 13.1 Down and off warm-up.

PULL-THROUGH

Stand on one foot with the other leg in front, knee extended. You should look as if you are going over a hurdle or kicking. Use hip extension to bring the leg down and through ground contact in a quick and powerful motion (figure 13.2) and return to the starting position. The arm on the same side starts in the air in a forward flexed position; the opposite arm is extended. As you pull the leg down and through, lift the opposite arm into flexion and pull the same side arm down into extension. This simulates a running movement. Perform a set of 12 repetitions with each leg.

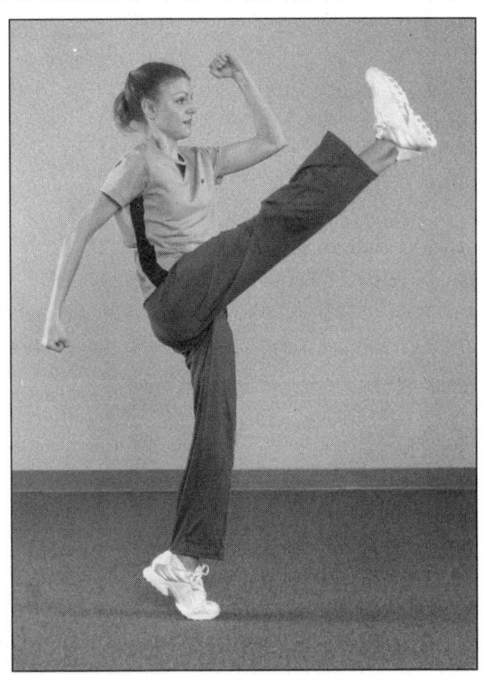

Figure 13.2 Pull-through warm-up.

AFRICAN DANCE

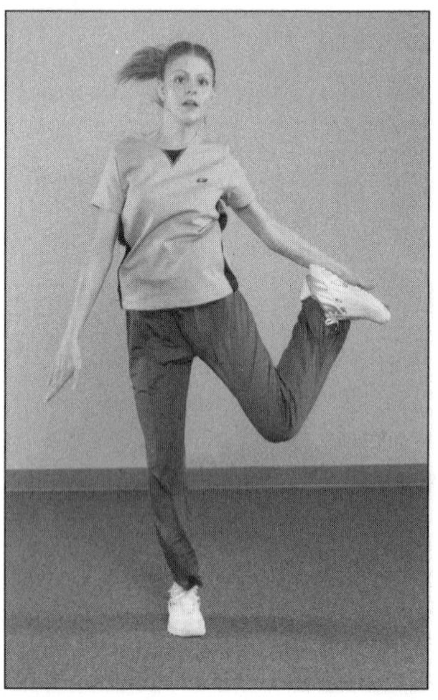

Run forward on a clear surface for 10 to 15 yards. With each step, bring the leg up behind you by flexing the knee and swinging the foot out and away from the body (figure 13.3). You should be able to touch your heel with the hand on the same side. This movement improves medial rotation of the hip and promotes quick firing of the hamstrings. Do this drill for 10 to 15 yards, alternating heels as you run, or do one side at a time for approximately 10 yards per side.

Figure 13.3 African dance warm-up.

DRUM MAJOR

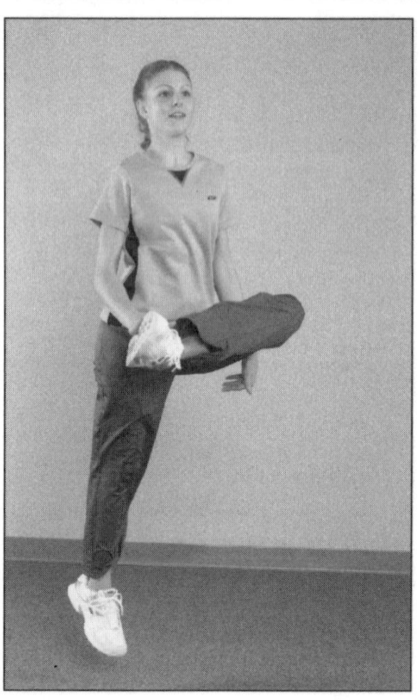

This running warm-up is the opposite of the African dance exercise. Pat your heel when the knee and hip are flexed and the foot is in front of the body (figure 13.4). This requires external rotation of the hip and complements the African dance because it also promotes hip mobility. Perform one set, alternating legs, or perform one set of 10 to 15 yards on each side of the body for comparison.

Figure 13.4 Drum major warm-up.

Squat

The squatting movement pattern is characterized not simply by a squatting movement but by the foot position. The foot position is described as a symmetrical double-leg stance. Each leg is in the same position and moves through the same pattern with respect to hip, knee, and ankle movement. Therefore, power, speed, and agility work to complement the squat movement pattern is not necessarily a complete replication of the squat movement pattern.

Any power, speed, or agility drill that complements the foot position or stance of the squatting movement pattern is also considered beneficial. Few athletic movements perfectly replicate a full-range-of-motion deep squat, but many athletic movements use the symmetrical stance position within sport-specific skills. If you have recently regained or improved your squatting movement pattern, these simple drills will complement not only the movement pattern but the posture and foot position necessary to develop power, speed, and agility within this movement pattern.

TUCK JUMP

Stand with your feet approximately shoulder-width apart in an erect tall spine position with your arms by your sides. Jump as high as you can, bringing your knees as close to your chest as possible. At the top of your jump and when the knees are as close as possible to the chest, quickly hug them by grasping the knees with the hands (figure 13.5). Quickly let go. Let both feet return to the floor for a stable landing. Perform 1 to 3 sets of 8 to 12 repetitions.

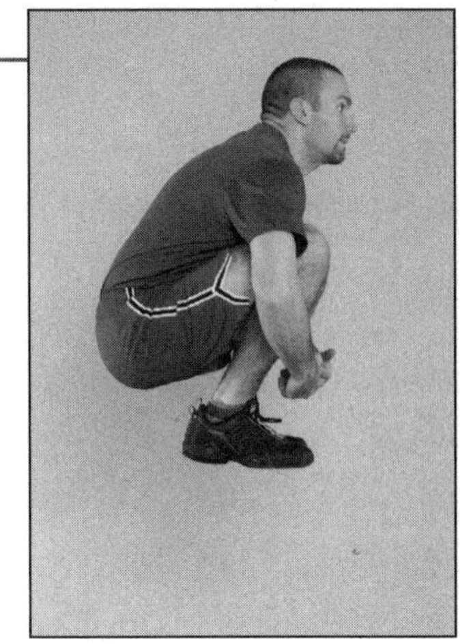

Figure 13.5 Tuck jump.

STANDING LONG JUMP

Stand in a relaxed and ready position (figure 13.6a). Use an exaggerated arm swing backward and then quickly forward and explode with your legs at the same time. Jump and propel yourself forward as far as possible (figure 13.6b). Land with a stable base and absorb the impact by allowing your body back into the ready position. Try to maintain your balance and turn and face in the direction you started. From the same foot placement of your landing or at the line where your heels hit, jump back toward the starting line, trying to exceed your previous jump, for 10 repetitions. Do 1 to 2 sets.

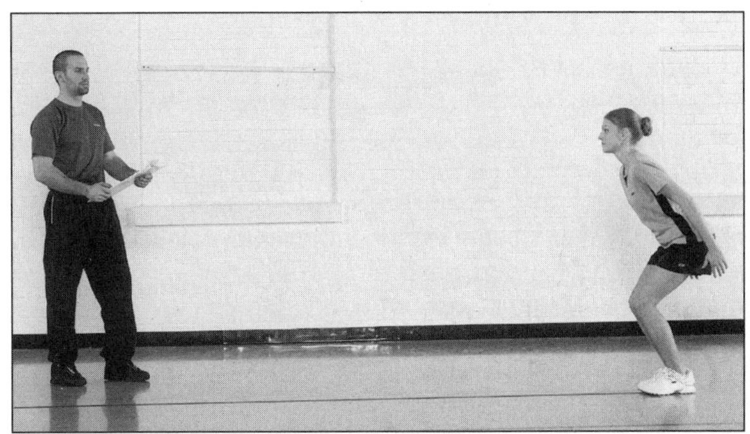

a

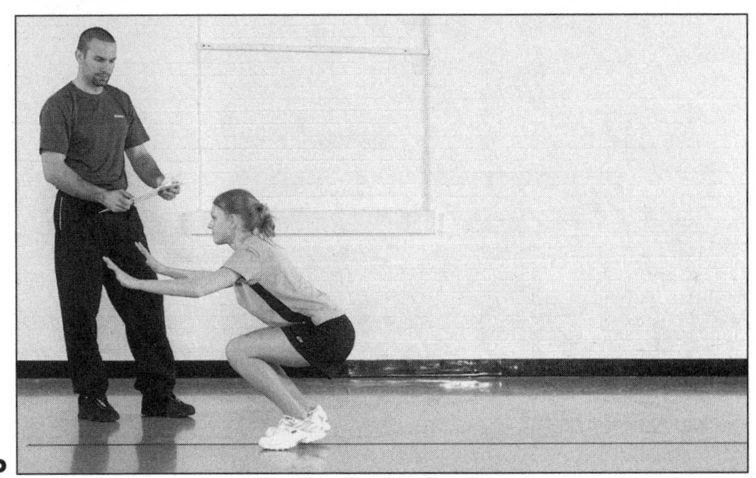

b

Figure 13.6 Standing long jump: *(a)* begin in a relaxed, ready position; *(b)* jump forward as far as possible.

PIKE JUMP

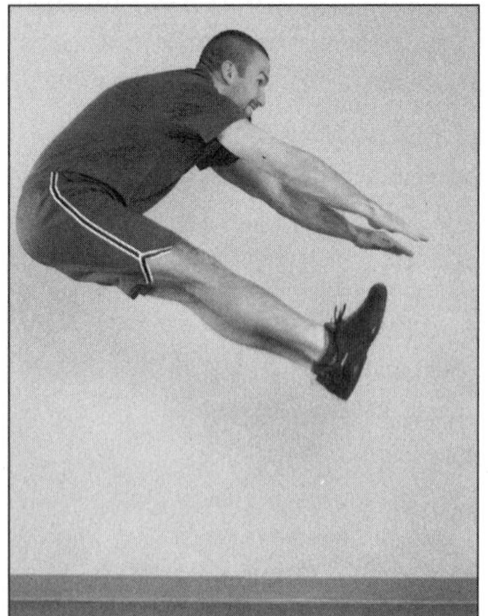
Figure 13.7 Pike jump.

This is a high-intensity jump and should be preceded by an adequate warm-up and stretching. Attempt it only if you are proficient with the tuck jump and long jump.

Assume the ready position with the feet shoulder-width apart, arms by the sides, hips and knees flexed and arms extended. Use a countermovement of the arms into exaggerated extension and then pull the arms forward and upward in an explosive movement (like a vertical leap). Keep the legs straight and together and try to lift them to the front, pulling them side by side (figure 13.7). You want to appear in midair as if you are doing a toe touch in a seated position. After the toe touch, let your legs fall back to the ground and land in the ready position and reset your feet. Perform 5 to 10 jumps but do not rush. Rest for 10 to 15 seconds between each repetition. Reset your body and try to jump higher with a cleaner and more fluid toe touch each time.

SQUAT STANCE MEDICINE BALL THROW

Use a 2-, 4-, or 6-kilogram medicine ball that bounces. Use a racquetball court or a hallway with walls made of cinder block. Stand in the center of the area, equidistant from each wall. Get in a squat stance, knees bent and spine erect (figure 13.8a). Turn the upper torso and shoulders and propel the ball against the wall hard enough so that it bounces back (figure 13.8b). Grab the ball slightly in front of your body and quickly propel it to the other side. As you catch the ball, come up out of the squat position a little but do not rotate.

Remember, this is a squat stance drill. Do not pivot on the feet and do not turn the squat into a lunge. Maintain foot, knee, and hip position. Rotate the shoulders only and thrust the ball with the arms. Maintain a stable squat base. You create power and rotation from the legs, but without changing the stance. Use the squat to generate kinetic linking and power to propel the ball.

a
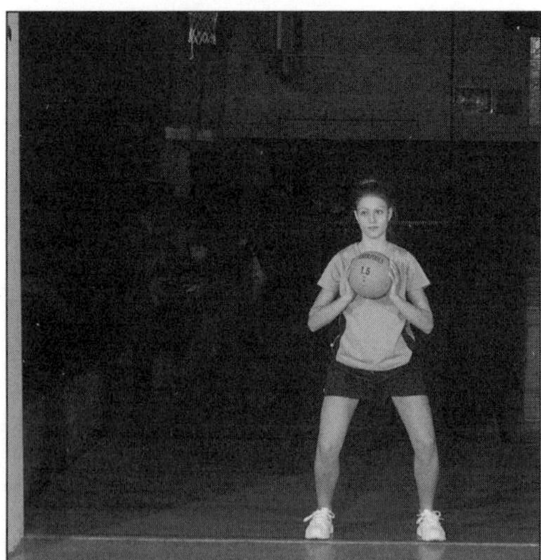
b
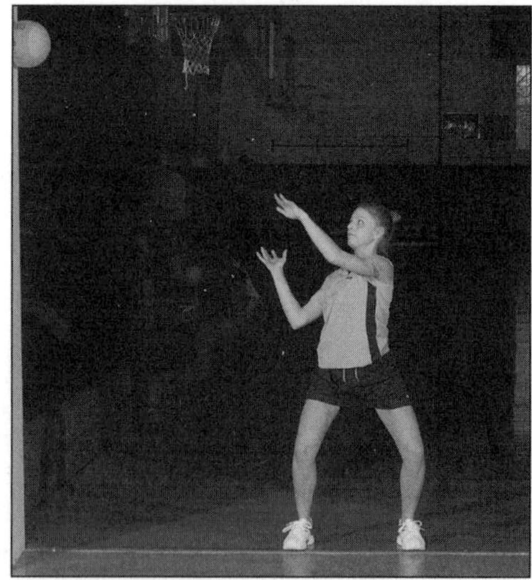

Figure 13.8 Squat stance medicine ball throw: *(a)* stand in a squat stance; *(b)* turn and throw the medicine ball to the wall.

If two walls are not available, stand to one side next to a block wall. Throw and catch the ball, moving farther away from the wall with each throw and catch. Examine left-right power by noting how far away from the wall you can move and still make perfect throws and catches while maintaining body position. If you note a left-right difference, work the weaker side more often.

Hurdle Step

The hurdle step is simply a single-leg stance with striding movement patterns. Compared to the lunge, it is a more upright pattern. The hurdle step is often used in jumping, kicking, and running. However, do not consider only the movement involved in the hurdle step, but also foot position. Of the three movement patterns, it is the only one that involves a single-leg stance. The squat stance involves a symmetrical double-leg stance. The lunge stance involves an asymmetrical double-leg stance.

The hurdle step is unique and gives you many opportunities to compare your stability and efficiency from one leg to the other. If you had difficulty in the hurdle step or your original movement screen and have improved your hurdle step through core training, mobility and stability exercises, and strength and endurance training, you can use these drills to add power, speed, and agility to a movement pattern that once gave you difficulty. These high-speed drills will help your brain recognize the improved movement pattern.

ALTERNATE-LEG BOUND

Find a suitable running surface with 30 to 40 yards of space. It is advisable to have another 5 or 10 yards of space to decelerate and gain control. Mark a starting line with a piece of tape and a second line 5 yards beyond the starting line.

From the starting line, start moving forward with slow and steady acceleration until you reach the second line. At that point, jump off one foot, stride through the air as far as possible (figure 13.9a), and land on the opposite foot (figure 13.9b). Continue striding as fast and as long as you can until you have performed two, three, or four stride movements on each side. Adjust the amount of strides by the space you have available. Mark the distance where you complete the drill. Walk back to the starting line. Stretch a little and rest for up to 2 minutes before repeating the drill. Each time you perform the drill, try to exceed your previous mark with the same number of strides. Perform 5 to 8 sets. As you become more proficient with the alternate-leg bound, you may want to expand the drill up to 100 yards.

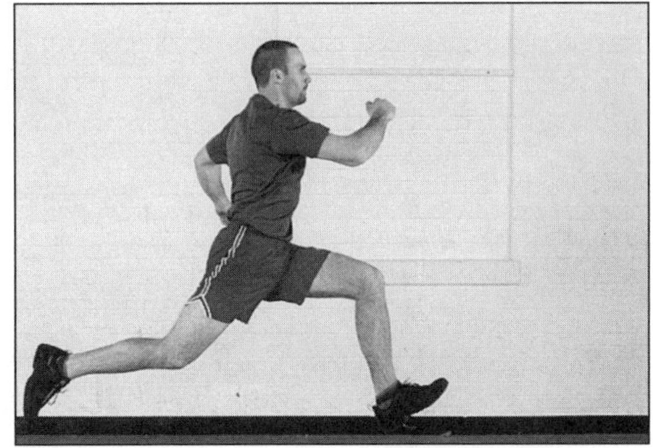

a

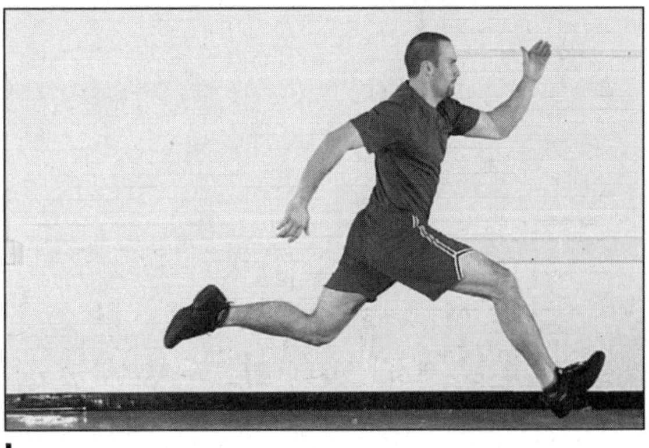

b

Figure 13.9 Alternate-leg bound: *(a)* stride through the air and *(b)* land on the opposite foot.

SINGLE-LEG BOUND

This drill will be performed in the same area and on the same surface as the alternate-leg bound. The level of difficulty is higher. Instead of bounding from the right to left leg, you will perform the entire drill on one leg, a hop. Find an area of 30 to 40 yards and mark a starting line and a takeoff point 5 yards beyond the starting line.

Get a running start from the starting line and take off from the takeoff point on your right leg (figure 13.10a). Pull your left hip and knee through to help propel forward. Land on your right leg (figure 13.10b) and jump again. It is normal and encouraged to have a cycle movement with your arms and nonjumping leg. This will help stabilize the core and add to the distance of the jump. Perform 4 to 6 single-leg hops and mark your distance for comparison to the left leg. After an adequate rest, perform a set on the left side and then alternate legs for 2 to 4 sets. Take special note of any significant difference between single-leg hops on the right leg and hops on the left leg. You may want to focus on the weaker side temporarily until you achieve balance and symmetry.

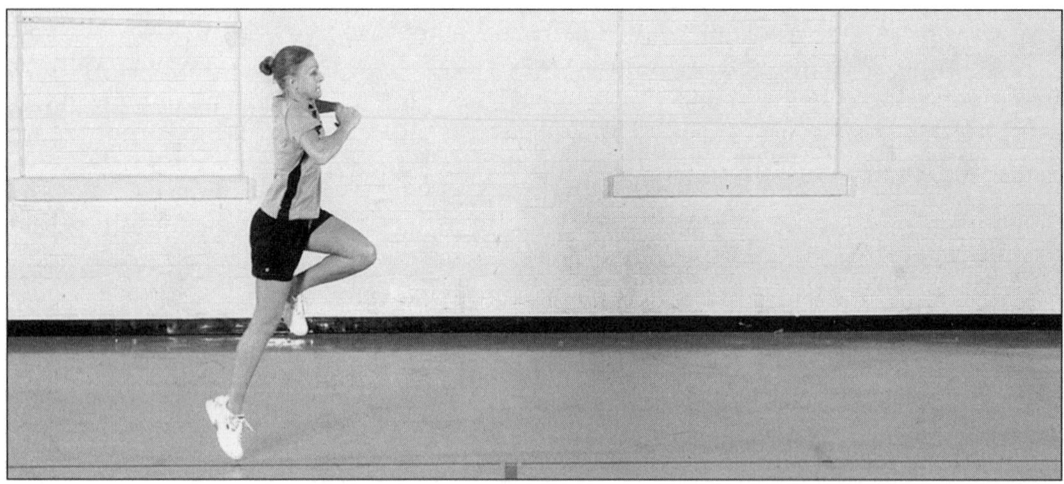

a

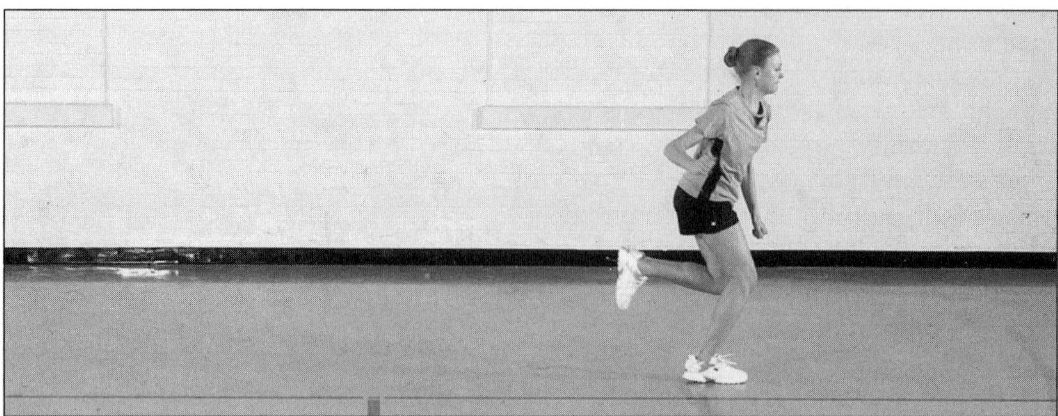

b

Figure 13.10 Single-leg bound: *(a)* take off from the right leg and *(b)* land on the right leg.

SINGLE-LEG PUSHOFF

Make sure you adequately stretch and warm up before this exercise. You will need a plyometrics box 6 to 18 inches high; a height at the level of or just below your kneecap is ideal. Stand facing the box. Get into hurdle step position with one foot on top of the box and one foot on the ground (figure 13.11a). The stride should be comfortable and not exaggerated. The leg on the ground should be directly under the body without excessive hip extension.

Jump into the air by pushing off the foot on the box (figure 13.11b). Land in the starting position with the same foot on the box and the same foot on the floor. Immediately repeat the movement for 8 to 12 repetitions. Use the arms. Perform 1 to 3 sets for each leg, alternating legs.

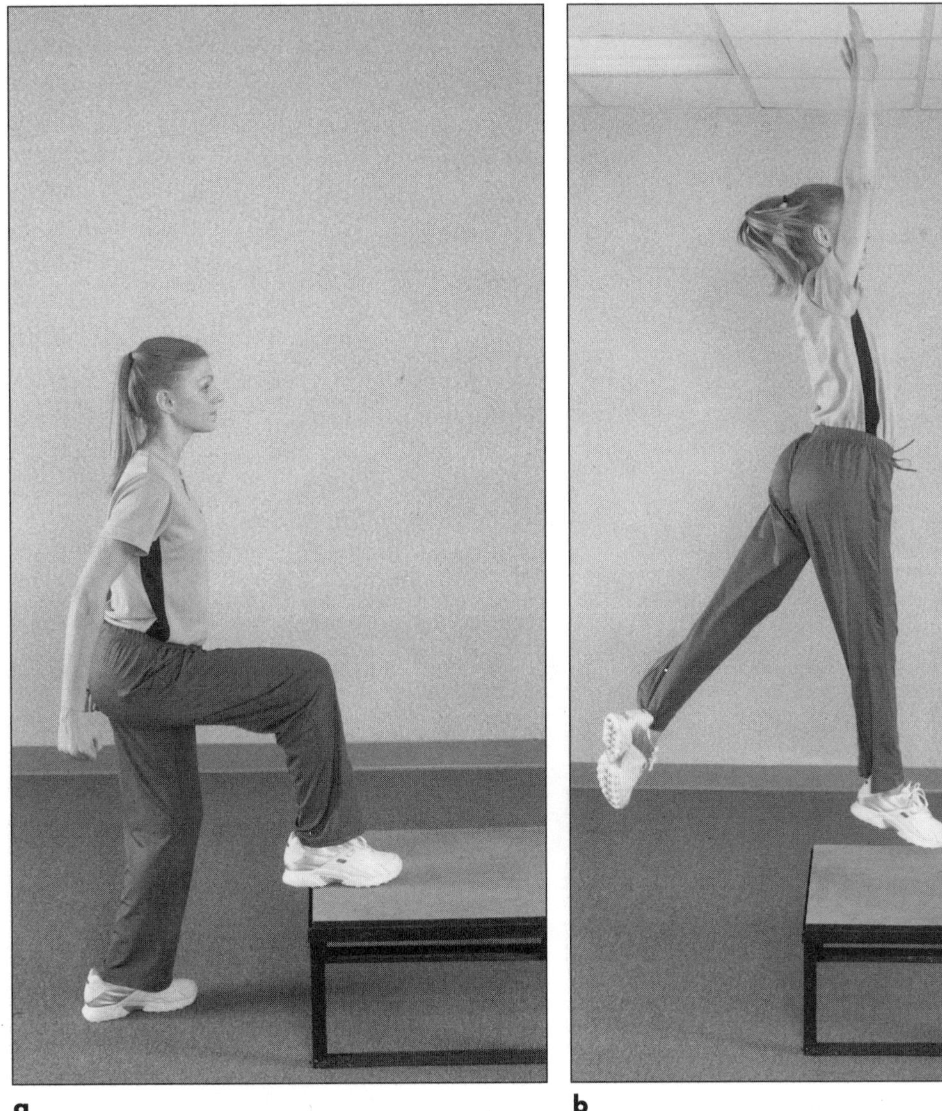

a b

Figure 13.11 Single-leg pushoff: *(a)* stand with one foot on the box and one foot on the floor; *(b)* jump up by pushing off the box.

ALTERNATE-LEG PUSHOFF

Use a plyometrics box 6 to 18 inches high. The box should be at or just below your kneecaps. Begin with the right foot on the box, left foot on the ground. Push off the box with the right leg and switch legs while in the air (figure 13.12a) so that you land with the left foot on the box and right foot on the ground (figure 13.12b). Immediately repeat the movement, switching legs again. Perform 12 to 16 repetitions for 1 to 3 sets.

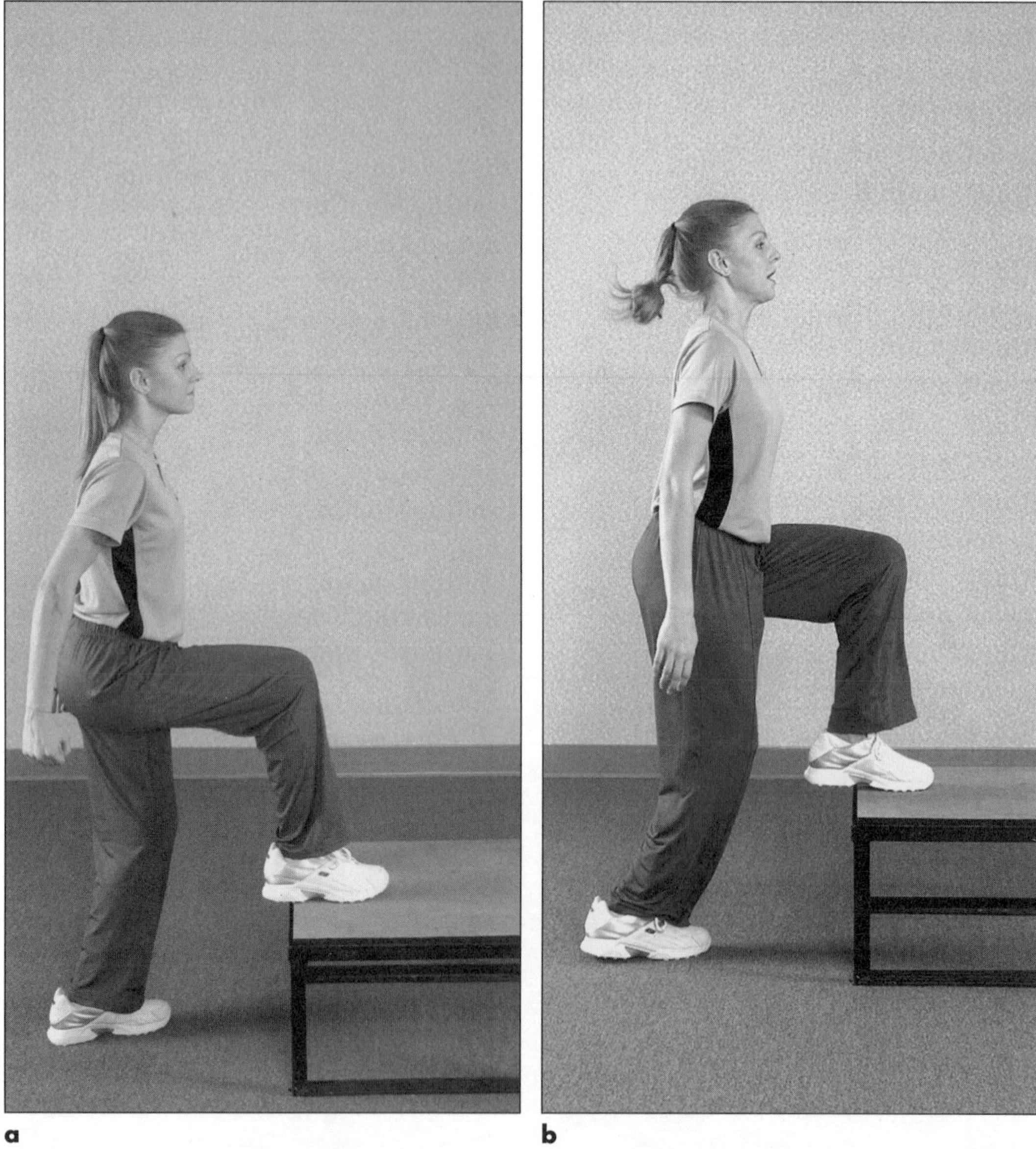

Figure 13.12 Alternate-leg pushoff: *(a)* jump in the air and switch legs; *(b)* land so the other foot is on the box.

HURDLE STEP MEDICINE BALL THROW

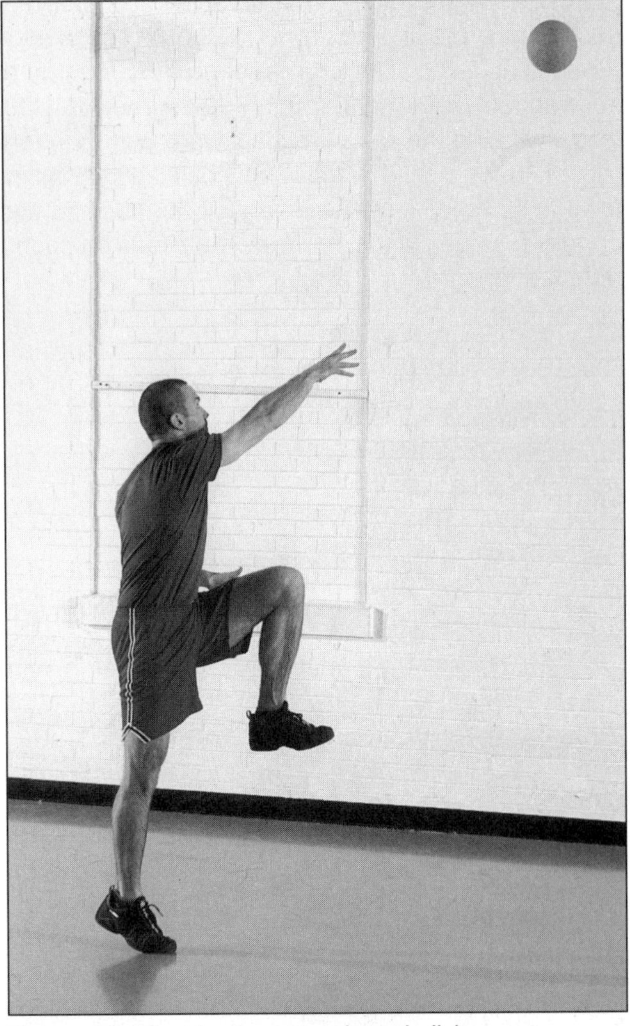
Figure 13.13 Hurdle step medicine ball throw.

Stand with your left side toward a block wall. Use a 1-, 2-, or 4-kilogram medicine ball that bounces. With the ball in your right hand, swing it down by your side and then up and across your body in a lift-type pattern toward the wall. Throw the ball against the wall; it should bounce back in the same diagonal downward pattern. When you lift the throwing arm up and across your body, lift the left knee up and forward so that it resembles a hurdle step (figure 13.13). Use the momentum in the left leg as a counterbalance to the arm crossing the body and propelling the medicine ball.

As you develop better coordination and power, move farther away from the wall so that you have to propel the ball farther and harder to get it to bounce back. The bounce back should follow the same path as the throw. Note any left-right differences. The spine should be tall and erect throughout the drill. If you observe a significant difference between the left and right side, always work the weaker side to develop improved power in the hurdle step stance. It is not uncommon to have better coordination on your dominant side; however, a little practice should improve stability and power in both directions.

Lunge

This is the third movement pattern to develop power, speed, and agility. The squat, hurdle step, and lunge have been used as a simple way to group movement patterns that share the same basic foundation. Consider the squat, hurdle step, and lunge not only as movement patterns but also as unique foot positions. The foot position of the lunge could be described as an asymmetrical double-leg stance. Legs are in opposing positions but both are in contact with the ground. The lunging movement pattern provides a stable, low center of gravity and is used in athletics for direction change, deceleration, and quick turning and cutting movements.

SPLIT-SQUAT JUMP

Start in a lunge stance with a tall spine and your rear knee approximately 6 inches off the floor (figure 13.14a). The front hip should be flexed at 90 degrees and the knee should be flexed at an angle of 90 degrees or greater. The rear hip should be in extension and the rear knee should be flexed at roughly 90 degrees or a little less. Explode upward into a vertical leap, swinging the arms first backward and then forward to help propel the body upward (figure 13.14b). Land in the same position with balance and control. Reset and jump again for 8 to 12 repetitions. Reverse your leg position and perform the same movement in the opposing lunge stance. Perform 1 to 3 sets on each side, alternating between the left and right leg forward.

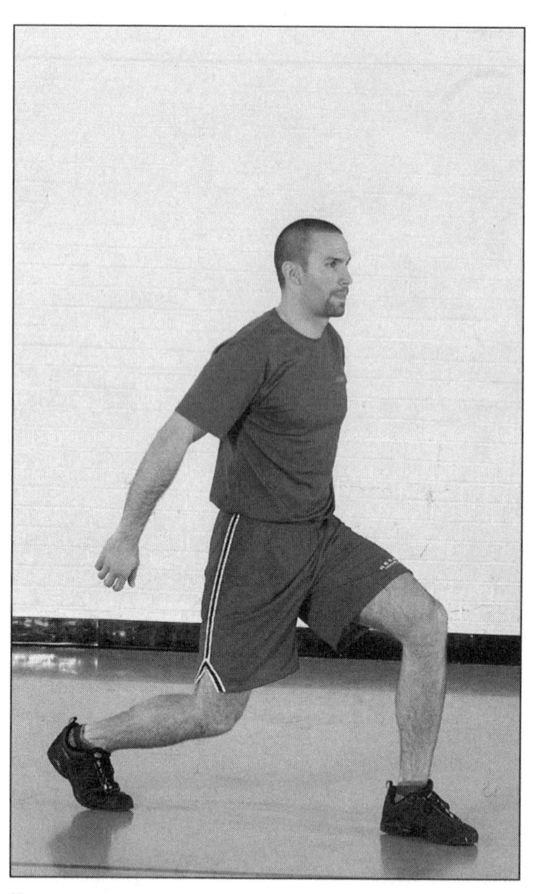

a

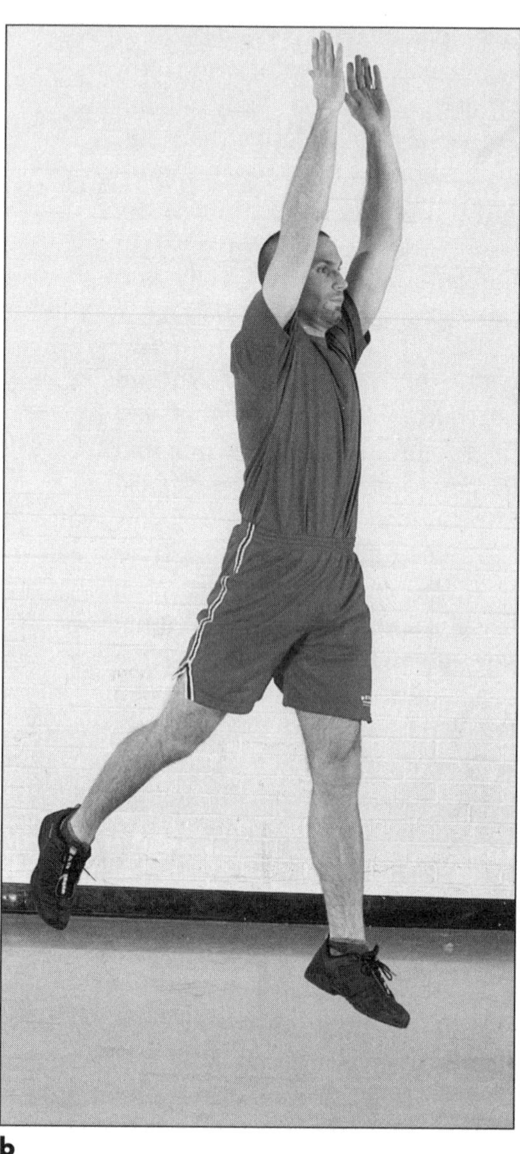

b

Figure 13.14 Split-squat jump: *(a)* begin in a lunge stance; *(b)* jump up.

CYCLE SPLIT-SQUAT JUMP

The starting position is in lunge stance with the exact same angles and upright body posture as in the split-squat jump (figure 13.15a). The major difference is that you will perform a cycle in the air so that you will land in the alternate or opposite lunge position (figure 13.15b). This cycle should be smooth and controlled. The greater your jump height, the more time you will have to perform the cycle. Use the same vertical leap propulsion of the arms with a countermovement backward and then a forward movement to pull you up. Land in a stable position and jump immediately, performing 12 to 16 repetitions for 1 to 3 sets.

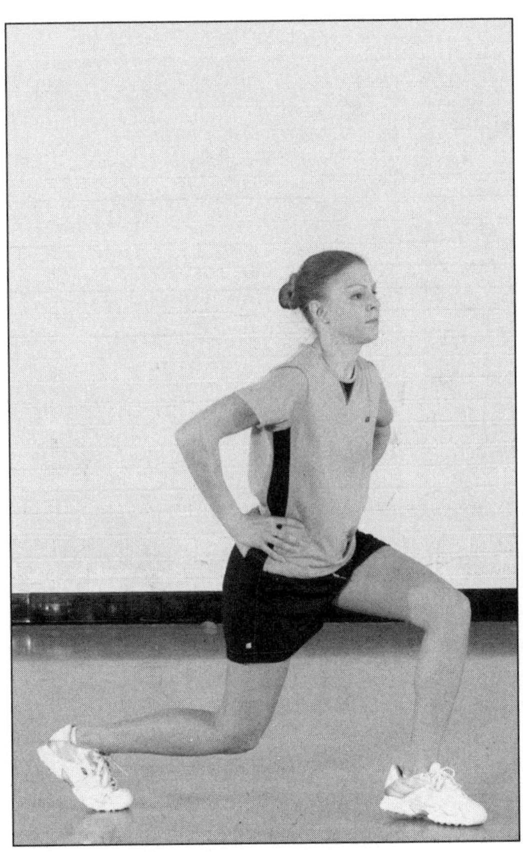

a

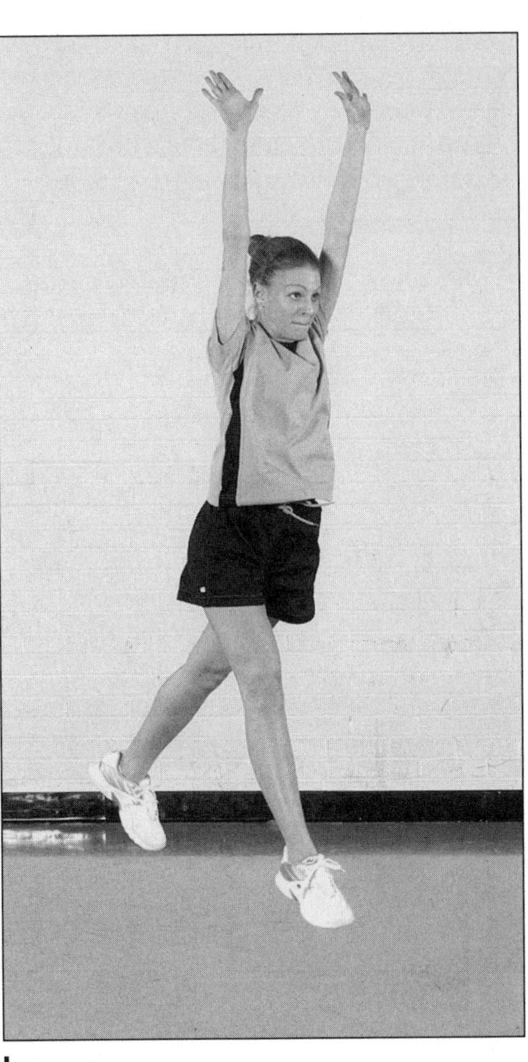

b

Figure 13.15 Cycle split-squat jump: *(a)* begin in a lunge stance; *(b)* jump up, switching legs while in the air.

DEPTH JUMP

You will need a plyometrics box 12 to 42 inches high. Start with one that is at or slightly below your kneecaps. Assume an upright stance on top of the box with the feet shoulder-width apart and the toes near the edge of the box. Step from the box (figure 13.16a), alternating your stepping leg between each repetition. Land on the floor with both feet (figure 13.16b) and, immediately upon landing, use your arm countermovement into extension and then into flexion to perform a vertical leap (figure 13.16c). Remember, this move is plyometric. You can use the energy stored in your body immediately gained upon landing and explode upward. If this drill is done correctly, your vertical leap will be higher with the depth jump than it is from a stationary starting position on the floor. The preload gained by your fall from the box stretches the tendons and also causes a stretch reflex through your muscles. Learn to use this movement to propel you higher. Perform a set of 20 repetitions, trying to jump higher and higher on each depth jump.

The depth jump does not use the lunge movement pattern, but it will prepare you for the next drill, which incorporates the lunge.

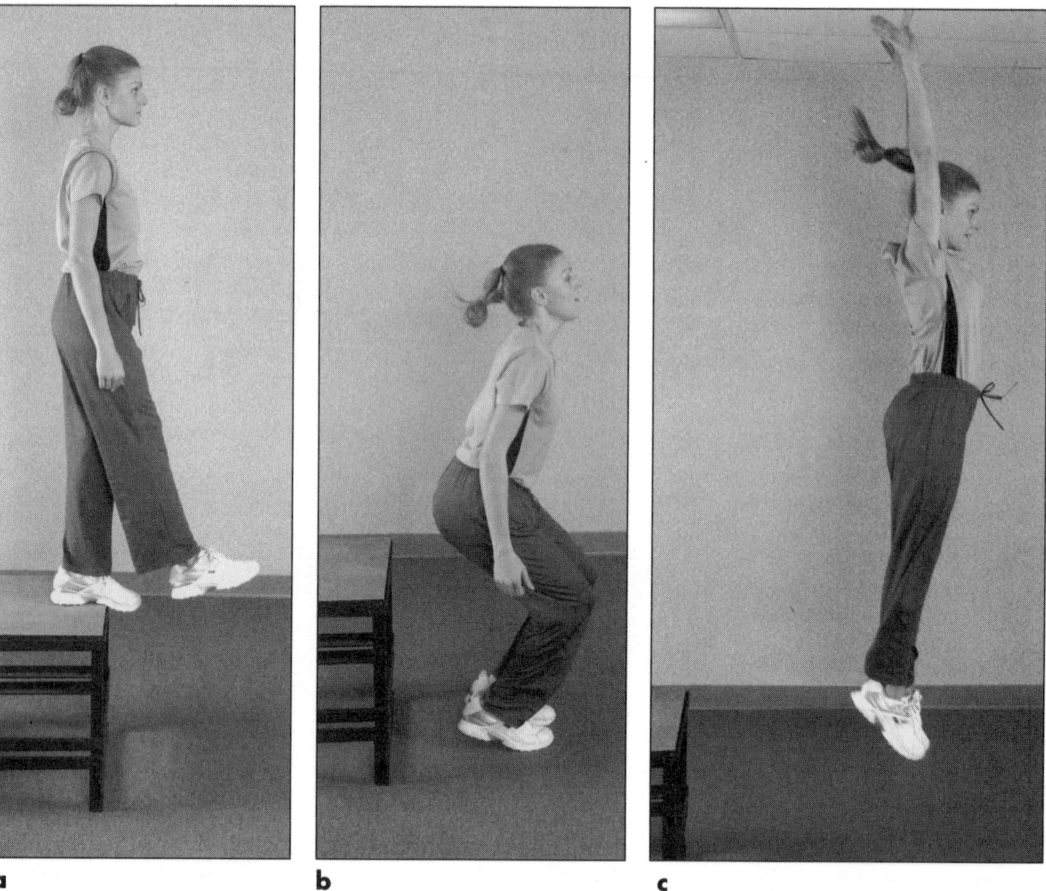

a b c

Figure 13.16 Depth jump: *(a)* stand on top of the box; *(b)* step off the box, landing on both feet; *(c)* immediately perform a vertical leap.

DEPTH JUMP WITH LATERAL MOVEMENT

The previous depth jump did not use the lunge movement pattern. However, it did show you how to pull and store your energy and reuse it. It also showed you how to change directions very quickly. You performed a falling movement, and upon landing you quickly reversed your direction to jump. Your brain can take what it learned from a vertical direction change and apply it to a lateral direction change.

Use the same plyometrics box you used for the depth jump. Drop off the box and land on both feet (figure 13.17a). Have a partner stand approximately 10 feet in front of you and indicate which direction you should sprint, left or right (figure 13.17b). Another way to perform this drill is to have your partner bounce a ball in the direction that you are to sprint; you try to retrieve the ball. You will not know what direction your partner is going to indicate, but try to react in enough time to still use the stored energy you gained from dropping off the box.

You and your partner may note that your ability to land and accelerate left may not be as good as your ability to land and accelerate right or vice versa. Work on the weaker side with extra drills. Perform 3 to 4 sets of 8 to 12 repetitions with a 50-50 ratio of left to right sprints, or have your partner create a bias toward your weaker side with 70-30 or 60-40 ratios of left-right sprints.

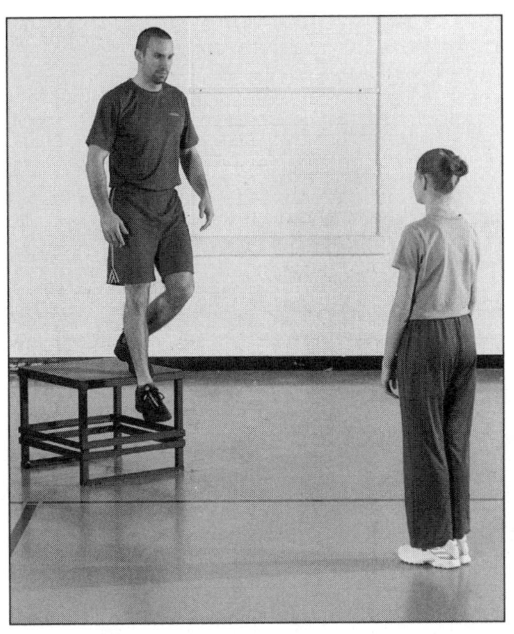

a

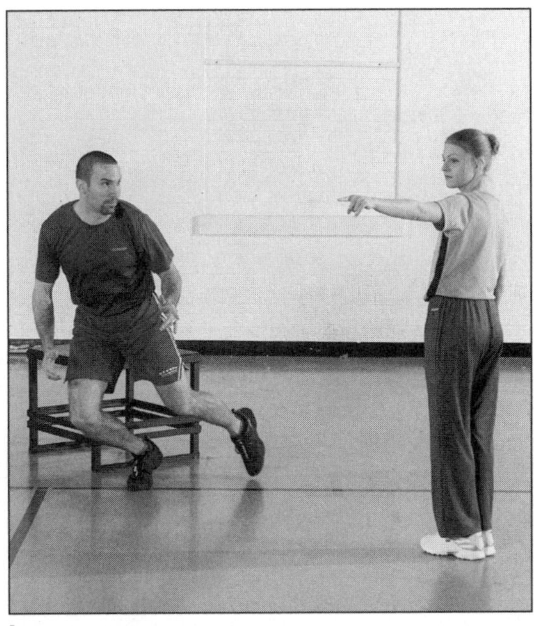

b

Figure 13.17 Depth jump with lateral movement: *(a)* drop from box, landing on both feet; *(b)* sprint in the direction indicated by your partner.

MEDICINE BALL LIFT THROW FROM A LUNGE STANCE

Use a 1-, 2-, or 4-kilogram medicine ball that bounces. Get into lunge position with a block wall to your left (figure 13.18a). The left leg should be forward, bent 90 degrees at the hip and knee. The right knee should be down.

Hold the ball in the right hand and swing it up and across the body toward the wall. Throw the ball out in front so that it bounces off the wall and comes back, but try not to bend, twist, or lose balance. Keep the spine upright and erect. Quickly pick up the right leg and step into a lunge position with the right leg forward (figure 13.18b). Allow the left knee to go down. Catch the ball and hold position. Focus on keeping the body low. Do not stand up and do not lean the trunk forward.

After making a successful catch, return to the original lunge position with the left leg forward and repeat. Use this drill to move down the wall in 5 to 7 catches. Reverse direction and repeat 5 to 7 catches going the other way. The farther you are from the wall laterally, the greater power you use in the throw. If one side is more difficult, spend more time working that side. Develop coordination, and power will come.

a

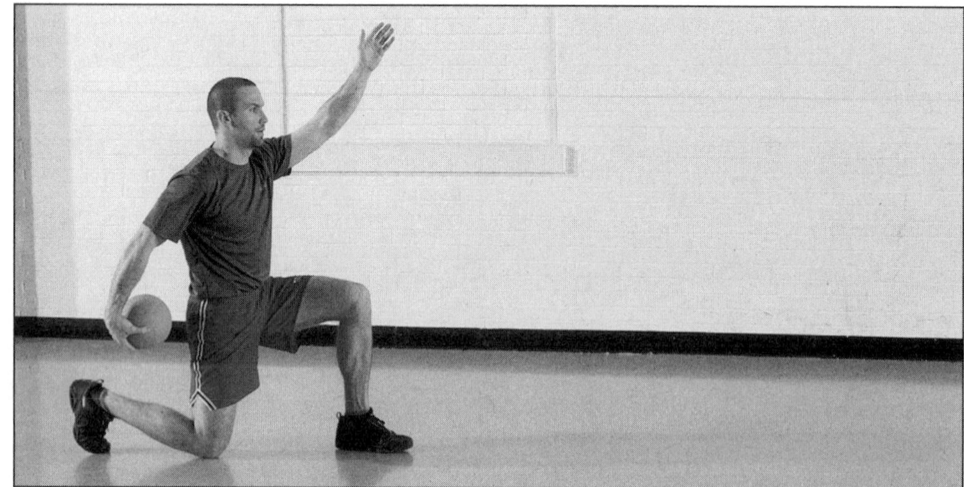

b

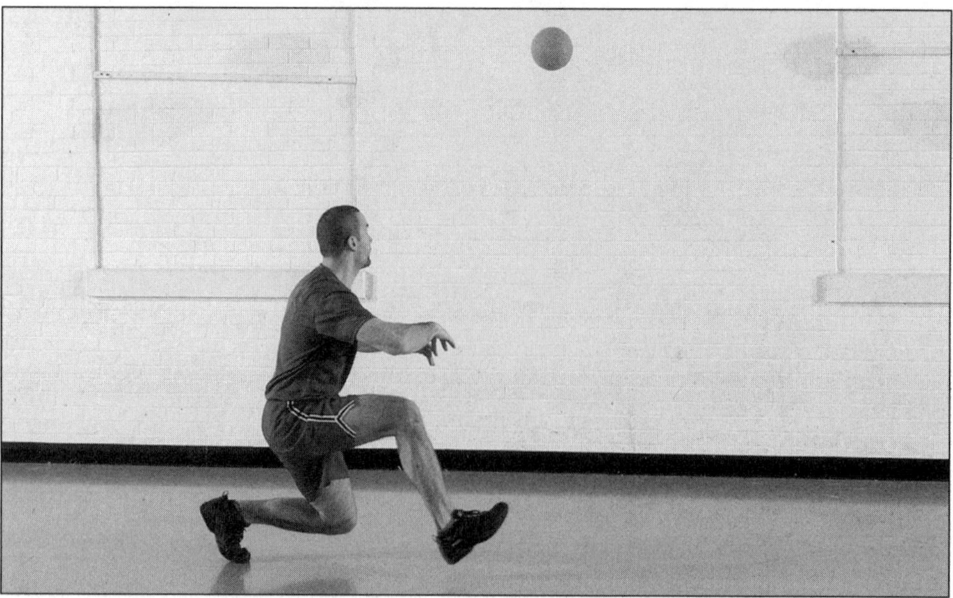

Figure 13.18 Medicine ball lift throw from a lunge stance: *(a)* begin in lunge position; *(b)* throw the ball and switch legs.

Speed Moves

Specific rope jumping techniques can complement basic movement patterns. Try some of these basic and advanced moves to develop a speed base. In the following section, Buddy Lee discusses some of the basic concepts of rope jumping in his jump rope training system. After Buddy Lee's primer on rope jumping, I will relate his jump rope moves specifically to the movement patterns we've covered so far.

Getting Started

Warm up with a slow jog in place before starting to jump. To avoid muscle soreness and injuries, stretch calves before jumping, during rest breaks, and after each jumping session. Perform slow stretching exercises for both the upper and lower body, particularly the neck, shoulders, torso, thighs, shins, ankles, and calves. This is especially important in the early phase of a jump rope program to avoid injury and muscle soreness.

Choose a lightweight speed rope. Detemine the correct rope length for your height by standing on the center of the rope and pulling the handles up to reach the chest, shoulder, or underarm. Adjust the rope as needed.

When jumping, hold the rope handles with a firm grip. Hold the elbows close to the sides. Make small circles with the wrists while turning the rope. Keep the torso relaxed and the head erect and focus on an object straight ahead to maintain balance. Jump only one inch, or just high enough to clear the rope. Use a light knee and ankle motion while jumping on the balls of the feet.

The key to effective rope jumping is to be light on the balls of the feet. Never sacrifice good jumping form for speed!

Mastering the Skill of Jumping

For the first two weeks, emphasize jumping technique, not speed or endurance. Rope jumping is a skill movement that requires proper timing and coordination of the rope swing with each jump. Practice jumping only high enough to clear the rope and landing lightly on the balls of the feet. Progress slowly as you focus on mastering the skill of jumping and be prepared to encounter snags with the rope. To avoid soreness, stretch before and after each jumping session. With practice, patience, and perseverance, you will soon develop the timing, rhythm, and form necessary for a jump rope training program for cross-training.

For the basic bounce step, with feet together jump only high enough to clear the rope (about one inch) and land lightly on the balls of your feet (figure 13.19). Each time the rope passes under your feet, it counts as one jump.

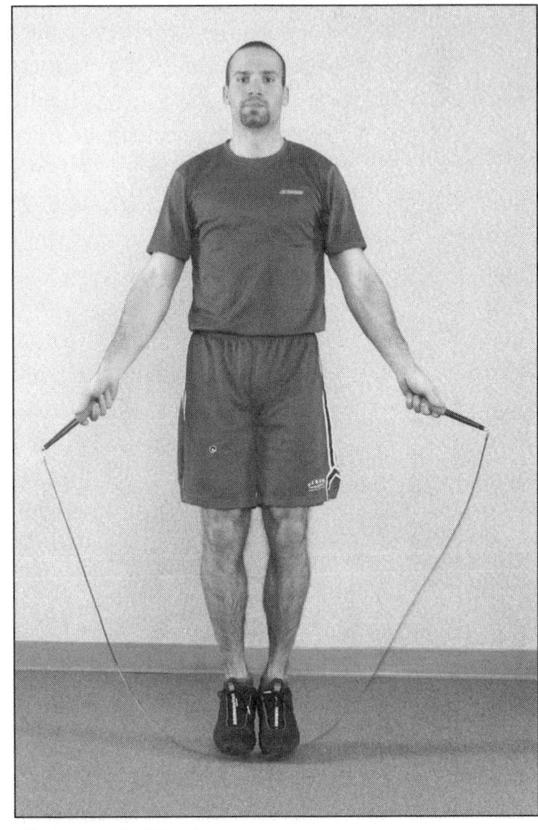

Figure 13.19 Bounce step.

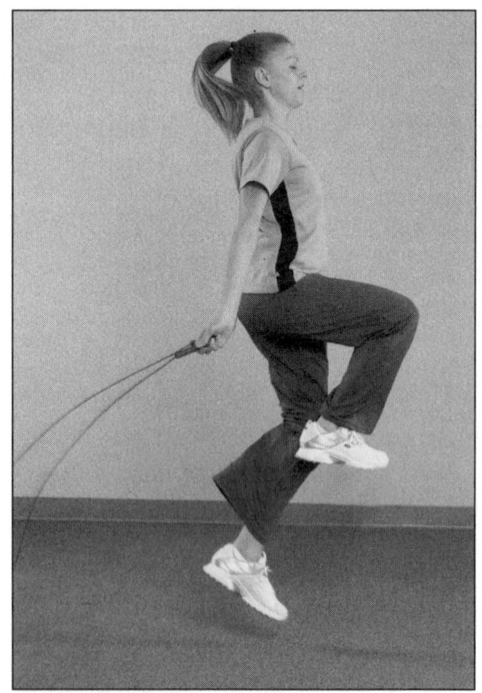

Figure 13.20 Alternate-foot step.

For the alternate-foot step or jogging step (figure 13.20), jump to clear the rope with alternating feet, lifting knees up, similar to jogging in place. Do not kick the feet back. To count jumps, count only right foot jumps, then multiply by 2 to get the total number of jumps.

Practice the basic bounce step and the alternate-foot step up to a 5-minute session twice a day for the first week. Depending on your skill level, begin with as few as 1 to 5 jumps or 5 to 25 jumps per jumping session, resting between each session. Shadow jumping—swinging the rope to one side of the body while jumping without the rope to practice rhythm and timing—may help you get the timing down if you are a beginner.

Goal 1 is to learn to perform the basic bounce step and alternate-foot step at least 50 times each without a miss. Goal 2 is to learn to alternate between the basic bounce step and the alternate-foot step. Perform 4 sets (a set is 30 to 60 seconds) of the basic bounce jump. Then perform 4 sets of the alternate-foot step. Perform as many jumps per set as you can without making a mistake. Alternate until you have achieved a smooth transition. Maintain rhythm and timing.

Once you can transition smoothly from the basic bounce step to the alternate-foot step, you are ready for goal 3: developing a jump rope capacity. Alternate between the basic bounce step and the alternate-foot step for a total of 100, 200, 300, 400, and 500 jumps without a miss. Get in rhythm by doing two bounce steps, then right foot followed by left, and create a four count. Goal 4 is to maintain a rope speed of at least 140 revolutions per minute (RPM), or approximately 2.5 turns per second. Ask someone to time you.

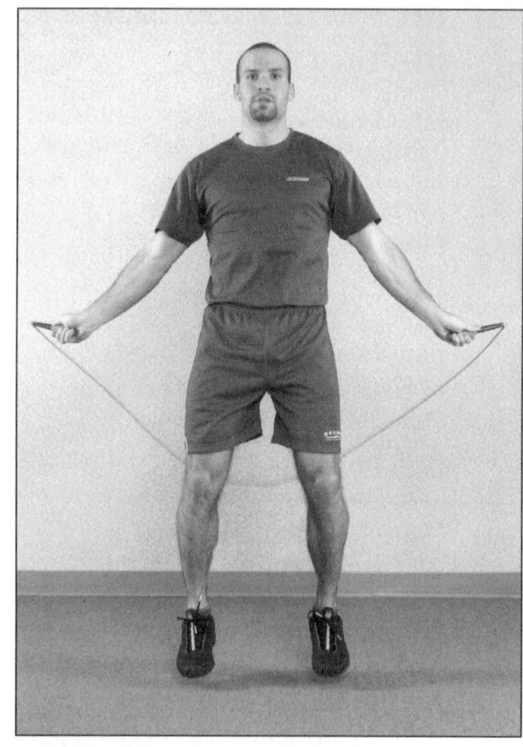

Figure 13.21 Side straddle jump.

Cross-Training Jumps

The following techniques will prepare you for jump rope conditioning programs for speed, power, and finesse. All of these techniques come from the two basic steps explained earlier: the basic bounce step and the alternate-foot step. It may help to try shadow jumping—swinging the rope to one side of the body while performing the skill without the rope—to practice rhythm and timing.

For the side straddle, begin with a basic bounce step (feet together) on the first swing. Jump with feet shoulder-width apart on the second swing (figure 13.21). Alternate back and forth, similar to a jumping jack.

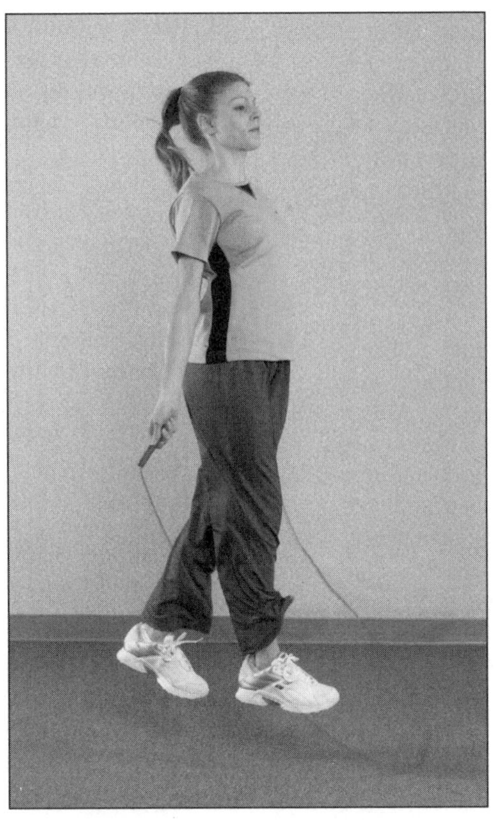

Figure 13.22 Forward straddle jump.

For the forward straddle, jump with one foot forward in a straddle position on the first swing (figure 13.22). On the second swing, switch feet, moving the other foot in front. Feet should be only a few inches apart. Alternate feet with each swing.

For the skier's jump, jump a few inches to the right on the first jump and a few inches to the left on the second jump, similar to a skier's slalom movement (figure 13.23). Keep feet together and torso straight ahead.

For the bell jump, jump a few inches forward, then a few inches back (figure 13.24). The result should look like the clapper of a bell swinging back and forth.

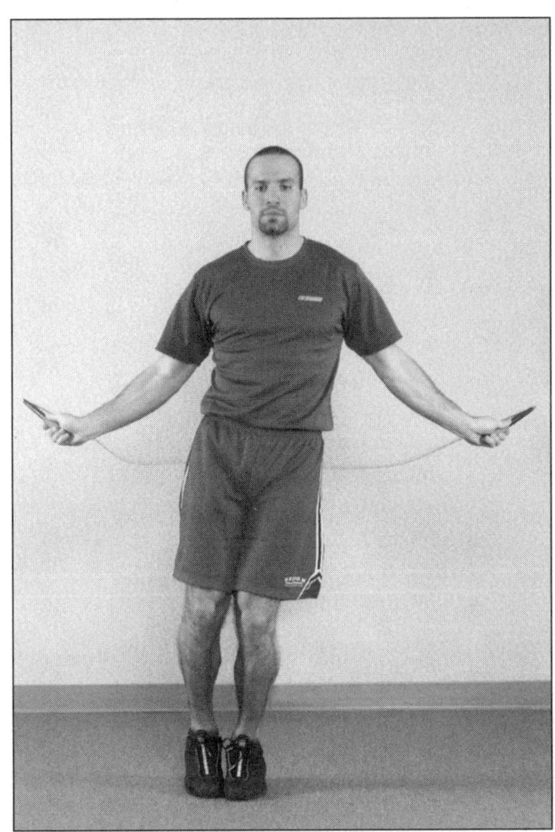

Figure 13.23 Skier's jump.

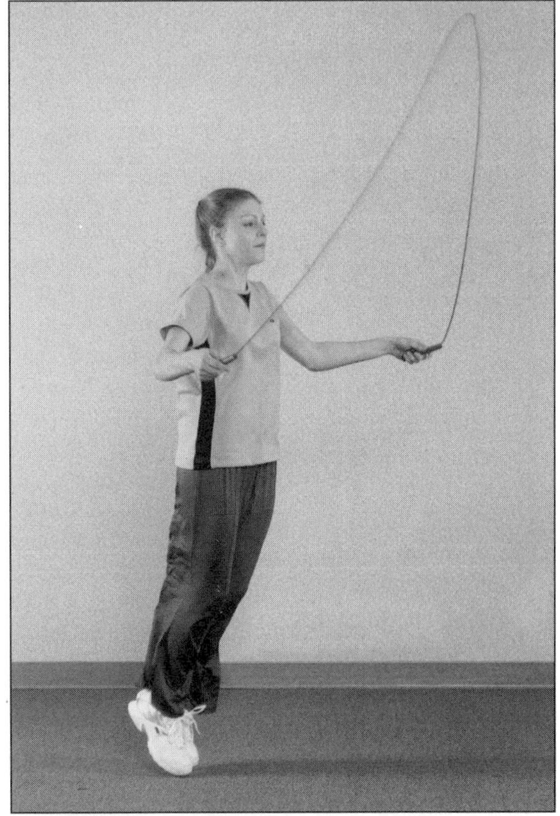

Figure 13.24 Bell jump.

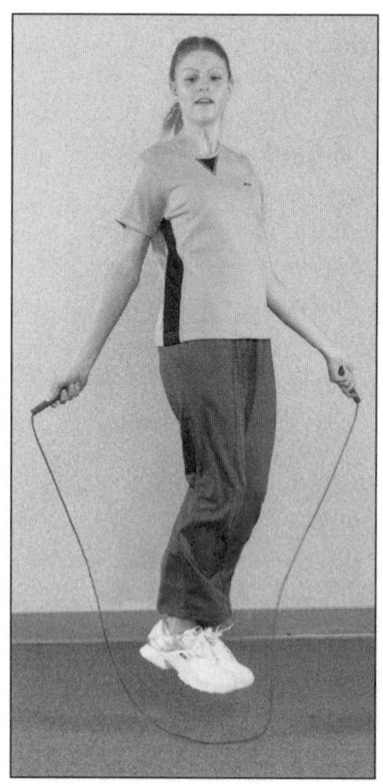

Figure 13.25 Twister jump.

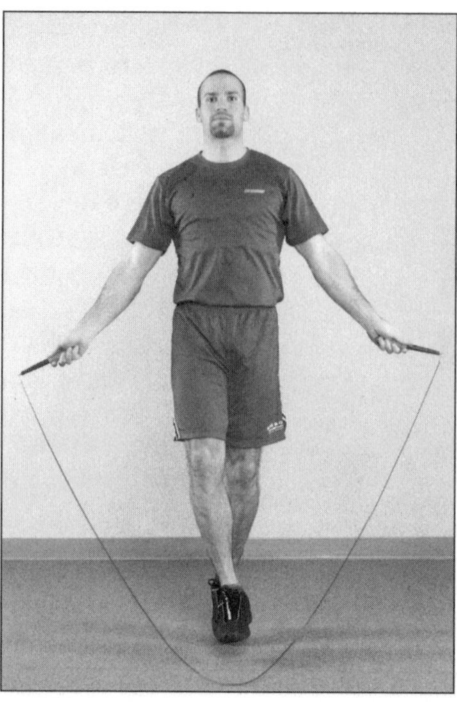

Figure 13.26 X-foot cross jump.

For the twister, bounce jump (with feet together) and twist the lower body to the right (figure 13.25). On the next swing, jump and twist the lower body to the left.

For the X-foot cross, jump to a side straddle (feet shoulderwidth apart) on the first jump. On the second jump, cross one leg in front of the other (figure 13.26). Jump to a side straddle again on the third jump. For the fourth jump, cross the other leg in front.

For the forward shuffle, extend one foot forward a few inches with the knee straight (figure 13.27a). Alternate feet and keep the upper body straight. To do a backward shuffle, extend one foot back, bending the knee at a 90-degree angle, alternating feet (figure 13.27b). The movement resembles a low kicking motion.

a

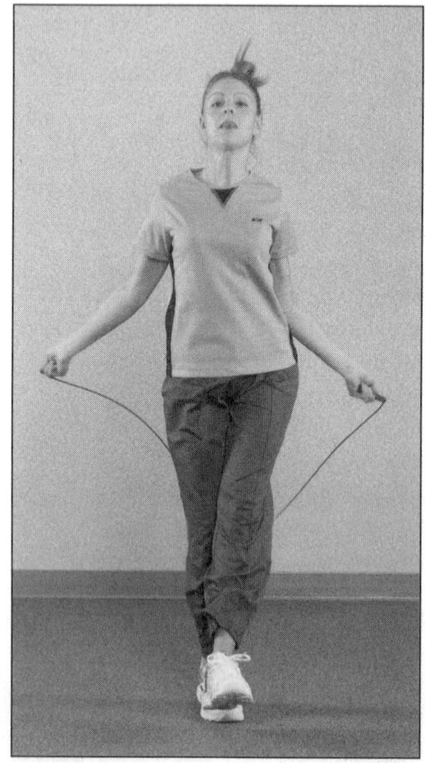

b

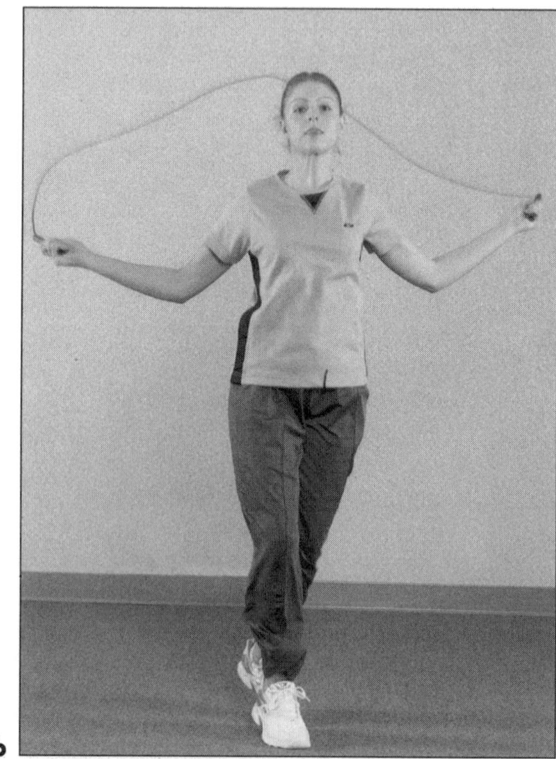

Figure 13.27 *(a)* Forward shuffle; *(b)* backward shuffle.

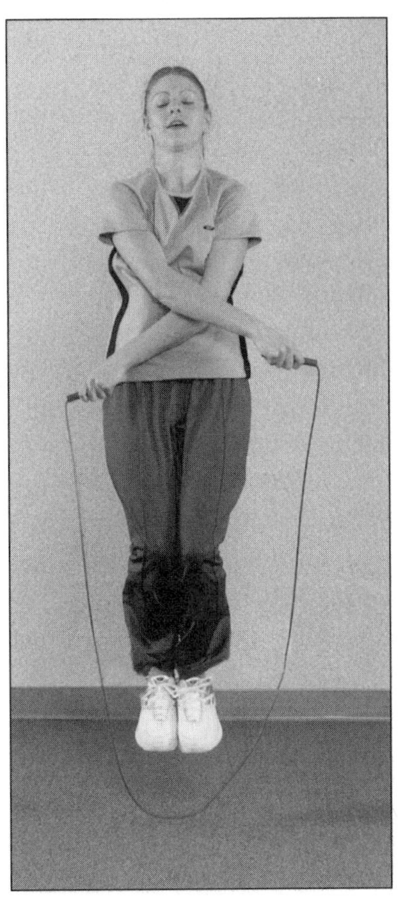

For the arm criss-cross, swing the rope around and cross the arms at waist level, extending the arms to the sides to create a wide loop to jump through (figure 13.28). Uncross on the second jump. Alternate on every other jump.

For the side swing to jump, swing the rope to the right and then to the left (figure 13.29). Open the rope by extending the right arm to the right. Jump over the rope.

For the power jump, with feet together jump a little higher than in the basic bounce step (figure 13.30). Turn wrists quickly to pass the rope under your feet twice in one jump. Keep the head straight and the torso relaxed for good jumping form.

Figure 13.28 Arm criss-cross jump.

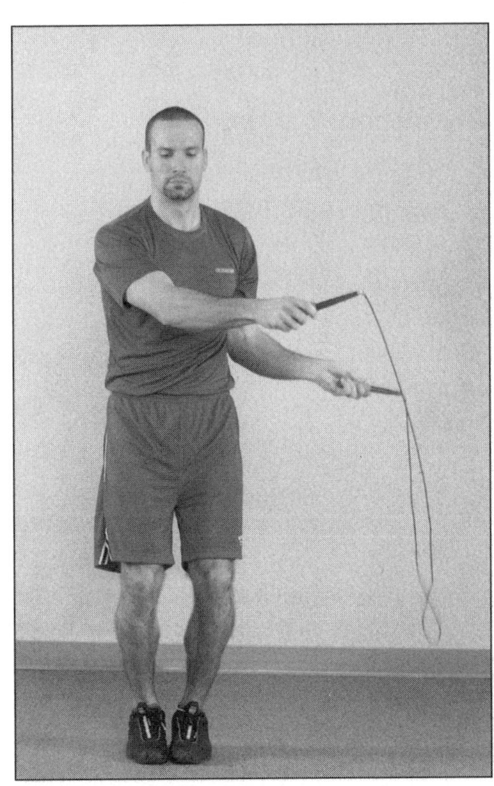

Figure 13.29 Side swing to jump.

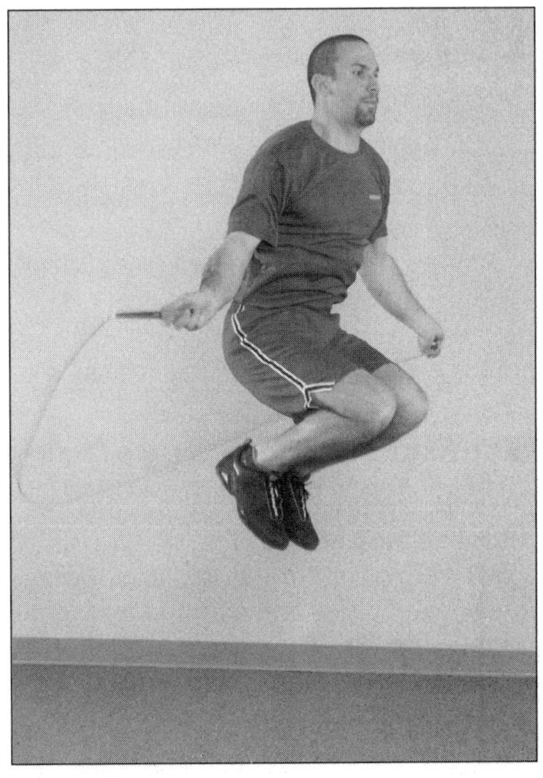

Figure 13.30 Power jump.

Conditioning

After mastering the skill of jumping and the basic jump rope techniques for cross-training, concentrate on improving endurance and increasing rope speed to 200 RPM. Depending on present jumping ability and conditioning, this phase may last from 4 to 6 weeks.

The first goal of the conditioning program is to perform 5 minutes of continuous jumping at a rope speed of 140 RPM. The second goal is to perform 10 minutes of continous jumping at 140 RPM. Use either the bounce step or the alternate-foot step or a combination. The goal is continuous jumping at a fast pace. The third goal is to work up to 180 to 200 RPM. The fourth and final goal is continual testing. You should know your 30-second max and your 1-minute max with respect to rope turns. Continually check these numbers and try to improve or maintain what you have.

Circuit Training

This circuit training program is for cross-training and is designed to develop anaerobic capacity, speed, quickness, agility, power, and strength while improving balance, coordination, rhythm, timing, and concentration, as well as foot, ankle, leg, and wrist strength for better sport performance.

To warm up the muscles, perform a slow jog or jump without the rope for 1 to 2 minutes. Stretch thoroughly, especially the calves.

For the next 6 minutes, perform all sports cross-training jumps at moderate intensity at a rate of 180 to 200 RPM or at 85 percent maximum heart rate (MHR).

The next 4 minutes are for moving through the circuit. Move through the entire circuit twice. Jump as fast as possible or at 95 percent or more of MHR. Alternate between these stations at high intensity. At each station, jump for 30 seconds, then actively rest (jog in place) for 30 seconds.

- Station 1, speed: alternate-foot step
- Station 2, power: power jumps (two turns of the rope per jump)
- Station 3, finesse: side swing to jump and arm criss-cross

To cool down, jog at a low intensity to lower your heart rate. Stretch thoroughly, especially the calves.

Progress at your own pace. Never overdo it. Too much jumping too soon can cause a number of ailments, such as shin splints, sore calves, and triceps and shoulder injuries. My goal is to keep you motivated and injury free so that you continue to use rope jumping as an integral part of your sports training program.

Get Specific With Rope Jumping

Some of the jump rope moves in Buddy Lee's system specifically apply to the three most basic movement patterns used in athletics: the squat, hurdle step, and lunge. Use the jump rope moves that address the area you have been working on to reinforce quickness, agility, and stamina in the movement patterns that cause you the most trouble. Combine these moves with stretching and core training. This recipe will reinforce better mechanics for your particular pattern problem.

Stretching and core training alone will not address quickness, speed, and speed endurance. Rope work alone may reinforce poor mechanics. Someone with limited movement patterns can still jump rope because it is a very tight and compact exercise that does not require maximum range of motion. Although poor movement patterns will not be addressed and may be reinforced, jumping rope is unlikely to cause more postural or mechanical problems. You are less likely to use poor posture and mechanics when jumping rope than when jogging or running. At higher speeds, the revolving rope will not allow poor posture or poor mechanics to any significant degree. If you do not jump correctly, you will probably not be able to turn the rope without hitting it or continually stopping and restarting. Jogging and running do not provide this extra level of qualitative feedback. Posture and mechanics can drastically change throughout a run. Jogging and running can actually create poor mechanics and posture. Stretching and core training create awareness of left-right differences and limitations and provide the opportunity to correct imbalances. Speed and quickness training creates motor learning opportunities, but you don't want to reinforce asymmetries and limitations. So balance the body and add speed.

To improve the squat, use the side straddle, skier's jump, twister (which is also good for torso rotation work), and the bell jump. For the hurdle step, try the *high stepper*—to execute this, do the alternate-foot step with an exaggerated hip and knee lift. The high stepper also is good for active straight leg raise work. Also use the *hip flexor,* a single-leg jump with the nonjumping leg held at 90 degrees at the hip and knee. Jump as fast as possible with minimal movement of the flexed leg. For the lunge, use the forward straddle and the X-foot cross.

Rope work lends itself to speed training because it is easy to count rope turns over time, which will demonstrate changes in performance. Keep records with the following information:

- Type of jump rope movement
- Number of sets
- Time for each set (30 seconds, 1 minute, and so on)
- Rest time between sets (30 seconds, 1 minute, and so on)
- Number of repetitions or rope turns
- Left versus right performance comparison, if applicable

A lot of elements can be modified, but change only one thing at a time. If you add a set, don't change anything else. You can extend jumping time or reduce rest time, but don't do both simultaneously. You can leave the time the same and increase rope turns. You can try to maintain the original number of rope turns (usually your fastest) over the rest of the sets.

Work on all three basic patterns—squat, hurdle step, and lunge—but focus on the problem area if one exists. Rope work provides many training options. An intense workout can be done in a short amount of time (see Buddy Lee's 5-minute speed program or the basic program in chapter 10). Rope work creates less jarring and pounding on the body than sprinting or conventional plyometrics. With rope work, movements are small and crisp and jumps are short and quick. Speed is the main emphasis in most rope jumping programs. Because jumping rope creates less stress on the body and emphasizes speed, it is one of the best choices for in-season and maintenance training.

Buddy Lee's Five-Minute Speed Program

Before starting this jump rope program, you must be able to perform 5 minutes of jumping at a rate of 140 RPM. This program is designed to produce a synergistic effect among an athlete's quickness, speed, strength, endurance, and timing. This synergy will create the edge in performance that makes the winning difference.

Warm up by jogging in place without the rope. To avoid muscle soreness and injuries, stretch the upper and lower body before beginning to jump, during the jumping session, and after each session, focusing on stretching the calves.

Jump as fast and efficiently as possible with a 10- to 15-second rest period between sets. Count jumps and try to achieve the same number or more in the next session:

1. Alternate-foot step: count to 50
2. Bounce jump: count to 25
3. Alternate-foot step: count to 50
4. Power jump: count to 25
5. Alternate-foot step: count to 50
6. Forward straddle: count to 25
7. Alternate-foot step: count to 50
8. Skier's jump: count to 25
9. Alternate-foot step: count to 50
10. Skier's jump: count to 25
11. Alternate-foot step: count to 50

Use this program two to three times per week.

Sprinting

Once a sound base of movement patterns, core training, and rope jumping has been developed, running sprints is the best choice to develop speed. Running and sprinting are fundamental human movements. Even athletes in sports that do not directly depend on running or sprinting can benefit from speed work. Running and sprinting reinforce a solid core and fundamental athletic coordination.

I feel that downhill sprinting is a natural and effective way to improve speed. The authors of *Sports Speed* state that "combined downhill-uphill sprinting has been shown to force runners to take more steps per second than flat-surface sprinting." Whereas uphill sprinting forces you to work harder (see earlier recommendations on uphill work, page 129), downhill sprinting forces you to work faster. The effect of gravity will pull you down the hill and assist your sprinting activity, so you will develop greater momentum. This extra bit of speed will force you to increase your stride rate and stride length.

Find a grassy area with an incline that does not exceed 3 1/2 degrees. A slope with a greater fall than this can put you at risk for injury and will not produce the desired results. You will also need about 20 yards to accelerate on a flat surface followed by the downhill slope, which ideally should be another 20 yards followed by a flat area to decelerate. Over a 5-week period, progress from 2 to 3 downhill sprints to 9 to 10 downhill sprints. Start with only a 10-yard acceleration before the downhill and slowly progress to 20 yards. Start with rest times of approximately 2 minutes and progress to 3 1/2 minutes when you get up to 9 to 10 sprints. Perform 2 to 3 workout sessions a week and let this be the first part of your workout following warm-up and stretching. Do not train downhill sprinting if you feel fatigued, tight, or stiff.

An analysis of correct sprinting form has allowed researchers to identify key factors contributing to efficient movement. It has also revealed a diversity of styles and techniques among champion athletes. This diversity suggests the need for athletes to improve their basic style without trying to mimic the exact technique of others.

Tips for Sprint Training

- Use your arms, but let them be loose and swing from the shoulder.
- Let your body lean, but do not bend. Your body should have a straight forward lean from the ground, not a bend forward at the hips. Most athletes exaggerate the lean a little. So lean, but do not force it.
- Don't run on your toes; run on the balls of your feet. Let the heel make contact and push off the balls of your feet.
- Don't overstride or try to pull the ground toward you. Let the foot land underneath you (your center of gravity). Placing the foot in front of this point will only slow you down. Push off the ground and use your extension.
- Do not understride and focus only on cadence. You will move fast but not cover much ground. Let your stride length and frequency create a smooth, complementary rhythm.

Agility

Propelling a stationary body into rapid movement and exerting maximal force require both strength and power (speed-strength). An athlete may be quite strong, yet lack explosive power and be incapable of sprinting a fast 40-yard or 40-meter dash. Speed and power training should involve movements that are similar to those in the sport (this is the principle of specificity).

The three drills in this section were chosen because they represent the type of specific quickness needed for most field and court sports. They give you a right-left comparison and can be tracked for time to demonstrate improvement. These drills can also be used as competitive games between two athletes, which will in most cases increase the workout intensity. The three drills also promote controlled direction changes and a low center of gravity. Each drill will use an elastic tether.

Tethered training with elastic tubing focuses specifically on one aspect of movement. It causes you to become more stable and controlled. The tubing actually is used to emphasize mistakes.

For example, consider a tennis player who needs to move quickly out of ready position, but who has the habit of standing up too straight and shifting her weight to her heels. She is going to lose precious seconds that she would have if she were to stand in a relaxed ready position with the weight shifted onto the toes.

Elastic tubing used around the waist in training pulls the athlete backward (into the mistake of resting on the heels). The brain automatically causes a weight shift forward into a more stable ready position. If the tennis player used tubing while hitting balls, she could correct her mistake.

Many drills can be done with tubing, but make sure the drill promotes good mechanics and weight shifting and results in better skill and performance. Any tubing work can create sweat. This book is not about sweat—it's about getting something in exchange for sweat. It's easy to dream up 20 or 30 different tubing exercises and play around, but don't waste time. Pick a few drills, such as the following three, and stick with them, working on time and technique.

Tubing can be dangerous when used incorrectly. It should be used to stimulate better movement patterns and to serve as a form of interval training. It is better to have 5 minutes of well-executed activity than 15 minutes of off-balance blunder (even if blundering burns more calories). Any work can harden the body, but only well-executed drills at or near the speed of competition will hone the neuromuscular system. In most cases (regardless of sport), the drills provided here will be sufficient. You need left-right directional balance, good mechanics, and the ability to perform and recover quickly. Don't complicate training with too many drills. Only a few are needed to establish a personal baseline, chart progress, and set training goals. Constantly changing to new drills can cause a loss in perspective.

The following three drills are excellent for developing agility, but the tubing causes a high level of energy expenditure, so fatigue will hit more quickly. Nearly all sports require a high level of agility, but it is equally important for athletes to be able to maintain agility throughout competition. If agility is lost quickly because of fatigue or poor body mechanics, then the athlete will never finish as well as she started. Use these agility drills to work multidirectional quickness, general coordination, and interval training at the same time.

HALF-MOON TUBING SHUTTLE

Place five buckets or baskets about 10 feet apart in a half-moon arc (figure 13.31). Place three tennis balls in each bucket, leaving the bucket at the starting point empty. Use an elastic tubing tether held by a friend or anchored to a stable and safe object. Attach the tubing to a belt so that the tubing is taut as you stand at the starting line. Go to any bucket and grab one ball. Bring it back to the starting point, drop it in the empty bucket, and go to another bucket. You can go to the buckets in any order. Do not throw the ball into the bucket at the starting point. Go back, stop, drop the ball into the bucket, and go to the next bucket.

Time the drill and compete with friends. This drill challenges multidirectional agility and quickness, as well as endurance. Create games with yourself and others by trying to maintain the same speed throughout four rounds. Keep a total score by averaging the times.

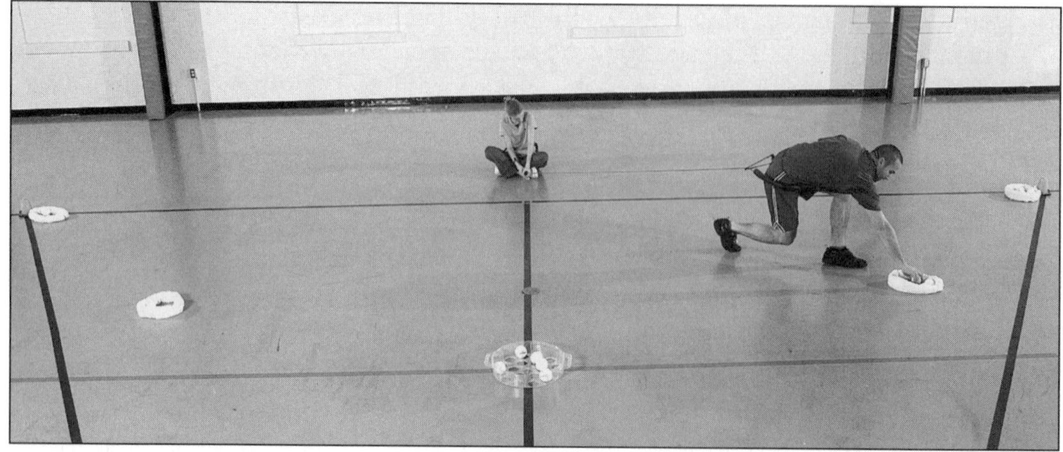

Figure 13.31 The half-moon tubing shuttle drill.

MIRROR DRILL

This drill requires four buckets, four tennis balls, a partner, and a friend to hold the elastic tubing. Place the buckets 6 feet from each other in a straight line (figure 13.32). You and your partner face each other on opposite sides of the line of buckets. Sprint laterally down the line using a lateral lunge or shuffle step until you reach bucket 4 at the end of the line. There are four balls in bucket 4; the rest are empty. Grab one ball out of bucket 4 and place it in bucket 3. Sprint back to bucket 4, grab another ball, and place it in bucket 2. Continue until each bucket has a ball.

Switch sides with your partner and complete the drill again. This drill can be done alone, but it is much more fun with a partner because you push a little harder when competing against someone else. Try to maintain your time or average for four rounds. Remember to note left-right differences.

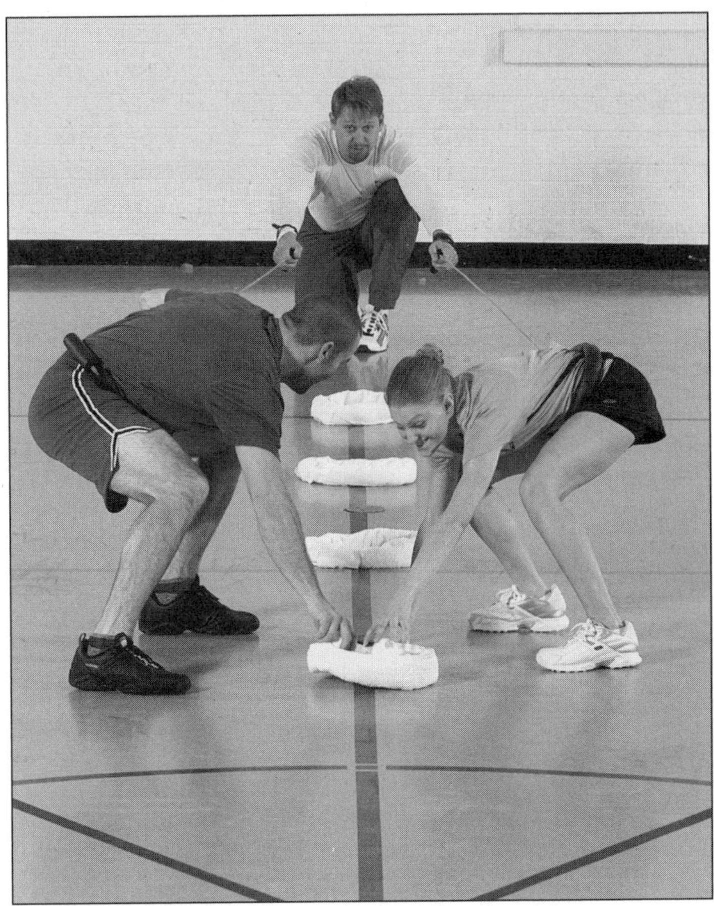

Figure 13.32
The mirror drill.

MEDICINE BALL MINI-TENNIS

Do not let the word *tennis* deter you from this drill. Even non-tennis players can get a great workout for both the upper and lower body and use many different movement patterns. This is an excellent conditioning drill that is both competitive and fun.

In the book *Power, Speed and Stamina for Tennis,* Jack Thompson and I proposed an effective drill for tennis called *medicine ball mini-tennis* that has excellent carryover into field and court sports. This drill requires a little equipment and time to set up but it is invaluable because it has many fundamental qualities. It is a competitive drill and creates an excellent interval training scenario. It isolates and equally challenges left and right movements of the body. It incorporates low center of gravity and the power stances of the lunge and the squat. It incorporates the upper-body movement patterns of chopping and lifting. It uses a medicine ball that allows for unrestricted movement at or near the speed of competition. It incorporates exaggerated weight shifting and assisted and resisted tubing work. In one direction the tubing will resist you, thereby increasing your strength and stability, whereas in the other direction the tubing will assist you by providing speed and causing you to demonstrate greater ability with control and deceleration.

You will need elastic tubing and an appropriate waist belt, a standard tennis court, and an inflatable medicine ball. The medicine ball should be 2 to 6 pounds or approximately 2 percent of the body weight of the athletes if they are equally matched.

Anchor the tubing to a fence on your right side at or near midcourt. Your opponent, who stands on the opposite side of the net, anchors his tubing to the fence on his left side at midcourt. Make sure the tubing is anchored to a stable object and that all attachments are secure and safe. You want a small amount of tension with minimal slack in the tubing when you are near where the tubing is attached, but you also want enough flexibility in the cord to allow you to reach the opposite side of the court. This requires a high-grade tubing; do not perform this drill if these standards cannot be preserved. An alternative is to have two partners hold the tubing, making sure there is minimal slack in the tubing at all times.

As you play mini-tennis, the tubing should be to your side and behind you so as not to obstruct medicine ball throws from the side in the chop and lift pattern (figure 13.33). The inflatable medicine ball allows you to adjust the game by inflating or deflating the ball. When you inflate the medicine ball, bounces are crisp, high, and fast, requiring more footwork and speed. Deflating the ball creates flat bounces that require more powerful and explosive movements of the upper body during the throw. Both methods are excellent. You just need to decide where you want to focus. Do you want to work the upper body with a deflated ball, or the lower body with an inflated ball? Or play the first 2 to 3 sets with an inflated ball and then deflate it for the next 2 to 3 sets.

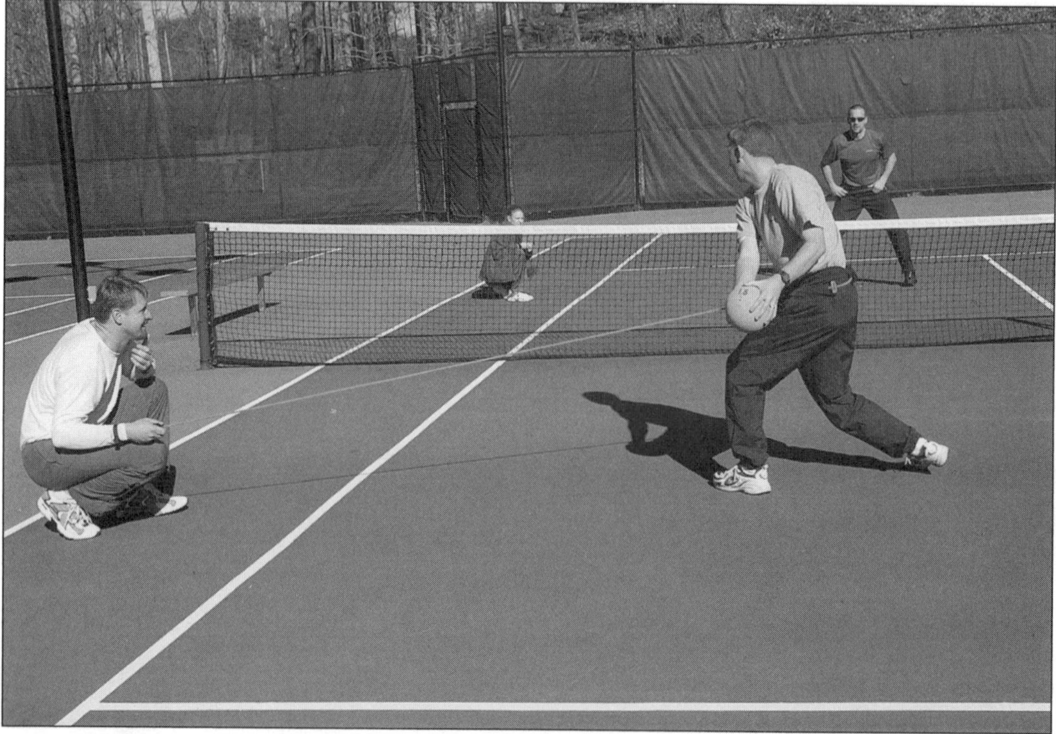

Figure 13.33 Medicine ball mini-tennis.

Although you are not using a racket, you will still use forehand and backhand movements. Every catch and throw with the medicine ball has to be with both hands on the ball. If both hands are not used in every catch and throw, a point is awarded to the other player.

All medicine ball throws should bounce within the front half of the tennis court. If you can get to a thrown ball before it bounces, you can return it however you please as long as it stays in play and will bounce within the front half of your opponent's court. You can rush the net to cut the ball off and return it quickly. If you throw the ball away from where the tubing is anchored, the tubing will act as resistance on your opponent as he chases the ball. If he returns it to you and you quickly throw it back toward where the tubing is anchored, your opponent will have to deal with the overspeed produced by the tubing and decelerate under control to catch and throw the ball.

Use the tubing and ball placement to score points. Failure to return the ball into the front half of the court constitutes a point. Rotate sides an equal number of times and score each game. If your opponent has less strength or power, you may want to offer him lighter tubing. If you are using tubing of the same size, it will increase your speed when changing sides of the tennis court. If you are using different strength tubing, take your tubing with you each time you alternate sides. You also can reduce the area of play to accommodate a less powerful athlete.

You can play medicine ball mini-tennis with an open or closed stance. An open stance is done from squat stance with your torso facing the opponent at all times. This requires you to rotate your shoulders and catch the ball on a bounce pass. You can return the ball either from a lifting pattern with an arc or a chopping pattern like a spike. Just don't get tangled up in the tubing. If the tubing presents a problem, move it a little farther backward on the fence behind the midcourt position.

If you choose to play with a closed stance, you step across your body with your front leg. If you are right-handed and are doing a backhanded movement, you will step across your body with your right leg. If you are performing a forehand, you will step across your body with your left leg. You will probably choose to use a combination of both. The squat stance keeps you in your ready position so that you have not committed to one side of the court or the other. The lunge stance gives you much more control accelerating and decelerating in one direction but causes you to commit somewhat to one side of the court or the other.

Enjoy this drill. Be competitive. Try to go longer and longer with the same intensity, and this naturally competitive form of interval training will help build your skills regardless of your sport. The upper- and lower-body workout is nicely balanced and the end result is an amazing amount of functional core training.

PART V

PERFORMANCE PROGRAMS

14

Rotation and Swinging

One of my favorite sports quotes of all time was spoken by golfer Lee Trevino: "It's the Indian, not the arrow." I am sure the statement is targeted at golfers who constantly upgrade equipment without ever looking at their swing mechanics, flexibility, core stability, strategy, or shot technique, but I think the statement applies to all athletes, especially those who use swinging or rotational movements.

Hitting a baseball or softball, swinging a tennis racket or golf club, and using a lacrosse stick or hockey stick are all swinging movements. Rotational movement is used in paddle sports, rowing, martial arts, and wrestling, in which a hip toss and twisting moves are used to defeat an opponent. You can see rotational and swinging movements in many different sports.

Often the focus is on the implement and not the athlete (in Lee Trevino's words, the arrow and not the Indian). It is easy to focus on the implement or the tool used in the sport, but don't forget to be fundamental in the way you balance the body and train the core. The more you train fundamental elements such as foot position, weight shifting, and weight transfer, the greater your endurance and stamina will be. This will allow you to train longer and hone specific skills. But if you focus exclusively on skill and do not work on the foundation, you will greatly reduce the volume of training you can perform before fatigue.

The supplementary work in this chapter focuses on the many components that make up swinging and rotational movements. Explore each activity to determine whether it relates to your sport. There are many other drills that also complement swinging and rotational movements, but the ones in this chapter are fundamental for multisport application to identify right-left asymmetry and can be modified to a wide array of athletic abilities and training intensities.

The movements tested in chapter 5—squat, hurdle step, lunge, active straight leg raise, and seated rotation—are all important for rotation and swinging, but squats and seated rotations are fundamental to rotation and swinging movements. Make sure these patterns are not limited and can be performed well, and that there is no asymmetry in the seated rotation.

STANDING MEDICINE BALL CHEST PASS

This test will quickly reveal any left-right power differences in the ability to rotate or swing. Train to get this difference within 10 percent, whether the sport-specific movement pattern requires symmetrical or asymmetrical movement.

You will need a space that is safe and free of obstructions and a medicine ball that is approximately 2 percent of your body weight (table 14.1). Draw or tape two lines on the floor that intersect to form a T. Stand at the intersection of the two lines with your feet on the left-to-right line, facing the intersecting line. Throw the medicine ball from a double-leg squat stance as far as possible without stepping (figure 14.1a). The throw will have some arc. Go for maximum distance. Perform 2 to 3 throws and record the best distance.

Now throw the ball down the right-hand line and then the left-hand line (figure 14.1b). Perform 2 to 3 throws on each side and record the best distance. Do not change foot position and do not step. When you throw to the left, you will propel the ball predominantly with your right arm. When you throw to the right, you will propel the ball predominantly with your left arm. Do not lose your balance and do not lean or shift weight. From the waist down, you should move very little. Stand in a bent-knee, bent-hip ready position approximately 2 to 6 inches lower than your normal standing height, feet shoulder-width apart. Heels should be planted on the ground.

Compare right and left throws to the forward throw. Right and left throws should each be at least half the distance of the forward throw. The difference between left and right throws should not be greater than 15 percent; if it is greater, work on the weaker side. The drills in this chapter provide right-left options and allow you to work each side equally or focus on a particular weakness in squat stance to one side or the other.

Don't worry about comparing scores with other athletes unless they are the same size and weight as you. The test is designed so the athlete throws a light ball as fast and as far as possible. Focus on narrowing left-right differences within 10 to 15 percent.

Table 14.1 Standing Medicine Ball Chest Pass: 2 Percent of Body Weight

Body weight (lbs)	Medicine ball weight in lbs (kg)
120	2.4 (1.0)
140	2.8 (1.0)
160	3.2 (1.5)
180	3.6 (1.5)
200	4 (2.0)
220	4.4 (2.0)
240	4.8 (2.0)
260	5.2 (2.5)
280	5.6 (2.5)

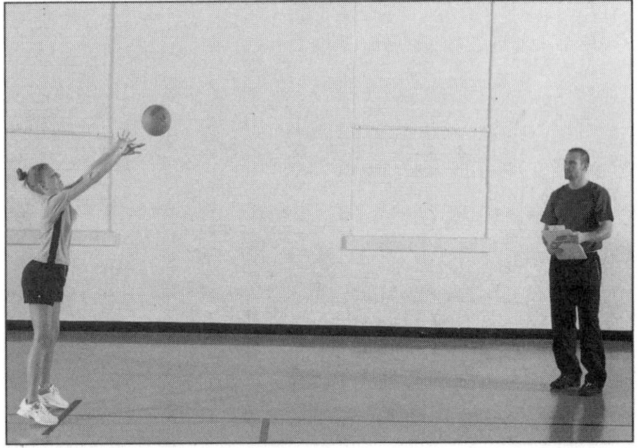

a

b

Figure 14.1 Standing medicine ball chest pass: *(a)* from a squat stance, throw the ball forward as far as possible; *(b)* throw the ball to the side.

Throwers and Strikers

Even elite throwing athletes can benefit from the fundamentals in a rotation and swinging program. Even though the ultimate goal for a thrower or striker is to throw or strike, it is vital to develop a fundamental base in rotation and swinging movements. Specific throwing and striking training (chapter 15) will build on what is gained in this chapter.

According to Chris Welch, president and CEO of Human Performance Technologies, Inc., throwing, striking, and swinging (in most cases) are the results of two types of force: *linear* and *rotational.* These two forces drive the different movement patterns for throwing and striking. Whether the athlete steps, strides, or keeps her feet planted, she shifts weight away from and then toward the target with the lower body. Also, a coiling movement is followed by an uncoiling movement that starts at the hips and then moves to the shoulders and arms. The weight shift is the trip hammer that sets the level of power. The goal is not to generate rotational power, but rather to transfer linear or weight-shifting power into rotational power. Imagine a short powerful movement being transformed into a big fast movement.

To visualize this concept, imagine an off-center playground seesaw. If you stepped off a box onto the short end, the short end would cover less distance going down than the long end would as it traveled up. You turned a short-distance force into speed because the long end traveled through a longer arc of movement in the same amount of time. Keep this in mind as you read chapters 14 and 15.

Because there are many similarities in the way power is generated for swinging and rotation movements and throwing and striking movements, it is extremely hard to separate the information or the conditioning programs. For practical purposes, we will say that rotation and swinging involve both arms working together, whereas throwing and striking focus all energy into the movement of one arm. Also, it is more common to have a dynamic lower body (which simply means taking a step) in a throw or a strike. Baseball players and lacrosse players often step before swinging. Hockey players are in constant motion when they move around the ice and strike the puck. In contrast, golfers have a static, planted position. Although there is not a step with the golf swing, a weight shift provides the linear component of power, which is transformed into rotational power. For our purposes, there is in most cases less movement of the lower body in a rotation or swinging activity.

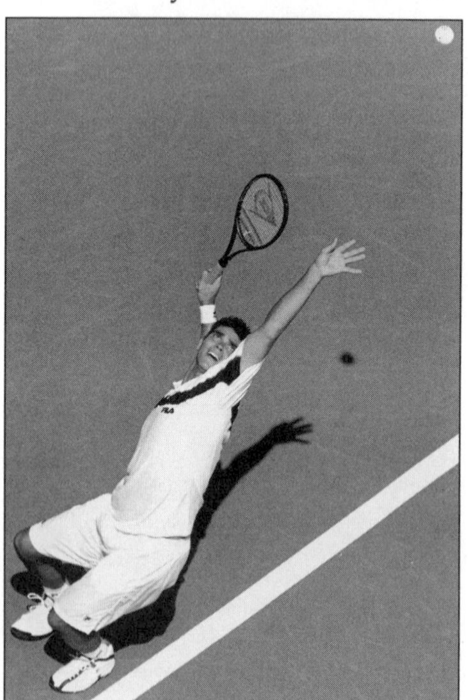

Athletes who perform swinging movements in sports such as tennis shouldn't focus on the implement used in the sport at the expense of movement fundamentals.

Another important element to consider in rotation or swinging is symmetry. Golfers, baseball players, and rowers are committed to a swing or rotation involving only one side of the body in one direction of movement. Lacrosse players, kayakers, and tennis and racquetball players use swings and rotations from both sides of the body. Whether the movements of the sport are asymmetrical (one-sided) or symmetrical (two-sided), it is important to first train symmetry. The body functions best from balance even if it is involved in asymmetrical activity.

Remember that you are not training for skill—you are complementing skill, laying the foundation for skill development and building the fundamentals of movement. The foundation of a skyscraper doesn't look impressive, but the end result is worth it. We will use the same chop and lift movement covered in chapter 9 and move into multidirectional movement.

Cable Column Work and Medicine Ball Work

For the standard chop with a stick, you will stand or kneel perpendicular to a cable column. In addition, you will throw the medicine ball with a bounce, which uses the chop pattern, perpendicular to a wall or partner. Imagine the body rotating to a perpendicular angle. If you rotate toward the cable column or away from the wall or partner, you will work on the follow-through of the movement. If you rotate away from the cable column or toward the wall or partner, you will work on the starting or initial phase of the movement. The same rules apply if you are in a scissors stance or squat stance doing medicine ball throws and chops. It is nearly impossible to create the full range of movement needed in swinging and rotational sport-specific patterns with any degree of accuracy with this method.

Some people use a cable column to try to replicate a sport-specific swinging or rotation movement, but this is the wrong approach. Instead, break the movement down into two or three patterns and then let the brain put those patterns together when the body performs the whole movement.

For example, imagine a baseball swing. Forget about the bat and forget about hand position for the moment. The movement is all about generating power from the ground up through the core. Consider the chop and lift (page 106) from a standing position. A right-handed person's first move is a chop down and across the body from right to left. Imagine a diagonal line across the body. Now perform a lift from right to left. The second diagonal line creates an X across the body. This X involves all the muscles used to create the arc of motion needed by the baseball bat.

The letter U represents a natural arc of motion. Swinging and rotation moves in tennis and hockey as well as other sports are more compact and use less range of motion than the baseball swing. The chop and the lift incorporate core stability and weight-shifting reactions needed to do these movements correctly.

The body can be rotated slightly to intensify the initial phase, follow-through, or final phase of the chop and lift, and doing so can be a useful way to test mobility and stability, body awareness, and coordination. As you reach back to go deeper or longer in the start position or push through to go deeper in the follow-through, you may have a tendency to compensate, lose the erect upright angle of the spine, or move into poor form. If this happens, go back to fundamentals. Keep the spine tall and erect. Let the arms do the work and rotate the torso as far as possible without losing erect posture so that the arms are not unnecessarily taxed.

Try not to rotate the hips and pelvis. Of course, the hips and pelvis rotate during a swinging movement in real sports activities, but this movement is a small arc of motion that is extremely quick and nearly impossible to train consciously because it occurs as a part of a larger movement pattern. If the hip turn has a large arc, speed or acceleration are compromised. A body cannot go faster and farther at the same time. The hip turn needs to be compact, solid, and explosively quick.

When the chop and lift is performed in a half-kneeling position and different foot positions, the hip muscles work isometrically (without joint movement) in the exact same sequence that generates the hip turn in free motion and sport movements. Don't train the hip turn alone. The muscle tension generated in the hips will create enough muscle memory to give you a quick and compact hip turn at the speed of competition. Keep the hips stable and the pelvis in line, and let the shoulders do the rotation.

Flexibility gained through the upper spine helps generate speed and uses some of the power created in the hips. This flexibility will also make the abdominal muscles and spinal muscles more reactive. Remember, a muscle gets feedback through stretch and tension. If adequate amounts of stretch and tension in the torso muscles cannot be generated, they will provide less feedback when it's time to stabilize and transfer energy.

Use these exercises to minimize hip turn and exaggerate shoulder turn. When fundamentals are lost or the muscles become stiff or weak, there is a tendency to exaggerate hip turn. This places unnecessary stress on the knees and also pulls the foot out of a power position, causing pronation on one or both sides. There may also be a tendency to reduce shoulder turn and try to make up the difference with exaggerated arm movements. Therefore, during the chop and lift there should be no hip or pelvis movement, a big shoulder turn, and adequate (but not excessive) arm movement.

These same rules apply to medicine ball drills. It is more appropriate to use a lighter medicine ball and generate greater speed than to use a heavy ball at slower speed. Use these throws in quick 8- to 15-repetition sets and try to hold fundamental posture at initial starting position from the waist down no matter what. This will be hard at first, and it will be possible only if the upper body is relaxed and the shoulders are allowed to turn. Keep the spine tall and breathe.

For the drill in the half-kneeling or lunge stance, narrow the base as much as possible. The narrow base demands that the core work harder to stabilize. A wide base allows compensation and can hide left-right differences. Allow the arms and hands to relax and stay flexible. Shake out the hands and arms before performing the drills and immediately after. Now is the time to use any core awareness. Don't tighten the body. Hold the core by relaxing breathing and holding the spine tall and by not allowing excessive hip or leg movement. In real-life activity, when the hips and pelvis are allowed to move a little, it creates quick, explosive, short-arc movements that generate a significant amount of power that the newly strengthened core can transmit to the shoulder turn and arm swing.

Don't be alarmed if performing the chopping and lifting movements temporarily reduces skill ability in a given sport. Golf is about tempo. Hitting a baseball is about timing. Controlling a putt is about feel or eye-hand coordination. Paddling a kayak through whitewater is about relaxing and allowing a quick, flexible core to react. None of this can be trained with a medicine ball. Feel and awareness has to be developed through practice.

Except for offseason training, I do not advise training with a cable column or medicine ball exclusively. In the offseason it's OK to go ahead and develop these fundamental patterns, but remember that a lot of time is needed for an athlete to get used to new core strength. It requires time spent looking at the fundamentals of a particular sport. Just because an athlete can whip around a medicine ball or pull on a cable column does not automatically mean that sport skill increases. It just means a more stable foundation has been laid.

During a competitive season or preseason, it is important to perform strength-training drills and skill drills that complement each other. Perform them on the same day, perhaps using one as a warm-up for the other. Find your own training style but stay symmetrical on lifts and stay consistent with skill and sport fundamentals.

As you train power, consistency in sports skill is more important than noticing vast increases in power. The power will come. As a matter of fact, some athletes may notice a reduction in power at first. But consistent training will lead to motor learning. The body will incorporate the newfound strength and coordination, but it takes time and feedback.

To gain extra strength in the hands, wrists, forearms, and shoulders, use the chop and lift patterns described in chapter 15 (page 190).

Tubing and Jump Rope Work

Tubing work for posterior weight shifting increases stability while allowing you to swing. Perform standing swinging and rotation work while tethered with light tubing that is anchored securely to a stationary object behind you. This will pull you onto your heels and cause you to shift your weight forward toward your toes. Bend your knees and relax. This will reduce hip turn but increase core stability and power transfer. As you swing, take a step forward to increase the tension on the tubing. Feel how it changes your swing. Perform a number of repetitions and make adjustments so that your mechanics look as though you are not tethered.

There is no set number of repetitions; this is simply a feel drill. Once you have a better feel, untie the tubing and perform your sport-specific swing. Note any differences in feel and performance. Swing 20 or 30 times, then go back to the tubing and perform 15 or 20 swings, then return to sport-specific swings. Go back and forth for a few sets. In most cases you should feel an increase in stability.

Two excellent jump rope techniques for rotation and swinging movements are the twister and the X-foot cross (see chapter 13, page 168). Two to 3 sets of 1 to 3 minutes for each move can complement a workout or a warm-up.

Heavy Versus Light

Research has been done on swinging and rotating with heavy and light implements. A standard example is a weighted baseball bat or weighted golf club. An athlete swinging one of these devices increases body awareness. The centrifugal force is greater and the inertia and momentum are different (usually more exaggerated) from the normal device.

Any changes in weight should be minute. Don't go overboard with using either heavy or light devices. Remember that weight and velocity have an inverse relationship: as weight goes down, velocity goes up, and as weight goes up, velocity must go down. So an athlete using a weighted implement should not try to swing or even expect to swing at normal speed. It's impossible. Use a weighted baseball bat or golf club or add weight to a sport-specific tool to improve awareness and expose fundamental flaws in mechanics.

Do not play with these implements or train with them for long periods of time. Use them appropriately to find a correct swing or turn. The feedback created through the use of weighted devices is going to be more appropriate if the athlete relaxes and uses it as a sport-specific warm-up. Swinging a light implement may require a much greater degree of skill and more supervision and coaching, but it will teach the athlete to move faster and get started more quickly.

Using a heavy or light implement can be compared to running up or down a hill. Both can improve running speed and technique, but each works differently. Running up a hill, which is like swinging a heavy implement, imposes greater stress on the body and should reinforce proper fundamentals. It slows things down enough for the runner to feel any flaws in flexibility, weight shift, or overall movement.

Running down a hill, which is like swinging a light object, allows the runner to go faster than normal with the help of gravity. This stimulates the neurological system. It exposes the brain to potential and allows the runner to feel faster movement than naturally felt in regular activity. It's not done for strengthening, but for coordination, timing, and relaxation.

One of the keys to moving faster than normal is to relax. When great athletes are in the zone they do not feel like they are moving faster—they feel like everything around them is moving slower. They reach this point through confidence, relaxation, breathing, and focus. When an athlete swings a light implement, she asks the neurological system to move a little bit faster. It is extremely easy to get sloppy when swinging a light implement. Therefore, it may be necessary to have a coach or training partner observe mechanics and fundamentals.

Swinging a light implement is not as popular as swinging a heavy implement, but it does have its benefits. Make sure movement planes are correct. Fundamentals should be sound and the body needs to be in the right position. Swinging a heavy implement allows the athlete to feel the arc of a motion. Swinging a light implement increases timing, coordination, and speed.

Paddle, Rowing, and Combative Sports

Chop and lift movements can be done on a stability ball or a Dyna Disc to simulate sport specificity in the actual position or posture of an activity. Sitting on a stability ball replicates a canoeing position; sitting flat or low on a Dyna Disc replicates kayaking.

Wrestlers, football players, rugby players, and participants in combative sports such as judo can use push and pull movements with a cable column to increase rotation, stability, and strength. For push and pull movements, create a specific situation. If part of the sport is to grab the clothing or garment of another athlete and push or pull, thread a towel through the handles of a cable column and use it to build grip strength while working on torso, core, and arm strength.

Use a lower-body position similar to that used in the sport. Do not arbitrarily stand or kneel. Use the position that would most benefit sport performance but also presented the most difficulty in movement patterns. For example, a wrestler who experiences problems with the lunge when his left foot is forward should try row and press movements on a double-handle cable column from a half-kneeling position with the right foot forward, then try the same exercise with the left foot forward. He should note any left-right differences in his ability to stabilize and lift weight to complete repetitions. You can follow the drills for chopping and lifting but use pushing and pulling. It is also appropriate to use angles. Pull from low to high. Push from low to high.

If standing perpendicular to a partner or wall when throwing the medicine ball or standing perpendicular to the cable column, use chops and lifts. If facing toward or away from a medicine ball partner, wall, or cable column, work on pushes, pulls, and throws. An excellent way to check rotational power is to perform the left-right medicine ball throw described at the beginning of this chapter in a squat stance. Other stances, such as a scissors stance or a lunge, can be used as well as long as right and left sides are compared.

15

Throwing and Striking

The great martial artist Bruce Lee once said, "I relax until the moment I bring every muscle of my body into play, and then concentrate all the force in my fist. To generate great power you must first totally relax and gather your strength, and then concentrate your mind and all your strength on hitting your target." I truly admire the wisdom in this statement, the way Lee uses the words *power* and *relax* in the same sentence. Only when you completely relax can your mind get out of the way and let your body do what it was trained to do.

Of course, you do need to train. Simply relaxing and performing power movements without a sound and stable base will not allow you to improve throwing or striking power. Bruce was considered a small athlete by American standards, yet he delivered amazingly powerful punches. Of course, he trained and put in many hours to create both mobility and stability within his body. He developed strength and used calisthenics, sparring, and weight training to complement both his endurance and explosiveness. Ultimately his skills were in the martial arts, and striking was a big part of that. Bruce realized it had little to do with arm strength and quite a bit to do with foot position, core stability, body mechanics, and a relaxed state of mind.

Throwing and striking are highly technical and require an advanced level of skill. Many times, using proper body mechanics will temporarily reduce power and you will have a tendency to do whatever it takes to throw, pitch, or strike with more velocity. This is the wrong approach. As proper fundamentals and good body mechanics are used, they become more familiar and natural. You will relax more when you get into these positions and perform these movements, and ultimately the power will come. Don't look at power as simply the ability to generate force with one throw, pitch, or strike; look at how long you can maintain a high level of force production.

Many times, you will be able to throw, strike, or pitch with great velocity whether you use proper body mechanics or not. But if you plan on doing this for some time and would like to enjoy a long, injury-free competitive career, do it right and do it a lot. Major league baseball pitcher Greg Maddux expresses this sentiment: "People judge too much by results. I'm just the opposite. I care about more than results. I'd rather make a good pitch and give up a bloop single than make a bad pitch and get an out."

The movements tested in chapter 5—squat, hurdle step, lunge, active straight leg raise, and seated rotation—are all important for throwing and striking. All the movements are important, but lunges and seated rotations are fundamental to throwing and striking. Make sure these patterns are not limited, can be performed well, and do not demonstrate asymmetry.

STEPPING MEDICINE BALL CHEST PASS

This test will quickly reveal any left-right difference in throwing or striking ability. Train to get this difference under 10 percent, whether your sport requires symmetrical or asymmetrical movement patterns.

This test is similar to the forward throw in the standing medicine ball chest pass (page 181). Use a medicine ball that is 2 percent of your body weight. Instead of a squat stance, as in chapter 14, throw forward using a step (figure 15.1). This will leave you in a lunge stance. Perform three forward throws stepping with the right foot, then three forward throws stepping with the left foot. Measure each throw and record the best. Look for differences between the left- and right-step throws. Work on any left-right differences greater than 10 to 15 percent.

Review the information in chapter 14 (pages 182 to 183). The fundamentals for throwing and striking are in the movements of swinging and rotation.

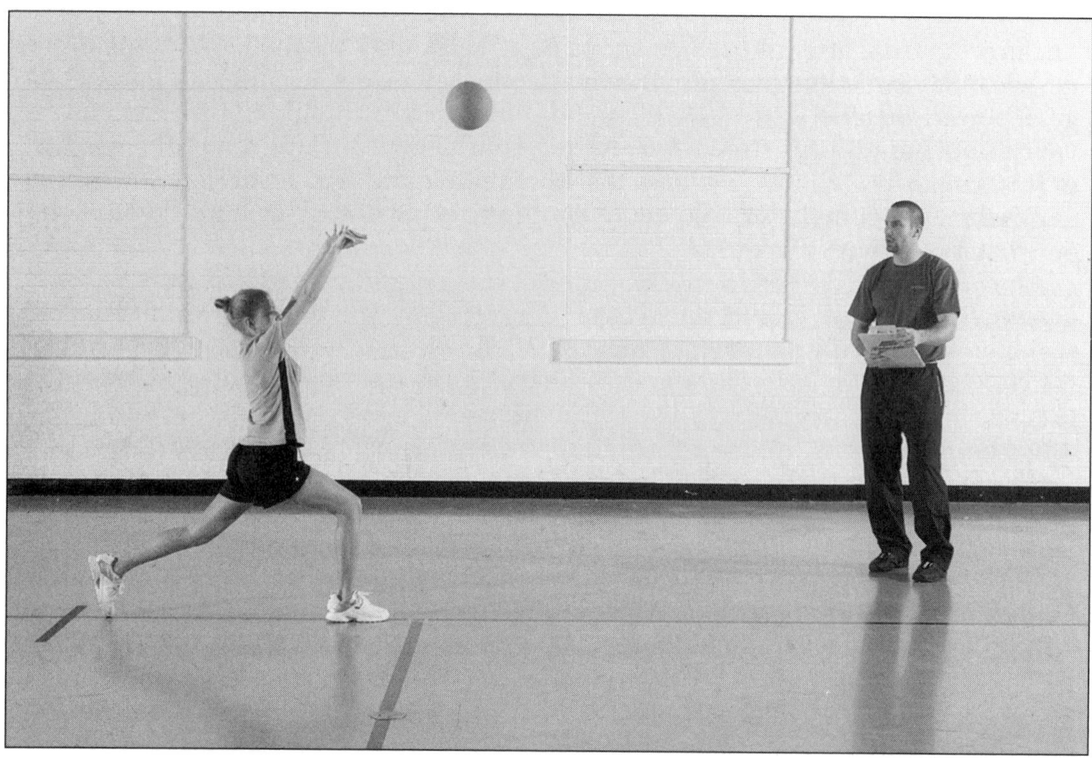

Figure 15.1 Stepping medicine ball chest pass.

Upper-Body One-Arm Movements

One-arm athletic movements are significantly more complex than often thought. To propel the arm for throwing, striking, and swinging, an athlete needs to have excellent coordination and linking of the lower body and trunk. Weight shifting, balance, and coordination are all important for what appears to be a simple upper-body movement.

Supplementary work for the upper body can reinforce movement patterns for upper-body activities such as the one-arm athletic movements of throwing, striking, and swinging with one arm (as in racket sports). Supplementary training for one-arm movements incorporates the entire body and will help prevent common imbalances associated with one-arm dominance. It will also help create a balance for activities that use a predominance of one movement pattern while neglecting other movement patterns. The use of contrasting movement patterns will help maintain movement balance and symmetry. It is important to use supplementary training methods for the upper body to maintain balance and general conditioning for the applicable movement patterns needed for sport-specific skill.

Throwing, striking, and swinging (specifically with one arm) are unique because all usually involve a step. If a step is not involved, a drastic weight shift is, so either way the athlete needs to train striding, stepping, or weight shifting.

When an athlete strides, he generates more hip speed, but striding also requires commitment. The athlete adds power to a certain direction of movement and is now committed to going in that direction. An athlete in a throwing, striking, or swinging sport or position who requires a step—whether an exaggerated step, as in pitching a baseball or swinging a racket, or a subtle quick step, as in throwing a quick pass or a short punch—needs to get the step right first. Here is how.

Medicine Ball Work

Get a medicine ball and find a hard cinder block wall. Start by standing 8 to 10 feet from the wall, facing it (figure 15.2a). Step toward the wall and throw the ball at the

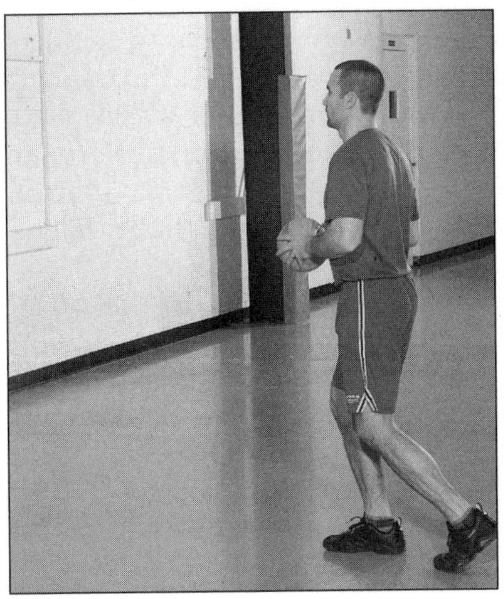

a

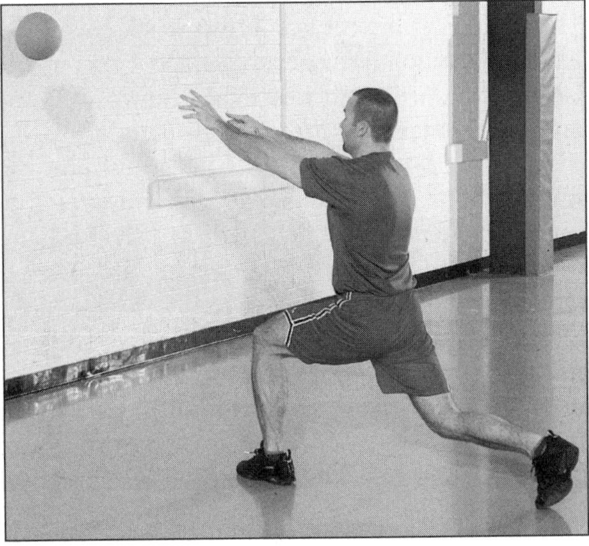

b

Figure 15.2 Medicine ball throw: *(a)* face the wall; *(b)* use a chest pass to throw the ball against the wall.

wall with a chest pass (figure 15.2b). Don't exaggerate the throw; exaggerate the step. Make the step a little longer, lunge a little deeper, and hit the ground hard with your front foot. Then perform an easy throw.

Note how power is generated from the ground up. Move back from the wall, but do not throw the ball harder: use the step to move the ball harder. This throw does not look anything like the throw or swing in a sport or the striking or punching done in competition, but it does create a link between the lower and upper body. Generate power low, bring it up into the core, and then direct it through the arms. It may help to perform the drill stepping on each side. Although a step on the nondominant foot may never be needed in the sport (for example, rarely will a quarterback be asked to throw with his nondominant arm), learning to step on the nondominant foot as if throwing with the nondominant arm may help the athlete learn to step more efficiently when throwing with the dominant arm. It also helps balance power.

Play a game with yourself. Start close to the wall, facing it. Take a step, throw the medicine ball in a chest pass, catch it when it bounces off the wall, then move back a little. Make sure to throw the ball high enough so that it comes back in the air. As you step back, you will have to throw the ball harder. Try not to throw it much harder with the arms, and exaggerate the step to generate power even if it takes a full lunge or if the foot slaps the ground and creates a lot of noise. Generate power from the lower body. Use a quick pushoff of the back foot to get power. Do this drill stepping with each foot. Perfect symmetry will probably never happen, but it's good training. Go immediately from this drill to your chosen throwing or striking sport and see what you've learned.

This is a great way to increase awareness of lower-body movements and improve hip turn. It is not necessary to exaggerate the step with a normal throw or punch. If you've gained timing, coordination, and power in the lower body through training, it's there. The brain has the input and it knows how to use it. Relax and perform throws, strikes, or punches. Evaluate both the quality and quantity of what you can do and how it is different.

Cable Column Work

The chop and lift cable column work covered in earlier chapters creates an excellent base for the following exercise, the chop and lift with independent arm movement. Use a standard high-low cable column pulley system, but instead of a stick use a large-diameter rope for a handle (see figure 9.2, page 103). The rope works each hand independently. The movement is spiral and diagonal and each arm follows a mirror image of the other. This exercise still uses the chop and lift pattern, but the hands, wrists, forearms, and shoulders are strengthened.

Previously, the use of the stick provided greater leverage so the core could be stressed without overstressing the arms. Now it's time to stress the arms. Use the foot positions that correspond to your problem. If your problem is resolved, then use the foot positions that correspond with your sport-specific movement. For example, if you're a pitcher and you do not have a movement pattern problem, then go to the hurdle step (single-leg stance) to improve your starting position stability. Use the half-kneeling position to improve lunge stability and the movement pattern for the pitching stride.

Tubing and Jump Rope Work

Use tubing to improve stride. Tubing can be used to resist or assist movement. Tubing work will help improve the stepping and lunging movement in throwing, striking, and swinging. The tubing goes around the waist to pull the athlete back and up. The tubing pulls against the natural lunging movement, which goes forward and down. The tubing reduces the effect of gravity and allows the athlete to exaggerate the stride. Take a little longer stride and drop the center of gravity a little deeper. You can use this type of lunge as a warm-up or as a dynamic stretch. You can also take advantage of the assistance and perform multiple repetitions of your throwing or striking movement pattern at half-speed.

Tubing work has many benefits. First, because the tubing assists the movement, the athlete can do more repetitions, which improves motor learning, making the increased leg action and hip turn feel more natural. Second, tubing work can be used to rehabilitate a leg that is weaker or deconditioned following an injury or surgery. Full-speed movement isn't needed; half-speed is a good place to start.

Remember, tubing work is not meant to train arm action; it's meant to train the power source, the legs and core. Hit a punching bag, throw a ball into a wall or to a partner, or hit a tennis ball (this drill works with any racket sport). Take a long, deep stride, perform the move, and reset. These moves also can be done with a cable column.

For the assisted lunge, the weight in the cable column will assist movement. Use a belt and a high pulley. Start at 10 to 30 percent of body weight. Face away from the pulley and step into a deep lunge. Gravity will not have the same effect it normally does. Because the task is easy, focus on lunge technique. The weight assistance will allow many repetitions. The multiple repetitions will develop comfort with a deep, full-stride lunge. Perform the lunge on both the dominant and nondominant sides. This is a great warm-up activity that reinforces form without taxing the legs.

For jump rope work, the forward straddle, arm criss-cross, and side swing to jump techniques will help build power and coordination. See chapter 13 for descriptions of the techniques.

16

Jumping and Kicking

Bruce Lee's advice to develop legs to their utmost strength and flexibility reminds us to develop strength and flexibility equally. There is no greater testament to the importance of balance between strength and flexibility than an athlete who is skilled at jumping and kicking movements. Of course, jumping and kicking require amazing amounts of strength and power throughout the legs. However, if you develop this strength and power and do not equally improve your flexibility or at least maintain what you have, your power will be wasted on overcoming your own tightness, or you will be able to generate more power than your range of motion will allow. Either way, you will hurt your performance or yourself.

I have discussed Bruce Lee's advice with many athletes. Many look at it, nod, and agree—but when I question them about what they read, they recount how Lee advocated strength training for the legs. They completely overlook, or at least minimize, the flexibility component of Lee's statement.

You likely have been working on your movement screen and have done everything in your power to maximize each of the movement patterns to allow your body to move freely. When propelling your leg through the air in a kick or propelling your body through the air with a jump, unrestricted and free movement is an asset. You want to minimize wasted energy every chance you get. Specifically working on your skill with your coach is one way to reduce wasted energy with your technique. But if you bring poor flexibility to the best technique in the world, you are still going to get wasted energy.

The movements tested in chapter 5—squat, hurdle step, lunge, active straight leg raise, and seated rotation—are all important for jumping and kicking. All the movements are important, but the hurdle step and active straight leg raise are fundamental to jumping and kicking. Make sure these patterns are not limited, can be performed well, and do not demonstrate asymmetry.

The vertical jump test (page 136) can give you an idea of your overall rank compared to other athletes. More important, you can look for performance asymmetry and compare the right and left single-leg vertical jump. Look for differences greater than 10 to 15 percent. Focus on training the weaker side and try to reduce the deficit. Perform the test periodically to assess single-leg power. Whether you are a kicking or jumping athlete, symmetry with your mobility, stability, and power will create greater balance in your performance.

On the surface, jumping and kicking movements may seem to have nothing in common, but this is not always the case. They are in the same chapter for a good reason. Jumping rarely requires an equal contribution from both legs, with both legs performing the same movement. A vertical leap, such as that used for testing, is an example of a perfect double-leg jumping situation. However, that particular movement rarely occurs in sports.

In this chapter we'll explore the fundamental movement pattern that links both jumping and kicking: the single-leg stance. The single-leg stance is best demonstrated in the hurdle step. In the single-leg stance, at some point in the movement pattern most (if not all) of the weight is shifted to one leg. Regardless of the kicking movement used in sport competition or combat, one leg usually remains on the ground (or at least the athlete drives from that one leg to generate the power for the kick). Most jumping movements for sport and competition also require the movement to occur predominantly off one leg. This leg is what we will focus on.

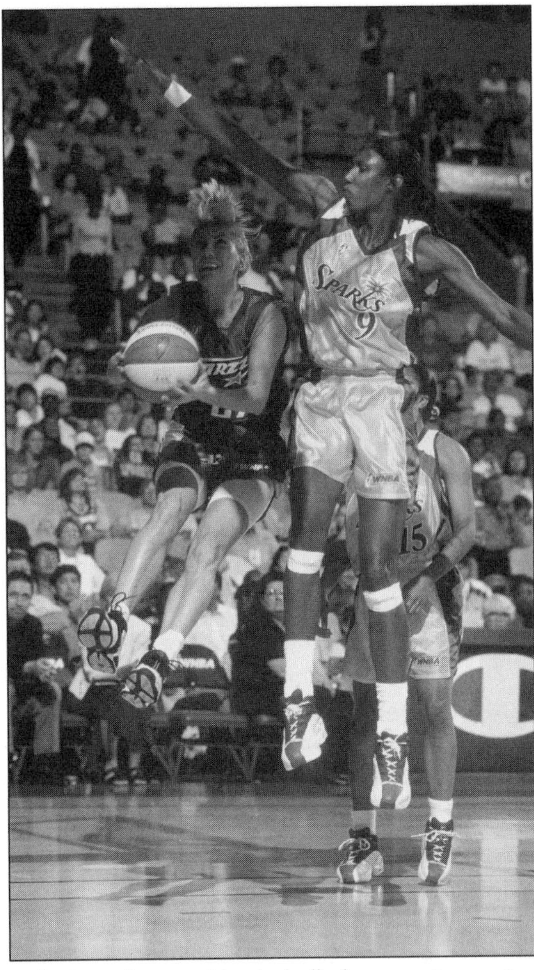

Today's professional basketball players get amazing height on their vertical jumps.

When observing impressive kicking and jumping movements, you may wrongly discern what initially caused the movement. When you focus only on the effect, you can forget the cause. Impressive kicks by different athletes, whether martial artists or football players, may look completely different. However, all kicks rely on the stability, strength, balance, and coordination of the standing leg to create a foundation of power.

Jumping is no different. We are often impressed by the height and hang time demonstrated by high jumpers and the aerial acrobatics of professional and collegiate basketball players. But if you focus on the result of the jump (the acceleration of the body upward or hang time), you will miss what caused the jump. The jump is a unified effort of both legs moving in different directions (much like a kick). The propulsion leg, usually the last one to leave the ground, generates the push in a jump. The true secret to jumping is creating pull with the other leg. Many natural jumpers do this without realizing it—they simply and naturally accelerate one leg up by flexing the hip and knee. The weight and momentum of this leg pulls the body up as the strength and power of the other leg pushes the body up. Both legs work together in opposite directions. This is similar to the description of a kicking motion. Because of this, these two activities have the same fundamental building block with movement.

Earlier we discussed movement patterns. The hurdle step movement pattern is a fundamental movement pattern that is used in most jumping and kicking situations. A double-leg jump may have a lot in common with the squat, and an off-balance jump may have more in common with the lunge. But for all practical purposes, the hurdle step and its mechanics demonstrate the movement patterns needed for correct jumping and kicking. The ability to separate the hips into opposite directions and maintain balance with an erect, elongated spine is the key.

An athlete may prefer to jump off one leg or kick with another, or a particular sport may dictate the movement (as with the specialty positions of punting and kicking in football), or an athlete may need to have a wide array of kicks (for example, a martial artist or soccer player). In any case, the athlete must have symmetry in this fundamental movement pattern. Even if the athlete never plans to kick with the nondominant leg, it is important to have balance between the left and right sides.

It is not necessary for a right-handed pitcher to throw an equal number of pitches with the left arm. He will always be extremely high in skill with the right arm and should never expect to be competitive with left-handed pitches. However, this is only true for the skill level of his performance. His left-right hip turn power, left-right shoulder turn power, and left-right leg balance and coordination should all be stable and symmetrical with respect to functional movements. The pitcher's arms will always be dissimilar, sometimes in form and definitely in function; however, the pitcher's body should never have to compete with imbalances in the core.

This same rule applies to the kicker. Every kicker has a favorite style and probably will never have to kick with the nondominant leg. But remember, this is a skill. The fundamental movement of separating the hips should be equal on the left and right. The ability to stand, balance, and demonstrate control on one leg should be similar as well. Starting with the hurdle step and eliminating any left-right imbalances will slowly develop the ability to stand on one leg.

Most kicking and jumping is done at extremely high velocity to propel the body, propel an object, or deliver a blow in the case of combative sports. There is not a lot of carryover from resistance training to the explosive movement needed in jumping and kicking. It is not appropriate to consider resistance training as a viable conditioning tool for the kicking (or pulling) leg in the jump. However, resistance training can be used to train the stable (or pushing) leg. The athlete must create balance, coordination, and control regardless of other body movements. Only from this stable base can the athlete achieve better jumping mechanics or kicking form.

This chapter lays the foundation for kicking and is equally beneficial to martial artists, soccer players, basketball players, volleyball players, and football players. When an athlete develops stability on a single leg, she can drive from that leg, whether she needs to jump or kick from that position.

Before continuing, please review the core training exercises for the hurdle step (chapter 7, page 68) and the strength-training exercises for the hurdle step (chapter 10, page 115). Most of these exercises are adequate for creating a functional base for jumping and kicking. For advanced training, try the following suggestions as well.

Practice

There is no substitute for practicing the particular jumping movement or kicking movement to address the individual needs of a sport or activity. However, the exercises presented in this chapter should provide a solid foundation and stable base. Many of these exercises can serve as excellent warm-ups before jump or kick training. Do not take them to the point where they cause fatigue or poor form. They will stimulate the solid mechanics needed to build better technique.

Single-Leg Pushes and Pulls

Use a standard cable column to perform pulls and pushes in a single-leg stance position. For greater stability and balance, you can push with both arms first then move to one arm as your balance improves. Pushing exercises should be performed on the same side as the standing leg. Pulling exercises should be performed on the opposite side of the standing leg. This is the natural reciprocal action of the arm and leg in both kicking and jumping. You will never see these drastic movements in real-life situations, but this exercise replicates the forces that go through the center of the body and create the core stability for lightning-fast movement.

SINGLE-LEG STANCE PUSH

Stand with your back to the cable column with the right leg down and the left leg flexed 90 degrees at the hip and knee (figure 16.1a). The spine should be held in a tall, erect position. Face forward. Use a very light amount of weight. Hold the hand, wrist, elbow, and shoulder in a comfortable position.

You can choose the direction of the cable. If you place the cable higher than the shoulder, push downward and don't allow the trajectory of the cable to change during the movement. For a more difficult movement, move the cable so that it is slightly lower than the shoulder but above the waist. Push upward.

As you push, let the body naturally react and create balance (figure 16.1b). You may notice an automatic slight bend in the right knee. This is good; never hyperextend the knee. Do not get shorter during the exercise. Do not crouch or flex the spine. If the body lowers at all, it should do so as the knee bends in an attempt to maintain balance (2 inches at the most). It may help to imagine holding a cup on your left thigh. The left knee needs to stay still so the cup doesn't fall during multiple repetitions of the single-leg push.

Perform this exercise equally on the left and right sides unless an imbalance is detected. Remedy the imbalance by performing multiple sets on the problem side, even if it requires using less weight on the machine. Make sure technique is good. Balance the body as quickly as possible. Use the single-leg stance push as part of a strength-training regime if jumping or kicking is part of your chosen sport or activity.

a

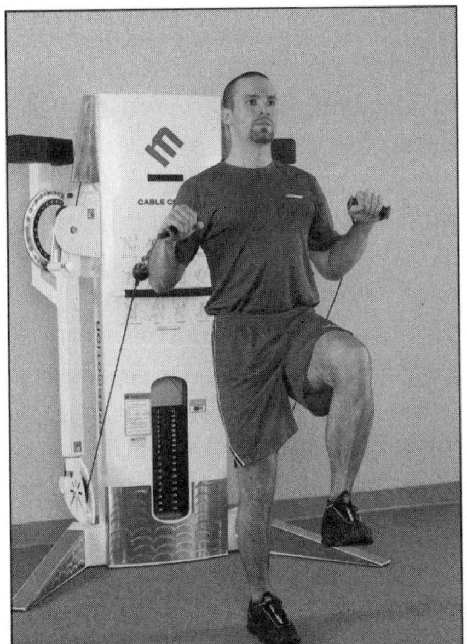

b

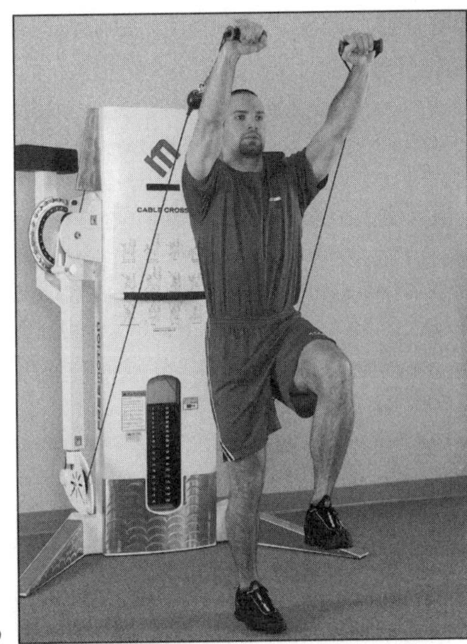

Figure 16.1 Single-leg stance push: *(a)* begin with back to the cable machine, one knee up; *(b)* push up.

SINGLE-LEG PULL

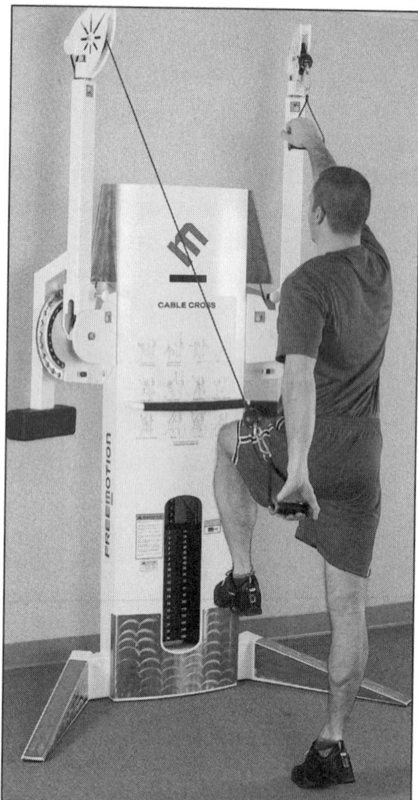

Figure 16.2 Single-leg pull.

Stand facing the cable column with the right leg down and the left leg flexed 90 degrees at the hip and knee. The spine should be held in a tall erect position. Face forward. Use a very light amount of weight. Hold the hand, wrist, elbow, and shoulder in a comfortable position.

Start with the cable column slightly higher than the shoulder. Pull down on the rope with the left arm (figure 16.2). To perform a row or pull-up, start with the cable column slightly lower than the shoulder.

Both the push and pull movements will create a rotation component that will make the body want to yield by bending or twisting. As the trunk is held erect and balance is maintained, the body naturally will use the strength of the core and the standing leg as a stable base to counteract any unnecessary rotation. A slight knee bend is the key. Try to relax. Remember, the core cannot react if the body is tense.

Perform this exercise equally on the left and right sides unless an imbalance is detected. Remedy the imbalance by performing multiple sets on the problem side, even if it requires using less weight on the machine. Maintain a tall, erect spine throughout the pulling movement, keeping the rest of the body relaxed. Pretend to balance a cup on the left thigh. Note left-right abilities, as well as endurance and strength.

Rope Jumping

Jump on one leg with the other leg held up and the hip and knee flexed to 90 degrees. Extra work with this drill will build a stable base and improve endurance for jumping and kicking activities. Train in intervals of 15 to 30 seconds per side with the single-leg jump and work toward symmetry between the left and right sides.

Rest for two, three, or four times the time for the rope jumping interval. For a 15-second jumping interval, rest for 30 seconds up to 1 minute before repeating the same amount of jumps in the next 15-second period. For a 30-second jumping interval, rest for 1 to 2 minutes. Be sure to look for left and right symmetry.

Timing jumping activities ensures that you do not waste energy. Jump as many times as possible in 15 or 30 seconds. Do not waste any movement or energy during the drill. Jump only high enough to clear the rope—no more. There is no extra credit for jumping higher than the rope. Keep the jumps quick and compact.

The forward shuffle and power jump help build power and coordination. See chapter 13 for descriptions of the forward shuffle (page 168) and power jump (page 169). Single-leg jumping is also an excellent way to improve power and control in jumping and kicking.

Medicine Ball Work

The medicine ball is lighter than the weight stack used with the cable column pull and press, so the movements are faster. Using an extremely heavy medicine ball in a single-leg stance is fruitless and can do little to improve the movement pattern. It is much better to use a ball that is a little too light than one that is too heavy.

For solo work, use a medicine ball that will easily bounce off a wall. (This drill requires an air-filled ball.) Play overhead catch, bounce pass catch, and over the left and right shoulder catch without losing balance. Stand on the right leg, holding the left leg up with the hip and knee bent to 90 degrees. Perform throws in different directions—overhead, left and right, and bouncing—trying to maintain an erect trunk without losing balance.

When possible, use a partner with the medicine ball drills. Do not perform a standard chest pass. Use bounce passes to make your partner reach high over his head and cross passes across your body from your left to his left (or from your right to his right). Performing these combinations while maintaining proper body mechanics helps improve core stability. Remember, work the right and left sides of the body. When in doubt, use a lighter medicine ball. As you gain the ability to maintain a stable body whether throwing or catching a medicine ball, you should grow to appreciate how many muscles it takes to maintain that stability when performing this type of movement.

The next level of conditioning allows dynamic movement. Do not bend or flex the spine. Instead, use the left leg (previously held in a stable position) as a counterbalance. This leg can help maintain balance when you catch the ball. Kick the leg into an extended position without touching it to the floor, and use it to help generate power in the core. Transfer this power to the arm throw to increase the velocity of the movement pattern. Teaching the body to transfer energy from the arms to the leg (as in a catch) or from the leg to the arms (as in a throw) helps to improve overall dynamics with jumping and kicking. These activities are designed to get the body to react in a certain way. Let them work. Concentrate on maintaining stability. Breathe and feel the move happen. The body will do the right thing if you let it.

For a forward chest pass, alternate leg kicks, beginning with one leg down and the other bent 90 degrees at the hip and knee. A chop throw with a bounce pass will provide right and left feedback. Stand on the right leg with the left leg bent 90 degrees at the hip and knee. Hold the ball over the left shoulder and throw down and across the body to the right. This is the chop. Perform the move as hard as possible.

Start slow and work up to the hand toss. The object of the hand toss is to bounce the ball over your partner's head. (The partner stands off your right shoulder, 10 to 12 feet away.) If this is not difficult, let some air out of the ball. Look at left-right differences in power and endurance. Fix the difference and maintain left-right balance.

17

Cutting and Turning

Most field and court sports require cutting and turning. The way you use your legs—specifically, your lunge movement patterns—will determine your ability to lower your center of gravity and decelerate and accelerate.

By now you likely have recognized left-right asymmetries within the lunge and other movement patterns and have taken the necessary steps to resolve any strength or endurance deficits you found. If you have taken rope jumping seriously, the quick, reactive movements you've been training for in rope work will complement your cutting and turning. These quick movements, added to core stability and better body mechanics, should reveal improved body mechanics with greater stamina in competitive situations. It is advantageous to have a reserve of energy in the second half or quarter of any sporting event.

You can use intervals throughout cutting and turning to develop conditioning intervals that will reinforce your mechanics, improve your endurance, and maintain the quality of your movement throughout a competitive event. I particularly appreciate the wisdom of John Wooden's approach to conditioning. He said that his team would always prevail against an equally skilled opponent because his team would be better conditioned. He was confident in his team's conditioning because of how they trained and the emphases he placed on quickness and execution throughout practice.

The movements tested in chapter 5—squat, hurdle step, lunge, active straight leg raise, and seated rotation—are all important for cutting and turning. Squats and lunges are fundamental to cutting and turning. Make sure these patterns are not limited, can be performed well, and do not demonstrate asymmetry.

The two fundamentals required for cutting and turning movements in athletics are a low center of gravity and control. The two work best together; however, control is needed even in situations in which a low center of gravity cannot be achieved, and a low center of gravity is safe and productive in situations in which control is not possible. The illusion of quickness is a demonstration of both of these factors. Quickness on the field or court often looks like above-average acceleration, but most of the time acceleration is not the key. Deceleration is the key because it sets up the rest of the movement. When one athlete is able to lose or break away from another athlete, it often is done with a cutting or turning movement. This movement is the result of deceleration or direction change followed by acceleration. It is important for athletes to train deceleration movements, whether they play soccer, football, or basketball or use deceleration to execute better moves, such as fielding a baseball or hitting a tennis ball.

It is ironic that quickness is often thought of as the ability to start a movement in a short amount of time. Actually, true quickness also includes the ability to stop a movement in a short amount of time. Quickness improves as deceleration develops because when an athlete is able to stop more efficiently and with better control, she has more time to set up, change direction, and accelerate in a new direction.

Deceleration Is the Key

Although there is no substitute for practicing particular cutting or turning movements to address the individual needs of a sport or activity, the exercises presented in this chapter provide a solid foundation and stable base. Many of these exercises can be used as warm-ups.

Remember that the secret to cutting and turning is deceleration. Practice feeling comfortable with deceleration moves. The exercises in this chapter will help stimulate the solid mechanics needed to build better technique. Cutting and turning moves will be quick and clean. Do not use these drills to the point that they cause fatigue or poor form.

Deceleration places much greater stress on the joints and muscles than acceleration. When an athlete tries to change direction without properly decelerating, his momentum may take him off line and put him off balance. This can either slow him down or increase the risk of injury. Training deceleration ultimately will reduce the risk of injury from deceleration-type movements such as landing, stopping, or changing direction.

TRIANGLE DRILL

Cutting and turning should be evaluated from the left and right sides dynamically or with linear movement followed by direction changes. The triangle drill is a good way to do this. This drill is effective because it forces you to turn or cut greater than 90 degrees five times in a tight pattern. To get an accurate representation, do two to three tests in each direction and average the times.

Use cones to create a triangle 10 yards by 10 yards by 10 yards. Sprint around the triangle twice (figure 17.1), sprinting past the start line to finish. Have a friend or coach time you. Take a long rest break (2 to 5 minutes), then perform the same drill in the opposite direction. This will assess ability in left and right cutting and turning. If there is a difference greater than 10 to 15 percent, work on the side with the slower time until both times are equal.

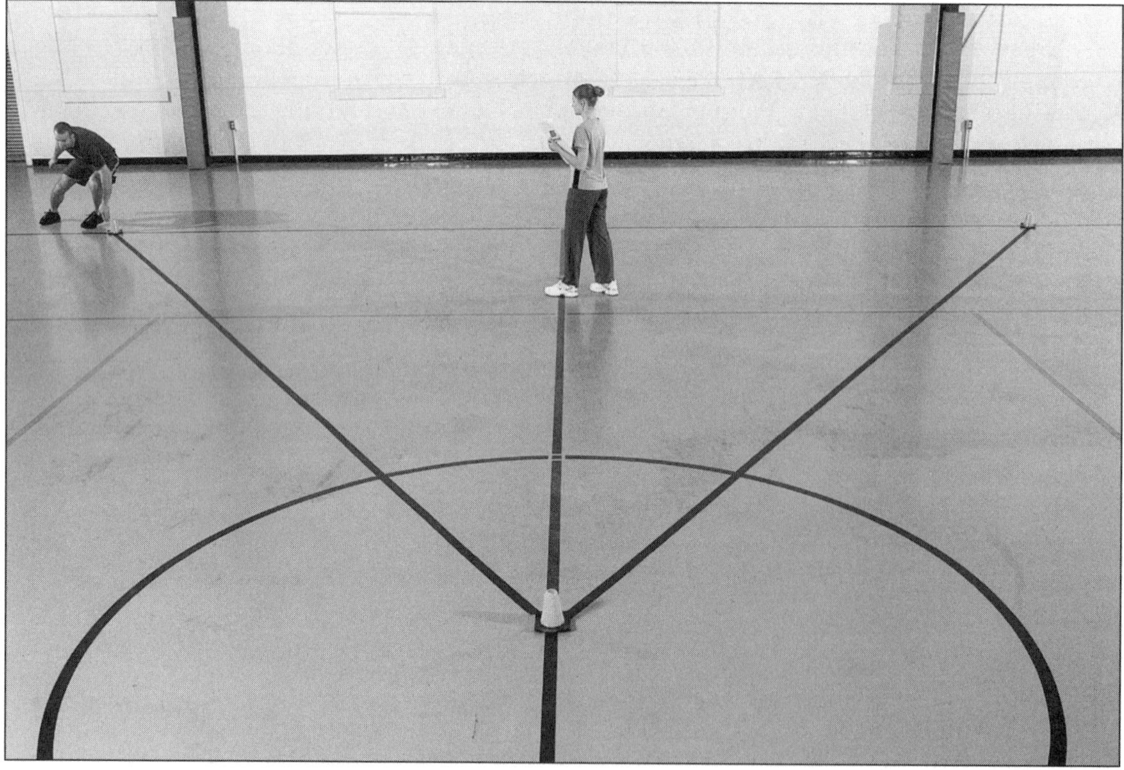

Figure 17.1 The triangle drill.

Medicine Ball Exercises

The squat is fundamental to training cutting and turning. An athlete who struggles with the squat doesn't need to worry, though. A leg-dominant person with strong or tight quads and hip flexors will struggle with the squat. The key is to work to improve the squat and then try this medicine ball drill to train core stability when the hips are extended.

Get into a tall kneeling position on a padded surface, keeping the body tall and fully extending the hips. Throw a forward overhead pass to a partner or at a wall. Next, try a bounce pass. Reach high for the bounce pass and allow the thighs to stretch. After a few throws, move backward 6 to 12 inches. You will have to throw harder and harder to maintain the throw and reach your partner or the wall. As you move backward, throw harder, but do it without sticking the rear out or flexing the spine. To check for left-right differences in core power, try chop passes to the left and right with a partner. This drill is not about taking away the legs: it's about extending the hips. This will help you lunge deeper and beef up the core, improving control.

To train cutting and turning, the lunge movement pattern must be solid. If the lunge test (see chapter 5, page 35) still causes difficulty on one side or both, fix that first. Once an athlete has mastered the lunge, he has the ability to keep the body low and maintain control. But before moving in this low stance, he needs to become comfortable holding a low center of gravity.

Medicine ball passes in a half-kneeling position are excellent for developing core stability while teaching the legs to relax and get low. For the medicine ball lift throw from a lunge stance in chapter 13 (page 164), you threw a medicine ball against the wall to your side from a half-kneeling stance, taking a step through, catching the same ball, resetting, and repeating. This drill improves starting speed but also helps the acceleration and deceleration movements needed for quick cutting and turning.

Here is another good drill. Get into a half-kneeling position facing a wall. Perform an overhead pass, throwing across one side of the body at the wall (figure 17.2). The ball should bounce off the wall and come back on the other side. Catch it, throw again,

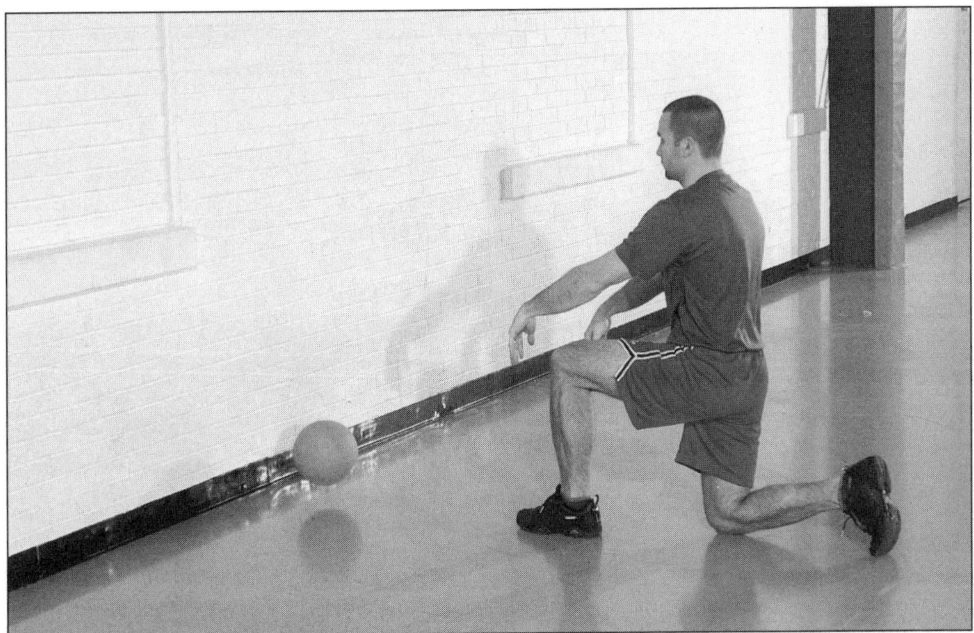

Figure 17.2 Half-kneeling medicine ball overhead pass.

and receive another bounce pass on the opposite side. Keep the spine tall and hold position while moving farther from the wall with each throw, producing great power without bending or twisting the spine. This exercise demonstrates core stability as well as the ability to hold a low center of gravity. If needed, allow the return off the wall to bounce before catching it.

The next drill is best performed with a partner. The partner may either train along with you or act as a coach. Partners who are not equally matched in ability should not try to train at the same time.

Get into a half-kneeling position with the left knee down and the right knee up. Narrow the base so that the left knee and the right foot fall in line about 6 inches apart (figure 17.3a). The partner, if training at the same time, can half-kneel to the left, facing the opposite direction, or stand on an elevated platform or step. A partner who is acting as a coach faces your left side. Using a medium to light medicine ball, throw a bounce pass to your partner, increasing speed with every second or third throw (figure 17.3b). Try to get a high bounce on the medicine ball so that your partner has to reach high.

a

b

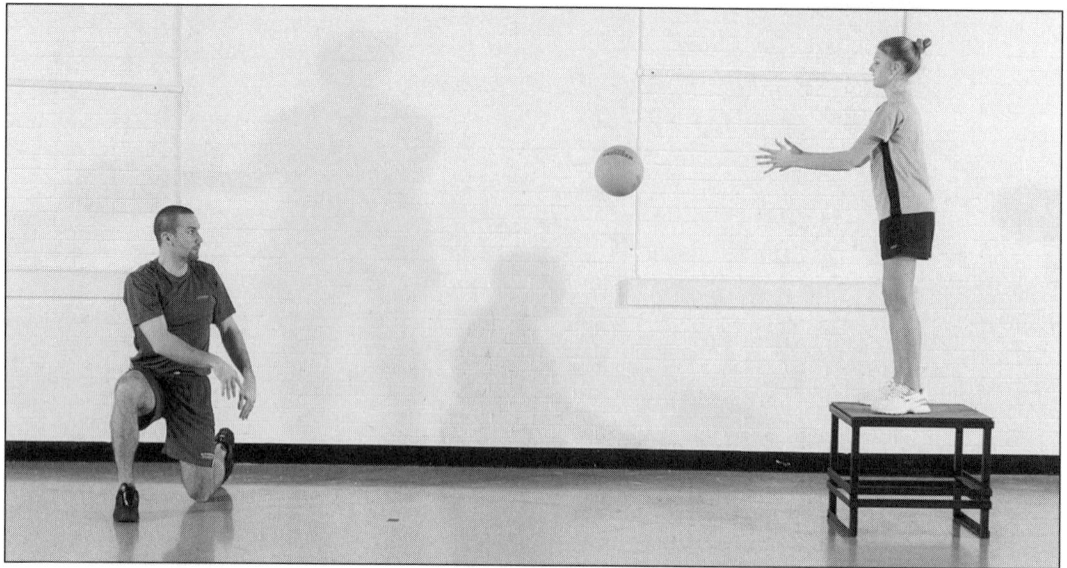

Figure 17.3 Medicine ball pass with partner: *(a)* begin in a half-kneeling position; *(b)* execute a bounce pass to your partner.

Your partner bounces the ball so that the ball passes in front of you over your right knee. Do not try to stop the ball. Place your hands on the ball as it comes by you. Go back into the chop and lift diagonal lifting pattern and then throw the ball down and across the body in a chopping pattern. You and your partner should aim for the same spot on the floor. A piece of tape on the floor can help. Note your ability to catch and throw the ball with the right knee down compared to ability with the left knee down. Approximately 20 throws on each side will show which is the strong side. Do not look at what the arms are doing. Keep a narrow base and maintain a long spine.

The next drill uses a similar movement pattern, but you will rise out of the kneel into a lunge. Maintain the lunge position but do not bear weight on the left knee; hover 6 to 12 inches off the ground (figure 17.4a). Maintain a narrow base as you throw and catch (figure 17.4b). The legs must be strong and the athlete must get comfortable and relax in this position. The only goal is to catch and throw. Do not allow any unnecessary body movement. Note any specific fatigue or poor technique on one side compared to the other. This position should become extremely comfortable for 30 to 40 throws to each side. Keep the hips squared to the front and allow the shoulders to turn. It may feel more comfortable at first to turn the hips, but this is poor technique. Keep the hips stable and do not rotate the pelvis in the throwing direction. This will help maintain core stability and build better body control for cutting and turning.

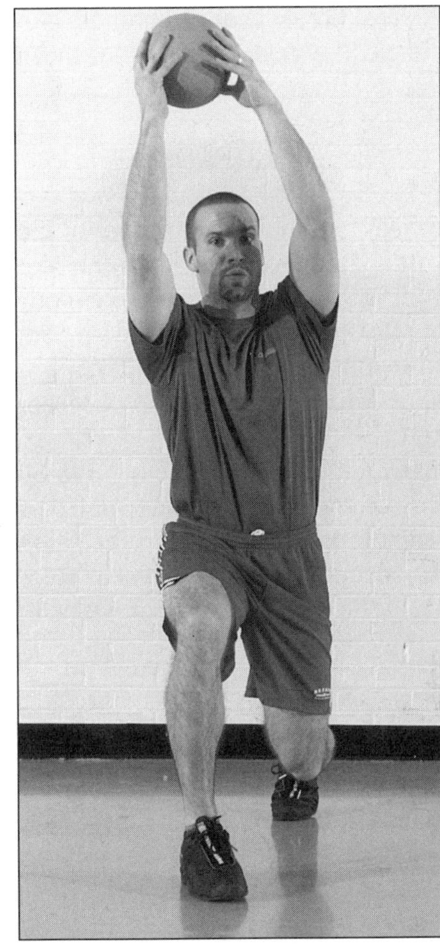
a

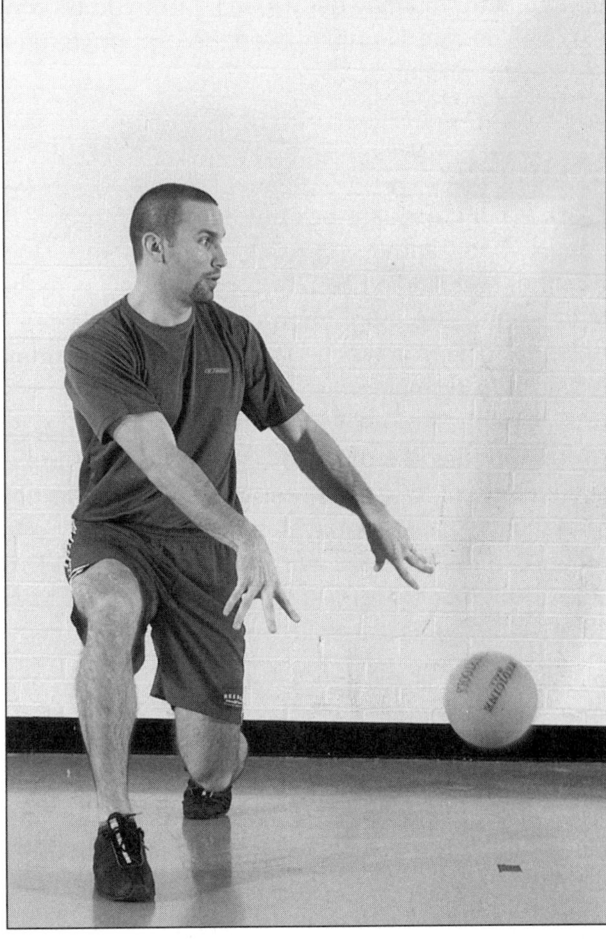
b

Figure 17.4 Medicine ball lunge and throw: *(a)* begin in lunge position with the down knee slightly off the floor; *(b)* throw the ball.

Jump Rope Training

The skier's jump (page 167), bell jump (page 167), and X-foot cross (page 168) build power and coordination. See chapter 13 for descriptions of the techniques.

After working with the rope to develop tempo and rhythm, try doing some high knee jogging with the jump rope. Lateral hopping is also an excellent drill that teaches management of the center of gravity and develops control.

HIGH KNEE JOGGING

Jump comfortably to get the rope turning. Pick up the tempo and start to lift one leg, going back and forth in a jogging motion while jumping over the rope. For the high knee jump, flex the hip to greater than 90 degrees. Keep the body tall through the spine.

Challenge yourself and see how fast you can turn the rope and alternate high knee strides. Train in intervals of 15 to 30 seconds. Perform as many jumps as possible in 15 to 30 seconds. Rest for two, three, or four times the time for the rope jumping interval. For a 15-second jumping interval, rest for 30 seconds to 1 minute before repeating the same amount of jumps in the next 15-second period. For a 30-second jumping interval, rest for 1 to 2 minutes.

Go as fast as possible and try to maintain the same number of jumps in each set for up to 5 sets. You may get winded, but try to relax on the rest break. Learn to breathe and exercise control. Do not tighten the legs or stiffen the back. Stay relaxed and fluid. That's the key to quickness.

LATERAL HOPPING

Mark a 1-inch-square box on the floor with tape. With feet together in the center of the square, begin turning the rope and jumping. Once you are comfortable, keep the feet together and bounce from one side of the box to the other without moving the upper body left to right. Use a tight and compact double-leg jump. It will look like a tight, compact downhill skiing position. This exercise is extremely helpful for core stability. As you progress, try jumping diagonally from corner to corner, or use any combination of corner or side jumps. Look forward or use a mirror. Stay relaxed.

Train in intervals of 15 to 30 seconds. Perform as many jumps as possible in 15 to 30 seconds. Rest for two, three, or four times the time for the rope jumping interval. For a 15-second jumping interval, rest for 30 seconds to 1 minute before repeating the same amount of jumps in the next 15-second period. For a 30-second jumping interval, rest for 1 to 2 minutes. Go as fast as possible and try to maintain the same number of jumps in each set for up to 5 sets.

SPLIT-STANCE LEG JUMP

The split-stance leg jump requires you to shuffle the legs between each jump—from left leg in front and right leg in back to right leg in front and left leg in back. It looks like a compact lunge and requires quickness on the toes. This drill teaches you to stay relaxed while moving extremely quickly in an alternate-leg movement pattern.

Train in intervals of 15 to 30 seconds. Perform as many jumps as possible in 15 to 30 seconds. Rest for two, three, or four times the time for the rope jumping interval. For a 15-second jumping interval, rest for 30 seconds to 1 minute before repeating the same amount of jumps in the next 15-second period. For a 30-second jumping interval, rest for

1 to 2 minutes. Go as fast as possible and try to maintain the same number of jumps in each set for up to 5 sets.

Tubing Drills

Tubing work is excellent for high-speed resistance. The pull of the tubing requires greater stability with speed and agility moves. That makes it an excellent way to overload the neuromuscular system and create heightened awareness with quickness and agility. When used correctly with safe connections and quality equipment, tubing can be a fundamental asset to motor learning and interval training.

STATIONARY FOUR-WAY RUNNING

This drill can be done inside or outside. Stand with the tubing around your waist with mild tension (not enough to pull you off balance, but enough to make you lean away from the tubing), facing away from where the tubing is anchored. Jog in place with high knees (figure 17.5). Try to run as though there is no tubing. Do not let the tubing pull you off balance or alter running cadence. Perform a 15-second high knee wind sprint, pumping the arms.

Rest for 15 seconds and rotate to the right so that your right side faces where the tubing is anchored. Perform another 15-second high knee wind sprint, then rest for 15 seconds. Rotate to the right again so that you face where the tubing is anchored. Perform a 15-second high knee wind sprint, then rest for 15 seconds. Rotate to the right again so that your left side faces where the tubing is anchored. Perform a 15-second high knee wind sprint. Your feet should remain in a 1-foot-square box for the entire drill.

Now you have faced every direction. The tubing has caused a weight shift forward, back, left, and right. You have now worked on deceleration, acceleration, right cutting, and left cutting, respectively. You managed the weight shift by working on control and balance. You can manipulate exercise time and rest time to make this an interval drill and work on running technique.

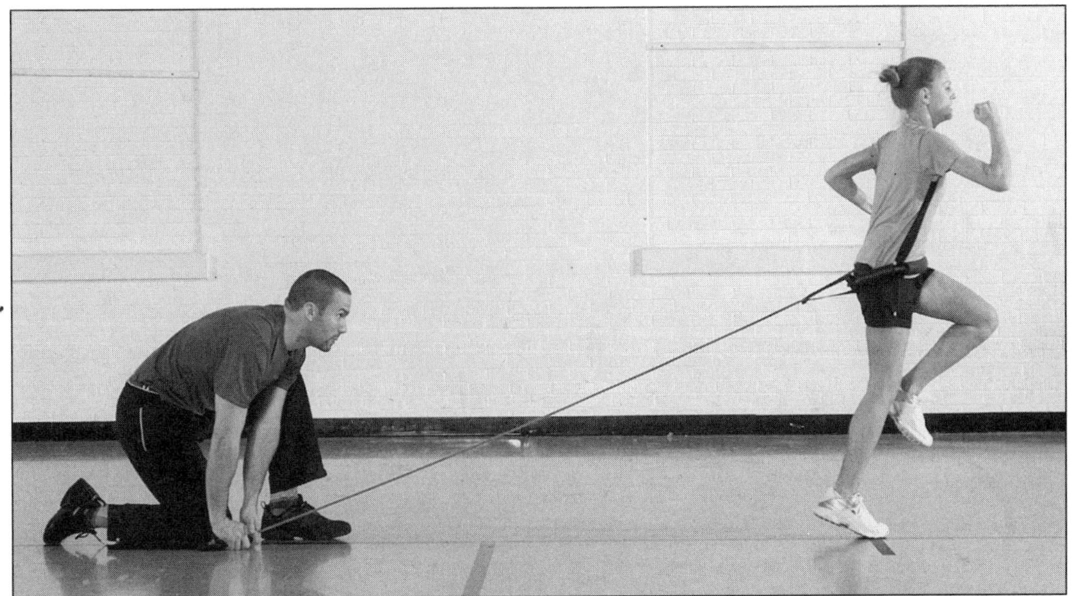

Figure 17.5 Stationary four-way running using tubing.

DYNAMIC FOUR-WAY BOUNDING

Bounding is jumping from one leg to another. Beginners should try to bound the length of their inseams. More advanced, experienced athletes should try to bound the length of their bodies or at least two-thirds the length of their bodies.

With the tubing secure around the waist, face away from where the tubing is anchored. Bound to the left and right with about one body length between where the left and right feet touch the ground. Rotate clockwise until you have performed lateral bounding in all four directions (figure 17.6). Use the arms as counterbalances and try to bound so that an observer would not think the tubing was creating much resistance. Use the same 15-second intervals as in stationary four-way running.

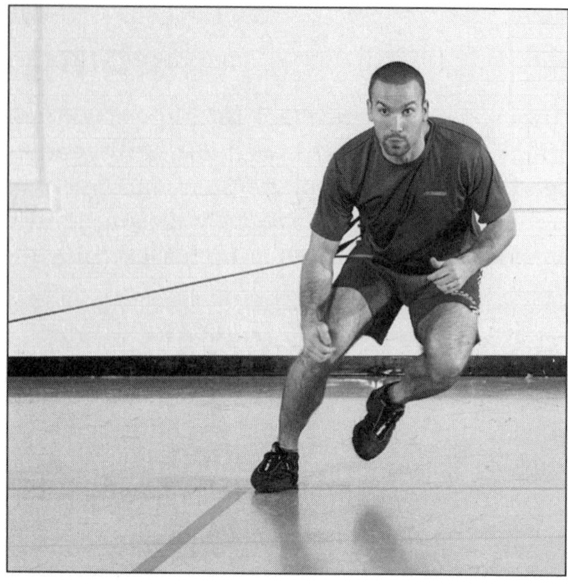

Figure 17.6 Dynamic four-way bounding with tubing.

FOUR-WAY HOPPING

Hopping is a double-leg jump that looks a lot like skiing moguls (figure 17.7). When running and bounding, alternate feet land with each step; hopping has a double-foot landing. Hopping is best performed at one-quarter to one-half of the body length and should follow the same format in all four positions. Use the same intervals as with stationary four-way running. When you begin it is OK to use sticks or ski poles to help with your upper-body balance. Eventually, you should be able to perform this without holding onto anything. Follow the same clockwise rotation for all four positions.

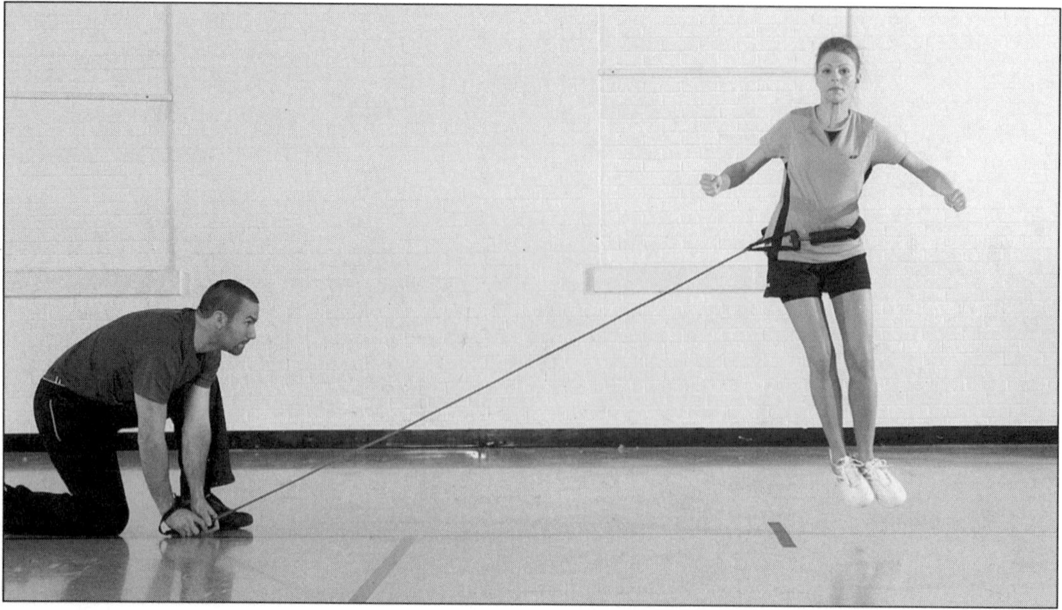

Figure 17.7 Four-way hopping with tubing.

18

Progress Evaluation

This book has asked you to look at your training and your body with a mixture of conventional and unconventional methods. The ideas in this book reflect a new trend in physical therapy, athletic training, and conditioning. Although more research is necessary to clarify and refine the study of movement and movement patterns, the concepts in this book are founded on well-accepted neuromuscular and kinesiological relationships.

The greatest difference between the approach of this book and that of other conditioning programs is that the screening of movement patterns is placed first and foremost. The ability to produce and perceive movement patterns free of limitation and asymmetry is the foundation of this program. Once you know this information, you can get results from many different programs; but you should not rate those results by one aspect of performance or sport skill. Fundamental movement patterns, general performance, and sport-specific performance should be considered together as interdependent characteristics of an athletic body in balance.

Use your own ideas on creating new ways to improve the function of the body . . . the hell with conventional methods and opinions.

—*Bruce Lee*

It's time to evaluate progress. I hope that you have patiently followed the recommended exercises, developing the body and improving performance step by step. If you've discovered your weakest link (or learned more about it), then this book has been worthwhile. If so, I assume that you've adopted a training regime that targets your weakest link. And because the weakest link limits the strength of the entire chain, any way you strengthen that part strengthens the whole.

With the movement screen, we first looked at extremes of movement (the first level of the performance pyramid) to find out what was physically available within the mobility and stability you currently possess. We then tested performance and looked at strength, power, and endurance, trying to determine what could be produced with what was on hand (the second level of the pyramid). We did not address sport skills (the third level of the pyramid) because your statistics and performance in your particular sport should provide feedback in that regard. I hope you discovered where in the pyramid your primary focus should be, although you should strive to improve them all. Your best investment is your greatest limitation.

The exercises in this book are designed to improve body awareness and create a feeling that comes through the natural and functional movements of the body. As an athlete becomes more conscious of the movements that feel natural as well as the ones that feel labored and difficult, she starts to relate the way a movement feels to the way she performs.

Two important keys to developing motor memory and reproducing a sport skill with consistency are the way a movement feels and the results it yields. If a movement feels natural and fluid but produces a poor result, the brain is not inclined to remember the way it felt. If a movement feels awkward, difficult, or labored but produces the desired result, the body desperately wants to remember it but may not be inclined to reproduce it consistently because it felt so unnatural. The goal, then, is to blend feel and performance into movement that feels natural and is consistently successful.

You need to make subtle changes until the movement feels more natural. While making these subtle changes, continue to move toward more natural movement until performance starts to diminish. Stop and work backward a little. This is how to develop motor learning.

Removing restrictions to functional movement and minimizing imbalances wherever possible improve an athlete's motor learning ability. Developing a strong core and creating strength in functional movement patterns generate correct movement with greater power for longer periods. This increase in endurance will provide more opportunity for motor learning during conditioning and skill training.

Ultimately, an athlete will return to practicing sport skills in his chosen sport. Chances are that he will train in much the same way he always has but with an increased awareness of body balance. He will treat injuries differently, listen to the subtle things his body says, and add quality to his training through greater movement awareness.

If you are like most people, you have been looking for small indicators of progress since starting this program. You wanted to see enhanced performance after the first stretching session or the first week of hill running or rope jumping. You wanted to see the whole game change after balancing the right and left sides of the body. Looking for enhanced performance is part of human nature, and it's OK.

To appraise what you've learned, ask yourself these questions:

- Did I identify a left-right imbalance?
- Did I find a major limitation?
- What is my weakest link?
- Was the weakest link a movement problem, performance problem, or skill problem?
- Has the weakest link improved?

Answering these questions demonstrates an appreciation of balance that few people have. Knowing weakness is one thing, but mapping it is the way to develop a complete training program. Remember that most athletes have a weakness at each level of the pyramid. Within each level, they have a particular aspect of performance that is lacking or could stand to improve. The balanced program is designed to keep your focus on your weakness. For example, consider a soccer goaltender who has just finished a winning season. He wants the next year of training to produce even better skills and more confidence. He decides to start with the movement screen. The screen reveals that he has a great hurdle step to the left and right; seated rotation also is above average both ways. He fails the forward lunge on the right leg, the active straight leg raise with the right leg up, and the squat.

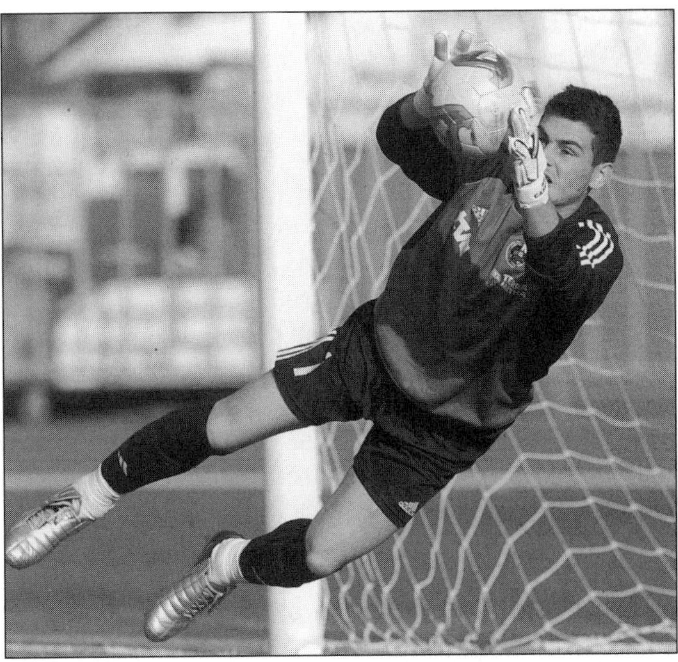

Even after a successful season, examine any weaknesses that exist and work to improve them before the next season starts.

Of the three screens that he failed, the lunge and active straight leg raise demonstrate asymmetry, which is a red flag when balance is the goal. If he is to improve in the squat to any degree, he must first resolve this asymmetry. He creates a 10- to 15-minute warm-up and cool-down to do every day regardless of the workout he has planned (skill drills, weight training, agility work, or whatever). The warm-up and cool-down involve stretching and foundation drills that target lunging and leg raising on the right. For two to three days a week, he does core training that targets the lunge and leg raise.

Next he performs strength and endurance testing and notices that his stats for the 1.5-mile run, sit-up test, and bench press are all average or above average. His 1RM squat, however, is below average. Instead of working on squat strength, though, he focuses on strengthening the lunge because he feels the left-right asymmetry is a strength problem as well as a flexibility problem. Because there is no strength training recommended for the active straight leg raise (there are only strength moves for the first three screens, the three basic foot positions), he continues core training to correct the active straight leg raise asymmetry. As he performs the lunge strength program, he notes a 25 to 30 percent difference between left and right lunges with the same weight. He decides to do 2 sets on the left side and 5 sets on the right for all strength-training lunge work.

Power, speed, and agility tests are all good except for the vertical jump, which is below average. Although vertical jumping is not a big part of his sport, out of curiosity he performs a single-leg vertical jump and discovers an underlying asymmetry. There is a 25 percent difference between his single-leg vertical jump scores, only this time the left leg is the problem. Initially this causes confusion because the left quads seemed stronger in the lunge; but he remembers that it's not about muscles, it's about movement. He had a lunge pattern problem on the right, not a weak right quad muscle. The lunge pattern requires hip extension on the left and hip flexion on the right. The active straight leg raise requires the same hip position. The core was the problem, not the quads. The single-leg vertical jump requires hip extension on the left and hip flexion on the right. Because this showed up as a problem in earlier tests, it makes sense that the left single-leg vertical jump is less powerful than the right. He decides that jump rope work targeting left-leg quickness and explosiveness will be part of his program. He follows the complete power, speed, and agility recommendations for lunging in chapter 13, paying special attention to left-hip explosive power in extension as well as all movements involving the right lunge position.

He has now mapped out the problems in the first two levels of the performance pyramid, giving him perspective of movement patterns and ability to generate power and efficiency in those movement patterns. Now he needs an appraisal of his sport skill. He talks with some of his teammates, who all compliment his performance. His coach is also very positive and complimentary, except for one thing. The coach points out that he fails to defend the goal to his right as effectively as he does to his left in competition. There is a 15 to 20 percent difference, but the coach quickly states that this is probably due to the fact that he is left-handed. The athlete knows that hand dominance isn't the key. Defending the right side of the goal usually requires a right weight shift starting with an explosion off the left hip. Testing revealed that the athlete has a small problem with this weight shift and explosion. Lunge movement to the right is fundamental to defending the right side of the goal. His stride to the right is not stable enough. He has proven this by testing right and left lunging ability in the weight room. Through testing, he has found the cause of his limitations on the field and is ready to work hard to improve.

Intelligent Training

Intelligent training is a combination of information and effort. Balancing the two is the secret to success. Unfortunately, this is difficult in our information junkie culture (or culture of junkie information). Many athletes who are serious about training peruse the Web, read articles, and skim books, constantly collecting information. But if the information is never assimilated into a plan or program, ultimately the effort spent on gathering information never has a practical application. Cardiac surgeons have more than enough information to condemn smoking, but some of them smoke nevertheless. The problem is not a lack of information—it's a lack of effort or application.

Of course, a mistake can be made in the other direction, when people blindly train without analyzing progress, potential, or alternative methods. Albert Einstein once commented that the definition of stupidity is doing the same thing over and over and over again and expecting a different result. Although information and effort should be balanced, the gathering of information should precede the application and effort. Once you think you have adequately researched and reviewed current training principles for your chosen activity, stop looking and start training. Most programs deserve at least 6 to 12 weeks of consistent adherence before you have the perspective to analyze their efficiency. It's your responsibility to objectively measure the things you wish to change.

One day, a high school student asked his coach how to become a better athlete. The coach dismissed the question, thinking the athlete was not serious about committing the appropriate amount of effort. The coach said, "Just do some push-ups and some pull-ups and run some sprints." This young athlete, Herschel Walker, had only a small amount of information, but he used that information to develop a strong, resilient, well-balanced body. He didn't have a lot of articles or equipment—he didn't even have a lot of coaching—but he had a small piece of information that seemed to make sense. You would be hard pressed today to find an athlete who would take that small amount of information and apply that much effort. The athletic state of mind should never be limited by time, equipment, or information.

This book has provided some basic information that has been used by elite athletes who have had problems with performance or who haven't responded to rehabilitation. You would be amazed at how much basic information is dispensed at the collegiate and professional levels simply because athletes have lost training focus and have gone off on unnecessary tangents caused by information overload or training overanalysis. Training is simple. Find the weak link and fix it. Maintain strength, work on weaknesses, and have a system to assess and reassess progress. Ultimately, every athlete will develop, refine, and implement a customized program.

Psychological Training

Training personality is simply the way an athlete prefers to train. Regardless of sport, athletes migrate to either consistency or variety. Some athletes like a consistent, regimented exercise program. They thrive on the routine and hate it when anything interferes with their workout schedules. They prefer certain equipment, training partners, facilities, and even clothes they wear while training. Any change in these things seems to throw them off. They may still train if things aren't perfect, but they aren't satisfied with the workout.

Some athletes prefer constant variety. They may work out extra long one day only to skip a workout planned for the next day. They may consistently give up workout sessions to do something more competitive, such as a quick game of racquetball or a round of golf. They like to mix it up and use multiple gyms or different pieces of equipment. Their training is defined by the fact that they like variety, so they can be inconsistent with one or more aspects of training.

Over time, both personality types offer advantages and disadvantages. Advantages often are obvious, but disadvantages may not be. Athletes who are too rigid and consistent may get stuck in a rut and not realize their full potential. Athletes who use too much variety in their workouts may not realize the benefits from one particular aspect of the program. Either way, it's important to know training personality as well as weak links. This knowledge allows an athlete to alter workouts to suit mental and physical limitations.

Competitive Training

John Wooden was perhaps the most cerebral coach ever, a man who preached discipline in an age of spontaneity. He never told his players to win, but simply to play their best within their own abilities. His wisdom and leadership allowed him to reach athletes such as Kareem Abdul-Jabbar and Bill Walton. He was a teacher whose striving for goodness deeply affected the players who played for him. Under Wooden, the UCLA Bruins won 10 national championships in 12 years, including 7 straight from 1967 to 1973.

The practices Wooden put his teams through were designed to be as competitive as the games the Bruins played against other teams. Bill Walton described the practices as "two hours of nonstop basketball, at the highest level, with the greatest players, and with the master sitting there, critiquing everything, never letting a single error go unnoticed or uncriticized, and yet always pointing out the positive things and building the team for the championship moment." During their run of 7 straight championships, the Bruins were so dominant that these practices often were more competitive than many of the real games.

Adapted from *ESPN SportsCentury*, edited by Michael MacCambridge, New York: Hyperion, 1999.

If you are extremely rigid in training, learn to mix it up or at least schedule some variety. Take a break. Explore various forms of cross-training. Lay off a day or two. Document any changes. If you use too much variety, you may want to set up a strict schedule and get a training partner who will help with consistency. Plan at least one or two consistent workouts per week and leave the third workout as a variety day. Work on strengthening weak links but do so any way that works. If quickness is a problem, try playing Ping-Pong, racquetball, or one-on-one basketball. Learn some basic boxing or martial arts and do some sparring. If endurance is a problem, take a bike ride or run or swim with someone who has greater stamina.

Competition is an excellent way to make training fit personality. Some athletes dread training and would much rather just go out and play. They love scrimmage sessions or competitive drills. These athletes will push harder to earn a point than they would to get another rep and would rather race someone than beat the clock. Most great athletes have forms of competition mixed in their training, whether they plan it or not. They love to play, not just in their chosen sports, but also in every aspect of their physical lives. This is good training because once an athlete learns to relax in competition, it doesn't necessarily matter what that competition is. Take on competitive events and go against someone equal or better in an area that stresses the weakest link.

It may work best to spend half of a workout on a competitive event and the other half on consistent training. Athletes who like a variety of activities may prefer to have the competitive portion of the workout first to get rid of some competitive energy, allowing a better focus on a more structured workout later.

Regardless of training personality, the way you correct weaknesses is just as important as how and when you work them. The best training program offers a variety of activities to prepare the body for the forces that will confront it in competition with enough consistency to get results. Keep records and track progress. Know tendencies and work in the opposite direction to create balance. Remember, you are what you practice most, so practice balance.

Basics of Skill

All athletes must ultimately study their skills. But in studying skill, don't overanalyze. Golf is probably the worst and the best example. Golf is a big business and often is looked at through a microscope. However, the best of the best did not get to the top by looking through microscopes. They did it by developing the fundamentals. As they rose through the ranks, they may have fixed little pieces of their games with in-depth analysis, only to find an extra shot or bit of consistency in one particular aspect of the game. A typical golfer who is looking at the overall fundamentals of golf needs to find something consistent with his swing and comfortable for his body. The problem is that most people are not conditioned, flexible, or aware of their body mechanics enough to be consistent and comfortable at the same time. They want to make a quick change, so they swing within their comfort zone but have bad mechanics—and consequently the swing suffers. Athletes who are having problems with a particular skill probably lack a fundamental. Microscopic analysis will not help.

A great way to solve problems is to ask, "Is this a static or dynamic problem?" Once a collegiate Division I lefty pitcher with left-shoulder problems came to my clinic. He was referred by a specialist in video motion analysis and had also been seen by some good sports physicians, physical therapists, and athletic trainers. The video specialist told me that he could not find any flaws in this pitcher's movement; the athlete had no history of injury or problems and his mechanics were nearly perfect, so the video specialist could not understand why the left shoulder hurt.

I took this young pitcher through a movement screen and strength test and saw no problems, no flaws, no asymmetries, and no significant limitations. Strength and performance were fine. I asked this young pitcher to come out to the gym and throw a tennis ball into a mini-trampoline to get an idea of the way he moved. The only flaw I could see was that he was not making enough use of the cocking motion most pitchers need. Because he was starting the pitch without getting into a full or cocked position, he had to exaggerate his follow-through to get the same distance to accelerate the ball. By reaching back just a little bit more in the start of his position, he was able to let his near-flawless mechanics take over. He started the pitch just a little bit earlier and therefore did not have to exaggerate the follow-through.

I am not a pitching expert, but this young man's problem was not a dynamic one. He had great pitching mechanics, good performance, and good movement patterns. He was simply starting his skill in the wrong position. If you start from the wrong place, then everything that occurs after that will be wrong.

Seriously consider the start position, finish position, and ready position—fundamentals. Are you in the best ready position? Do you shift weight correctly? Does fatigue show quickly by a change in posture, breathing, stance? Where is your focus? An athlete who does not start in the right place cannot end in the right place without major compensations in movement.

When altering skill, change only one thing each day and be sure to change the right thing. Use video and coaching. Read books and watch others. Keep notes. See which changes create the best results and jot down how you feel when you are trying to make those changes. If you reproduce the feel, you can reproduce the movement. If you cannot reproduce the feel, the movement will not happen. Remember, feel tells the brain where you are and what needs to be done. The language of movement is written in feel, not in words or pictures. Relax and try not to become frustrated. You've got to put in the time, but stop once you're fatigued and frustrated. When the body is tired, the brain is going to learn the bad stuff that you want it to forget.

Conclusions

I have maintained a general approach in this book. I have not talked specifically about one sport because conditioning and competition are fundamental to all athletics. Skill considerations, body type differences, and different physical attributes all play a large role, but this book is designed as a conditioning guide for athletes in many different sports. My purpose is to show that great athletes and great conditioning programs are more alike than different.

The information in this book is 10 percent innovation (the philosophy and techniques are based on movement fundamentals), 10 percent inspiration (the underlying theme is directed toward finding balance and harmony between the body and conditioning), and 80 percent incorporation (most of the exercises and drills are not new but are grouped in an efficient and effective way to provide specific results with minimal redundancy and wasted time).

The quotes in this book are designed to keep you focused on your goals. I have had the opportunity to work or be a guest in many elite college and professional training facilities. Almost all of them use quotes from athletes, coaches, and philosophers strategically placed throughout the rehabilitation or exercise area to state a training or motivational virtue. Use these quotes as you train to keep your thoughts and feelings about your training directed toward your larger goals.

The weight room can be the launching pad for a great athletic career or the path down an unnecessary tangent. Throughout my career I have seen good athletes get involved in conditioning, only to get distracted. Goals must be set in the weight room, but when those goals don't improve sport-specific performance or when they hurt fundamental movement patterns, pursuing those goals is worthless.

I would like to leave you with a few catch phrases that may help you remember some of the things covered in this book.

- **Go light and do it right.** When strength training with weights or using a medicine ball, it is better to have proper technique and good movement patterns than it is to stack up greater weight. When someone wins a world championship and a microphone is thrust in his face, he is never asked how much weight he can lift. It's about doing it right.
- **Go fast but make it last.** This refers to speed endurance. If speed training, try to speed up recovery. Try to produce multiple bouts of fast and efficient movement. It's not just about one blistering 40, but about how many 40s can be produced within 80 percent of the maximal 40. The same holds true through a quarter-mile, a shuttle run, or other speed, quickness, or agility drills. If speed is not present at the end of a competitive event, not many people will remember how fast the athlete was at the beginning.
- **Be quick but don't forget to stick.** Quickness is two-, three-, and four-step movements; it is also powerful movements of the trunk, torso, and arms over a very small period of time. If the athlete cannot maintain control and keep a stable base with the ability to stop and quickly change directions under control, then quickness is going to work against the athlete and ultimately may cause injury. *Sticking* is the ability to abruptly stop and control motion, and *quickness* is the ability to abruptly produce motion. One cannot exist without the other. Remember, it's the ability to stop under control—not start more quickly—that allows an athlete to put a move on an opponent and set up and execute more skillful and controlled movements.
- **Control breath and maximize rest.** Martial artists and marathoners may not seem to have a lot in common, but the elite ones are there because they learned to control their breathing. Breathing is involuntary, but if it changes it's a dead giveaway that fatigue has set in. The fatigued athlete slumps forward and starts breathing through the mouth. Learn to control breathing by slowing down the rate or number of breaths and increasing breath volume or depth. When not competing or during rest breaks, control breathing and learn to relax the body. Make the most of any rest break. Let opponents fidget, talk, fiddle with equipment, and not pay attention to their bodies. They will pay for this wasted time when the activity starts again. Breathe in through the nose, out through the mouth, deep and clear. Stand up straight when breathing. Remember, what's not done in training will not be done in competition.
- **Balance is the base.** If you work on balance (everything from standing on a wobble board to skipping rope on one foot), you will develop a stable base. In a deeper sense, the training base should come from balance. Continually push to balance strength and flexibility, speed and endurance, and power and agility on the left and right sides of the body. It's important to build training on top of balance. Training built on top of imbalance will only increase the imbalance. Even the best training in the world will yield poor results if placed on top of a faulty foundation or unstable base.
- **If you can't test it, don't train it.** This should be obvious. In this book, I have not suggested training anything that cannot be tested in some fundamental way. There is no reason to get bogged down with fancy equipment or multiple tests. Have

one or two good tests that demonstrate what needs to be worked on and frequently retest. If retesting reveals negative results, figure it out. If retesting reveals positive results, figure it out.

- **Relaxation is the foundation.** The mark of a champion is control during competition and relaxation in the presence of stress. This does not mean champions are not trying as hard as they can, but they compete in a relaxed, fluid fashion. There is no unnecessary tension, so there is no wasted energy. One of the best foundations for competition is relaxation. Relaxation can be trained through competitive events pairing up athletes of equal ability. Instead of trying harder, athletes should relax.

- **Make your plan and work your plan.** This is not my phrase—it's my father's. I have heard him say it all of my life, and the older I become the more sense it makes. In short, this is about achieving a goal through aiming and analysis. Someone can have the best intention and ability in the world, but if she doesn't know where the target is she can't hit it. Making a plan means taking aim and constructing a sequence and methods that will take you to the target. Working the plan means analyzing progress or failure along the way. All athletes can win with their A-games, but sometimes they have to win with their B- or C-games. The original plan will not always work, in competition or in training, but that's not what the quote is about. My dad did not say "Make the plan work"—he said "Work the plan." Working the plan is about being as objective as possible. It is about being flexible and working it out so that you stay on track. You need to construct a general plan of attack, but if you are rigid in your ideas you will not learn the important lessons that training and conditioning can teach. Manipulate all that is necessary to hit the target. Reconstruct your plan whenever you feel your results are not optimal, but be patient. Slow, steady progress is how the great ones did it, and you can't hope for better than that.

Always have a solid, objective rationale for manipulating your program and reconstructing your plan. Constantly test yourself and reinforce the productive things you are doing while exposing the nonproductive things. Remember to set realistic goals. Good plans implemented to achieve unrealistic goals are a waste of energy.

I hope this book provided a fresh perspective to training and that it will complement the training investment you have already made. Sport enthusiasts often believe that sport is a metaphor for life and that the positives of sport are displayed in life. Courage, perseverance, enthusiasm, focus, and fairness are all prized in life and in the athletic arena. If sport is the metaphor for life, then training must be the metaphor for lifestyle. The greatest minds have always regarded a balanced approach to lifestyle to be the most favorable. Achieving balance in training will be both challenging and rewarding and will demonstrate the benefit of approaching all things with balance. The following words of legendary football coach Paul "Bear" Bryant are simple and profound, and his esteem for learning reflects my sentiments in writing this book: "No coach ever won a game by what he knows. It's what his players have learned."

Bibliography and Sources

Anderson, B. 2000. *Stretching.* Bolinas, Calif.: Shelter Publications.

Baechle, T.R., R.W. Earle, and D. Wathen. 2000. Resistance training. In *Essentials of strength training and conditioning* (2nd ed.), edited by T.R. Baechle and R.W. Earle. Champaign, Ill.: Human Kinetics.

Chu, D.A. 2001. Explosive power. In *High-performance sports conditioning,* edited by B. Foran. Champaign, Ill.: Human Kinetics.

Cook, G. 2001. Baseline sports-fitness testing. In *High-performance sports conditioning,* edited by B. Foran. Champaign, Ill.: Human Kinetics.

Covey, S. 1997. *The seven habits of highly effective people.* Thorndike, Maine: G.K. Hall.

Dintiman, G.B. 2001. Acceleration and speed. In *High-performance sports conditioning,* edited by B. Foran. Champaign, Ill.: Human Kinetics.

Dintiman, G.B., R.D. Ward, and T. Tellez. 1998. *Sports speed* (2nd ed.). Champaign, Ill.: Human Kinetics.

Earle, R.W., and T.R. Baechle. 2000. Resistance training and spotting techniques. In *Essentials of strength training and conditioning* (2nd ed.), edited by T.R. Baechle and R.W. Earle. Champaign, Ill.: Human Kinetics.

Harman, E., J. Garhammer, and C. Pandorf. 2000. Administration, scoring, and interpretation of selected tests. In *Essentials of strength training and conditioning* (2nd ed.), edited by T.R. Baechle and R.W. Earle. Champaign, Ill.: Human Kinetics.

Jones, C. 1999. *What makes winners win.* New York: Broadway Books.

Knapik, J.J., B.H. Jones, C.L. Bauman, and J.M. Harris. 1992. Strength, flexibility, and athletic injuries. *Sports Med* 14(5): 277-288.

MacCambridge, M. 1999. *ESPN SportsCentury.* New York: Hyperion.

Pauole, K., K. Madole, J. Garhammer, M. Lacourse, and R. Rozenek. 2000. Reliability and validity of the T-test as a measure of agility, leg power, and leg speed in college age males and females. *J Strength Cond Res* 14.

Plisk, S.S. 2000. Speed, agility, and speed-endurance development. In *Essentials of strength training and conditioning* (2nd ed.), edited by T.R. Baechle and R.W. Earle. Champaign, Ill.: Human Kinetics.

Potach, D.H., and D.A. Chu. 2000. Plyometric training. In *Essentials of strength training and conditioning* (2nd ed.), edited by T.R. Baechle and R.W. Earle. Champaign, Ill.: Human Kinetics.

Sahrmann, S. 2002. *Diagnosis and treatment of movement impairment syndromes.* St. Louis: Mosby.

Semenick, D. 1990. Tests and measurements: The T-test. *NSCA J* 12(1): 36-37.

Index

Note: The bold **f** and **t** following page numbers refer to figures and tables, respectively.

About the Author

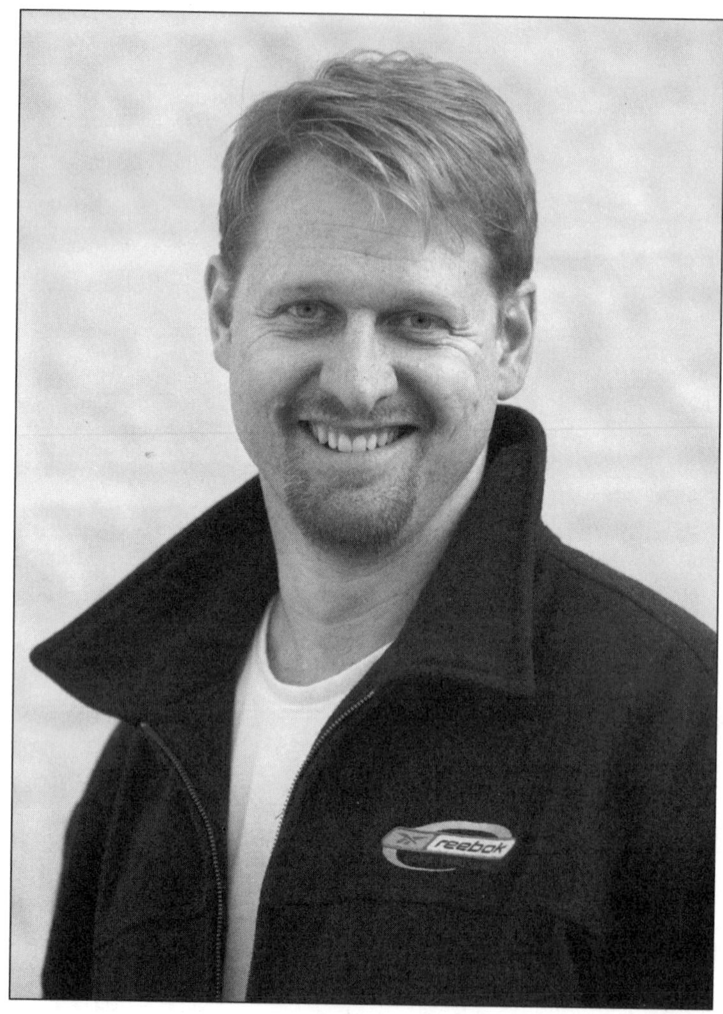

Gray Cook is a physical therapist, board certified in orthopedics. He also is a certified strength coach with experience in several sports at the youth, college, and professional levels. Cook is a nationally recognized lecturer and consultant to the NFL, NBA, NHL, and WNBA as well as numerous college sports medicine and conditioning facilities. His innovative research and applied work are found in many rehabilitation and conditioning publications.

Cook is the director of orthopedic and sports physical therapy at Dunn, Cook & Associates. He also serves as the creative director of sport-specific training for Reebok® and is Reebok's® first master coach.

Cook received his graduate degree in physical therapy educatior at the University of Miami School of Medicine with a focus on orthopedics and sports rehabilitation and research in motor learning. He is a faculty member of the North American Sports Medicine Institute and is the co-developer of the course titled Functional Exercise Training and Rehabilitation. He lives in his hometown of Danville, Virginia.